# BASIC TRAUMA NURSING SKILLS

By
## Linda B. Chitwood, RN, CRNA, MS and
## Jon P. Carson, RN, BS, EMT

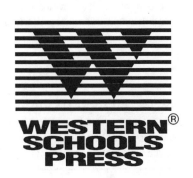
WESTERN®
SCHOOLS
PRESS

21 Bristol Drive
South Easton, MA 02375
1-800-618-1670

## ABOUT THE AUTHOR

**Linda B. Chitwood, RN, CRNA, MS,** has been a practicing nurse for many years. She is currently president of Media Medical Inc., a health-care media service, based in Memphis, Tennessee. She has many years experience writing for the medical profession. She has published articles in *Health Care News* and *Nursing.* She has written on many subjects, such as anesthesiology, gynecology, pediatrics, and pain.

## ABOUT THE SUBJECT MATTER EXPERT

**Jon P. Carson, RN, BS, EMT** is currently the nurse manager for the trauma admitting area, shock trauma and trauma assessment, and manager for memphis MEDCOM, the EMS Telecommunications Resource Coordination Center, both located at The Elvis Presley Memorial Trauma Center (a level 1 trauma center), a division of The Regional Medical Center at Memphis (Tennessee). He has been a nurse in an emergency/trauma setting for the past 18 years. He is a CEN, ALCS and BTLS provider, BTLS instructor. He is the author of one and coauthor of two journal publications.

**Copy Editor:** Barbara Halliburton, PhD

**Typesetter:** Gwen Nichols

**Graphic Artist:** Kathy Johnson

**Indexer:** Sylvia Coates

**Proofreader:** John Wolf, MA

**ISBN** 1-878025-66-X

**Library of Congress Catalog Card Number** 94-61993

Western Schools courses are designed to provide Nursing professionals with the Educational information they need to enhance their career development. The information provided within these course materials is the result of research and consultation with prominent Nursing and Medical authorities and is, to the best of our knowledge, current and accurate. However, the courses and course materials are provided with the understanding that Western Schools is not engaged in offering legal, nursing, medical, or other professional advice.

Western Schools courses and course materials are not meant to act as a substitute for seeking out professional advice or conducting individual research. When applying the information provided in the courses and course materials to individual circumstances, all recommendations must be considered in light of the uniqueness pertaining to each situation.

Western Schools course materials are intended solely for *your* use, and *not* for the benefit of providing advice or recommendations to third parties. Western Schools devoids itself of any responsibility for adverse consequences resulting from the failure to seek nursing, medical or other professional advice. Western Schools further devoids itself of any responsibility for updating or revising any programs or publications presented, published, distributed or sponsored by Western Schools unless otherwise agreed to as part of an individual purchase contract.

# IMPORTANT: Read these instructions *BEFORE* proceeding!

Enclosed with your course book you will find the FasTrax answer sheet. Use this form to answer all the final exam questions that appear in this course book. If you are completing more than one course, be sure to write your answers on the appropriate answer sheet. You have the option of faxing the FasTrax answer sheet to 508-230-2679 and within 48 hours get your course results automatically faxed back to you or you may elect to mail the FasTrax answer sheet to Western Schools and get your course results within 7–12 business days. Full instructions and complete grading details are also printed on the FasTrax instruction sheet, please review them before starting. *If you are mailing your answer sheets to Western Schools, we recommend you make a xerox copy as a backup.*

## ABOUT THIS COURSE

A "Pretest" is provided with each course to test your current knowledge base regarding the subject matter contained within this course. Your "Final Exam" is a multiple choice examination. **You will find the exam questions at the end of each chapter.**

In the event the course has less than 100 questions, mark your answers to the questions in the course book and leave the remaining answer boxes on the FasTrax answer sheet blank.

## A PASSING SCORE

You must score 70% or better in order to pass this course and receive your Certificate of Completion. Should you fail to achieve the required score, we will send you an additional FasTrax answer sheet so that you may make a second attempt to pass the course. Western Schools will allow you three chances to pass the same course...*at no extra charge!* After three failed attempts to pass the same course, your file will be closed.

## RECORDING YOUR HOURS

Please monitor the time it takes to complete this course using the handy log sheet on the other side of this page. See below for transferring study hours to the course evaluation.

On the back of the FasTrax instruction sheet there is additional space to make any comments about the course, the school, and suggested new curriculum. Please mail the FasTrax instruction sheet back to Western Schools in the envelope provided with your course order.

## COURSE EVALUATIONS

In this course book you will find a short evaluation about the course you are soon to complete. This information is vital to providing the school with feedback on this course. The course evaluation answer section is in the lower right hand corner of the FasTrax answer sheet marked "Evaluation" with answers marked 1–25. Your answers are important to us, please take five minutes to complete the evaluation. Thank you.

### TRANSFERRING STUDY TIME

Upon completion of the course, transfer the total study time from your log sheet to question #25 in the Course Evaluation. The answers will be in ranges, please choose the proper hour range that best represents your study time. You MUST log your study time under question #25 on the course evaluation.

## EXTENSIONS

You have 2 years from the date of enrollment to complete this course. A six (6) month extension may be purchased for $25. If after 30 months from the original enrollment date you do not complete the course, *your file will be closed and no certificate can be issued.*

## CHANGE OF ADDRESS?

In the event you have moved during the completion of this course please call our student services department at 1-800-618-1670 and we will update your file.

## NO RISK GUARANTEE

All Western Schools courses are backed by a No Risk Money Back Guarantee. If you're not satisfied with the quality of the course materials, you can return them unmarked within 30 days for a full refund (less shipping and handling). This does not apply to software courses.

Western Schools guarantees you will receive credit for this course from your state board or regulatory agency, or we will give you a full refund.

*Thank you for enrolling at Western Schools!*

WESTERN SCHOOLS
21 Bristol Drive, South Easton, MA 02375
(800) 618-1670

# BASIC TRAUMA NURSING SKILLS

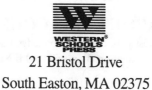

WESTERN®
SCHOOLS
PRESS

21 Bristol Drive
South Easton, MA 02375

Please use this log to total the number of hours you spend reading the text and taking the final examination (use 50-min hours).

| Date | Hours Spent |
|------|-------------|
| _____ | _____ |
| _____ | _____ |
| _____ | _____ |
| _____ | _____ |
| _____ | _____ |
| _____ | _____ |
| _____ | _____ |
| _____ | _____ |
| _____ | _____ |
| _____ | _____ |
| _____ | _____ |
| _____ | _____ |
| | **TOTAL** [ _____ ] |

**Please log your study hours with submission of your final exam. To log your study time, fill in the appropriate circle under question 25 of the FasTrax® answer sheet under the "Evaluation" section.**

Please choose the answer that represents the total study hours it took you to complete this 30 hour course.

A. less than 25 hours

B. 25–28 hours

C. 29–32 hours

D. greater than 32 hours

# BASIC TRAUMA NURSING SKILLS

## WESTERN SCHOOLS' NURSING
## CONTINUING EDUCATION EVALUATION

Instructions: Mark your answers to the following questions with a black pen on the "Evaluation" section of your FasTrax® answer sheet provided with this course. You should not return this sheet. Please use the scale below to rate the following statements:

| | | | |
|---|---|---|---|
| A | Agree Strongly | C | Disagree Somewhat |
| B | Agree Somewhat | D | Disagree Strongly |

The course content met the following education objectives:

1. Relates the importance of maintaining an open airway and lists specific techniques for opening and securing the airway.

2. Names the different types of shock and lists common causes of shock in the trauma patient.

3. Differentiates between the basic structures and functions of the head and identities common causes of trauma.

4. Differentiates between the basic structures and functions of the spinal cord and spinal column and how to initiate appropriate intervention for the patient who has spinal trauma.

5. Describes the basic structures of the thoracic cavity and describes how to initiate appropriate interventions for the patient who has thoracic shock.

6. Recognize common causes of trauma to abdominal organs.

7. Differentiates between the basic structures and functions of the musculoskeletal system and how to initiate appropriate intervention for the patient who has orthopedic trauma.

8. Discusses how to assess a burn patient, plan intervention, and transport the patient to the appropriate facility.

9. Recognizes common causes of trauma to the genitourinary system.

10. Describes the basic structures and functions of the eye and recognizes common causes of trauma.

11. Differentiates between structures of the face and neck and how to initiate intervention for the patient who has maxillofacial trauma.

12. Describes changes in anatomy and physiology that occur with aging and recognizes common causes of trauma in the elderly.

13. Describes the normal alterations in anatomy and physiology that occur during pregnancy and recognizes common causes of obstetric and gynecological trauma.

14. Describes the normal anatomy and physiology of infants and children and recognizes common causes of trauma in this age group.

15. Shows how to plan nursing intervention when several patients are present at the trauma scene.

16. The content of this course was relevant to the objectives.

17. This offering met my professional education needs.

18. The information in this offering is relevant to my professional work setting.

19. The course was generally well written and the subject matter explained thoroughly? (If no please explain on the back of the FasTrax instruction sheet.)

20. The content of this course was appropriate for home study.

Please complete the following research questions in order to help us better meet your educational needs. Pick the ONE answer which is most appropriate.

21. What was the SINGLE most important reason you chose this course?

    A. Low Price

    B. New or Newly revised course

    C. High interest/Required course topic

    D. Number of Contact Hours Needed

22. Where do you work? (If your place of employment is not listed below, please leave this question blank.)

    A. Hospital

    B. Medical Clinic/Group Practice/ HMO/Office setting

    C. Long Term Care/Rehabilitation Facility/Nursing Home

    D. Home Health Care Agency

23. Which field do you specialize in?

    A. Medical/Surgical

    B. Geriatrics

    C. Pediatrics/Neonatal

    D. Other

24. For your last renewal, how many months BEFORE your license expiration date did your order your course materials?

    A. 1–3 months

    B. 4–6 months

    C. 7–12 months

    D. Greater than 12 months

25. **PLEASE LOG YOUR STUDY HOURS WITH SUBMISSION OF YOUR FINAL EXAM.** Please choose which best represents the total study hours it took to complete this 30 hour course.

    A. less than 25 hours

    B. 25–28 hours

    C. 29–32 hours

    D. greater than 32 hours

# CONTENTS

# PRETEST

Begin by taking the pretest. Compare your answers on the pretest to the answer key (located in the back of the book). Circle those test items that you missed. The pretest answer key indicates the course chapters where the content of that question is discussed.

Next, read each chapter. Focus special attention on the chapters where you made incorrect answer choices. Exam questions are provided at the end of each chapter so that you can assess your progress and understanding of the material.

**The answer choices for the following questions are:**

  **a. True**    **b. False**

1. Trauma care in the United States costs $40 million annually.

2. Drugs, firearms, and alcohol are three significant contributors to trauma.

3. Assessment of the airway is NOT part of the initial evaluation of the trauma patient.

4. To assess the status of the trauma patient's airway, the nurse should look, listen, and feel for respirations.

5. Cardiac tamponade is a collection of blood and fluid in the pericardium that constricts the heart and restricts its contractility.

6. Cyanosis is a late and ominous sign of hypoxia.

7. Hyperventilation is often used in patients with head trauma to increase pco2.

8. The most likely person to have a spinal cord injury is a married man 55–70 years old.

9. Three of the six thoracic injuries considered immediately life-threatening are flail chest, hemothorax, and diaphragmatic hernia.

10. Treatment of an open pneumothorax includes turning the patient onto the affected side.

11. Emergency treatment of eviscerated abdominal organs includes stuffing the organs back into the abdominal cavity.

12. Impaired blood and nerve supply makes dislocation of the hips or knee joints a serious emergency.

13. "Rule or nines" is a standardized method for the assessment of burn patients.

14. Signs and symptoms of genitourinary trauma include pelvic pain, blood at the meatus, and hematuria.

15. Nursing comfort measures for patients with ocular trauma may include a well-lit room, elevated head of bed, and frequent questioning.

16. When faced with a patient who is bleeding from the neck, the nurse should compress the trachea against the cervical spine.

17. Air embolism is one complication associated with jugular vein injury.

18. The most common causes of accidental death in the elderly are motor vehicle accidents, falls, bicycle accidents.

19. During artificial ventilation of the pregnant trauma patient, until a cuffed endotracheal tube is in place, a second rescuer should apply cricoid pressure.

20. In infants and children with trauma, femur fracture coupled with blunt trauma to the spleen and head injuries is known as Waddell's triad.

21. A crisis is defined as a sudden event that causes substantial damage to property and harm to people.

22. The first rescuer arriving at a disaster scene should transport as many injured as possible to the hospital.

23. In general, before approaching a family about organ donation, the nurse should allow the family to grieve, express anger, and confront the tragedy of their loss.

24. Nurses caring for trauma patients may find that the patients' families react with anger, frustration, and hostility.

25. The use of seatbelts reduces mortality and serious injuries from car crashes by 50%.

# INTRODUCTION

Most nurses will be called on to evaluate trauma patients at some point, whether it be at the scene of a traffic accident or at the bedside of a patient who has fallen. Basic trauma nursing skills therefore are essential to the practice of nursing. The intent of this book is to introduce nurses to fundamental assessment skills and basic nursing interventions for the care of trauma patients. Because accidents are the leading cause of death in children and the fourth leading cause of death among all Americans, basic trauma skills are essential to nurses. These skills influence the survival and outcome of trauma patients, because those who receive skilled care in the first hour after injury have the highest survival rates.

This second edition of *Basic Trauma Nursing Skills* reviews basic anatomy and physiology and then presents an overview of the mechanisms of injury associated with trauma. It also describes common trauma and reviews assessment of trauma patients. New to this second edition are sections in each chapter that focus on nursing strategies and interventions. These interventions are based on common nursing diagnoses often seen in trauma patients. Just developed in recent years, the nursing diagnosis is the fifth component of the nursing process. The nursing process is well suited to trauma care because it facilitates decision making amid often chaotic circumstances. This edition also incorporates guidelines for advanced cardiac life support. As before, each chapter concludes with a summary, a listing of the critical concepts presented in the chapter, and a glossary of terms unique to the chapter.

Topics covered in this course include shock; trauma involving different body systems; and trauma care in special circumstances, such as in pregnant patients, infants and children, and the elderly. A separate chapter presents basic facts on organ donation. Other chapters review nursing care of burn patients, assessment and triage of disaster victims, and evaluation of victims of family violence.

This book is neither designed nor intended to be a complete or advanced curriculum in trauma nursing. It is a basic review of the signs and symptoms of trauma and of initial nursing interventions to be used as the patient is transported to a hospital for definitive treatment by a trauma team. It is not targeted strictly to practicing emergency or trauma nurses. Rather, it was created to meet the needs of nurses from all educational backgrounds who need an introductory course to develop their knowledge of trauma nursing. For those who wish to learn more, a selected reading list offers guidance; for those who desire to further develop their skills, an appendix lists agencies that can provide hands-on learning experiences.

# CHAPTER 1

## TRAUMA TODAY

## CHAPTER OBJECTIVE

After completing this chapter, the reader should be aware or the prevalence of trauma; the cost of treating trauma; and the impact that swift, skilled intervention has on the outcome of traumatic injuries.

## LEARNING OBJECTIVES

After studying this chapter, the reader should be able to

1. Differentiate between level 1, level 2, and level 3 trauma centers.

2. Recognize the significance of the "golden hour" in trauma care.

3. Indicate common causes or traumatic injuries.

4. Recognize current concerns about the delivery of trauma care in the United States.

## INTRODUCTION

Trauma is a wound or injury caused by energy in motion. In the United States, care of trauma patients costs more than $40 billion annually; when lost pro-

ductivity is included, the cost increases to $200 billion (Sheehy & Jimmerson, 1994). This chapter presents the statistics associated with trauma and explains the importance of skilled care in the first hour after the injury. It also describes the professionals and facilities developed to meet the needs of trauma patients, notes future trends in the delivery of trauma care, and introduces use of the nursing process in the care of trauma patients.

With an understanding or trauma and the development of basic skills, nurses can have a significant impact on the outcomes of trauma patients. As health care providers, nurses also have a commitment to prevent accidental and intentional injuries.

This chapter describes the causes of trauma; the following chapters discuss intervention for specific traumatic injuries. The final chapter gives guidelines for preventing trauma before it happens and for directing trauma patients to rehabilitation.

## TRAUMA STATISTICS

A child at play, a woman driving a car, a man at work, no one is immune or invulnerable to trauma. Traumatic injuries can happen to anyone, at any time. Trauma is sudden and generally unexpected. Accidents and assaults end lives, and other lives are changed forever in just that one instant.

Although no one is immune to trauma, traumatic injuries are often associated with certain activities and behaviors, and certain types of trauma tend to be clustered in specific populations. Consider the following examples: More than 50% of fatal automobile accidents occur on weekends. The typical patient with a spinal cord injury is a young man 19 years old, injured during the summer months. Men are injured by trauma more often than women or children are. Knowledge of the statistics of trauma may help you draw conclusions about the nature and type of injuries likely to occur in a trauma patient.

## General Statistics

- In the United States, 1 in 4 persons is injured every day, for a total of 57 million injuries; 150,000 persons die every year from injuries (*Introduction: Injury Pervention*, 1990).

- Violence has become a significant public health problem in the United States. Juveniles are increasingly responsible for the increase in violent crimes. Every year, about 1 million teenagers are raped, robbed, or assaulted by their peers.

- Annual costs for medical care and time lost from work for trauma patients are about $200 billion.

- Accidents are the greatest killers in the first 44 years of life. Accidents are the leading cause of death in children.

- Two-thirds of deaths from injuries are considered accidental. One-third are intentional in the form of homicide or suicide.

- Falls are the leading cause of nonfatal injury, whereas motor vehicle accidents are the leading cause of fatal injuries.

- Men are far more likely than women to be injured.

- The elderly and children are particularly vulnerable to fatal injury. Extremes of age often coincide with a poor prognosis.

- The lower a person's socioeconomic status, the greater his or her risk for homicide, assault, pedestrian fatality, and home fires.

- Native Americans have the highest death rate from unintentional injuries. Blacks have the highest homicide rate. Whites and Native Americans have the highest suicide rates.

- Approximately one-half of all fatal injuries involve the use of alcohol. Most of the fatalities are due to motor vehicle accidents, homicides, suicides, drownings, falls, and fires.

- Drugs, alcohol, and firearms contribute significantly to the prevalence of trauma in the United States.

## Motor Vehicle Accidents

The following information is from the Insurance Institute for Highway Safety's *Facts, 1993* (Fleming, 1993).

- In 1992, a total of 39,235 persons died in motor vehicle accidents. This number has decreased over the past few years, partly because cars are safer (e.g., many have air bags).

- Fifty-three percent of fatal motor vehicle accidents occur on Friday, Saturday, and Sunday.

- Frontal impacts account for 51% of the deaths of passengers; side impacts account for 30%.

- Sixty-nine percent of the drivers of passenger vehicles who are fatally injured between the hours of midnight and 3 a.m. have a blood alcohol level of 0.10% (the legal limit in many states) or higher.

- Drivers less than 30 years old account for more than half of all drinking drivers who are fatally injured in crashes.

- Fifty-three percent of all the deaths of occupants in passenger vehicles occur in crashes that take place between 6 p.m. and 6 a.m.

- Occupants of small passenger vehicles are injured more often and more severely in crashes than occupants of large vehicles are.

- After occupants of motor vehicles, pedestrians have the highest death rate. Most of the deaths are in elderly men.

## Falls

Falls rank second to motor vehicle accidents as the cause of injury. Children younger than 5 years and adults are the primary groups involved in falls (Campbell, 1988). In children, falls occur most often in the summer months and are from urban high-rise multiple-occupant dwellings; the victim is most often male. Because of the weight of a child's head, head injuries are common. Adults frequently land on their feet when they fall from heights, and these falls are usually related to occupational accidents or to escapes from fire or criminal activity.

Russell (1989) provides the following information:

- Falls in the elderly, especially women more than 75 years old, result in hip fractures.

- About 12,900 deaths each year are due to falls.

- About 11 million minor injuries each year are caused by falls.

## Drownings

Russell (1989) reports the following:

- About 31,500 near-drownings occur each year. Annually, more than 6,000 persons die of drowning.

- Children less than 4 years old are at the highest risk; swimming pools are the drowning site for many of these children.

- Males are four times more likely than females to drown.

- Most drownings in adults involve alcohol.

## Firearms

- The United States leads all countries in the world in homicides. By the year 2000, homicide deaths by firearms will overcome motor vehicle accidents as the leading cause of death in the United States (Centers for Disease Control and Prevention, 1994).

- Gunshot wounds are the second leading cause of death from injury. Each year, 31,500 deaths and 65,000 injuries are caused by firearms. Most victims are male.

- Most suicides and homicides are committed with firearms.

- Homicide is the leading cause of death in black men 15-34 years old.

- Three-quarters of homicides caused by firearms involve handguns; 60% of suicides are due to a firearm. A substantial proportion of all traumatic spinal injuries are caused by firearms.

- Most homicides are committed with a firearm, occur during an argument, and occur among persons who are acquainted with one another. Homicide rates in the United States far exceed those of any other developed country.

- Firearms are becoming the leading killer of children. In the United States, a child is killed by a gun every 2 hr.

## Burns

- Burns cause more than 1 million injuries each year.

- Children and the elderly are injured most often.

- About one-half of all fires involve cigarettes.

## Recreational Activities

- Children are often injured in bicycle accidents. Males are six times more likely than females to be hurt in a bicycle accident.

- Bicycle accidents are responsible for 649,536 visits to emergency departments each year. Deaths caused by bicycle injuries occur most often in July and August.

- Most deaths due to bicycling accidents occur between the hours of noon and 9 p.m.; the peak is between 3 p.m. and 6 p.m. In 1992, a total of 716 bicyclists were killed in crashes with motor vehicles. None of the 716 wore a helmet (Fleming, 1993).

- Football accounts for 229,689 visits to emergency departments each year, baseball for 285,593, and swing sets for 102,232 ("Wreakreation," 1994).

- In-line skating is expected to account for 83,000 visits to emergency departments in 1994 ("Wreakreation," 1994)..

## Violent and Abusive Behavior

- Violence is being characterized as the number one public health problem in the United States.

- According to a 1994 Justice Department study of 11 states (Thomas, 1994), 10,000 females less than 18 years old reported rapes in 1992. Almost 40% of those were less than 12 years old; most were attacked by their fathers, family members, or friends. Authorities think that only 30% of rapes are reported.

- According to current estimates, 4 million women are beaten each year by their spouses or boyfriends (Vachss, 1993).

- A total of 2.9 million instances of child abuse and neglect were reported in 1992; about 2,000 children are known to have been killed by that abuse. Reports of child abuse increased 50% between 1985 and 1992.

# THE GOLDEN HOUR

R. Adams Cowley is noted for his development of the concept of the "golden hour." He found that the survival of trauma patients was highest when skilled intervention began in the first hour after the injury occurred. During this hour, the patient should be resuscitated and transported to the appropriate facility for surgery or other necessary treatments.

The American College of Surgeons (ACS) notes, however, that "no matter how efficient the prehospital system may be or how skillful the resuscitation in the emergency department, definitive care must be provided promptly by a surgeon skilled in trauma for the patient to receive optimal benefit" ("Resources for Optimal Care," 1990). This means transporting trauma patients to the facility that can most appropriately treat their injuries. Determination of this need is based on the type of trauma but also involves consideration of other factors, including the patient's age and medical condition and the estimated time to arrival at the appropriate facility. Figure 1-1 is an algorithm used to determine a trauma patient's need for transport to a trauma center.

Interestingly, the proliferation of cellular telephones among the public may enhance trauma care by improving response time. Facsimile (fax) machines also mean that data such as electrocardiograms and the results of some other diagnostic studies can be transmitted instantly from an outlying hospital to a receiving trauma facility.

# DELIVERY OF TRAUMA CARE

According to a report from the ACS in 1990, 500-1,000 persons per 1 million population are injured each year. Delivery of care to these patients must be strategically planned to prevent costly duplication of services and to reduce the drain on health care resources. In order to meet these goals, health care institutions are ranked into three categories according to the services provided and the personnel available at the facility. A number of standards are applied before designation is determined, but in general, facilities are classified as level 1, 2, or 3.

- **Level 1:** A level 1 facility is a regional trauma center. All staff personnel and services required by trauma patients are available around the clock. A surgeon and anesthesia team are in the hospital 24 hr a day; specially trained nurses and support staff are ready at all times. Level 1 facilities also offer outreach and educational services to other health care professionals in the area.

- **Level 2:** A level 2 facility is the most common trauma facility; many community hospitals serve as level 2 trauma centers. Operating facilities and surgeons are immediately or rapidly available.

- **Level 3:** A level 3 facility is generally a small rural hospital with limited staffing and resources. Personnel are generally on call or in house to meet the immediate needs of a trauma patient before the patient is transferred to a level 2 or level 1 facility if the nature of the injuries so dictates.

The ACS ("Resources for Optimal Care," 1990) has identified three phases of death due to trauma:

1. The first peak is within seconds to minutes of injury. Invariably these deaths are due to lacerations of the brain, brainstem, upper part of the spinal cord, heart, aorta, or other large vessels. Any decrease in the number of these deaths will require effective programs to prevent these types of injuries.

2. The second peak of deaths occurs within the first 4 hr after injury. Death is usually due to intracranial hemorrhage, hemopneumothorax, ruptured spleen, lacerations of the liver, fractured femur, or multiple injuries associated with significant blood loss. These patients benefit most from regionalized trauma care.

3. The third peak occurs days or weeks after the injury and most often is due to sepsis or multiple organ failure. These patients also benefit from a trauma center. Concentration of the expertise of surgeons and physicians in one center allows a rational therapeutic approach that improves patients' outcome.

Measures to reform health care most certainly will have an impact on the delivery of trauma care. Insur-

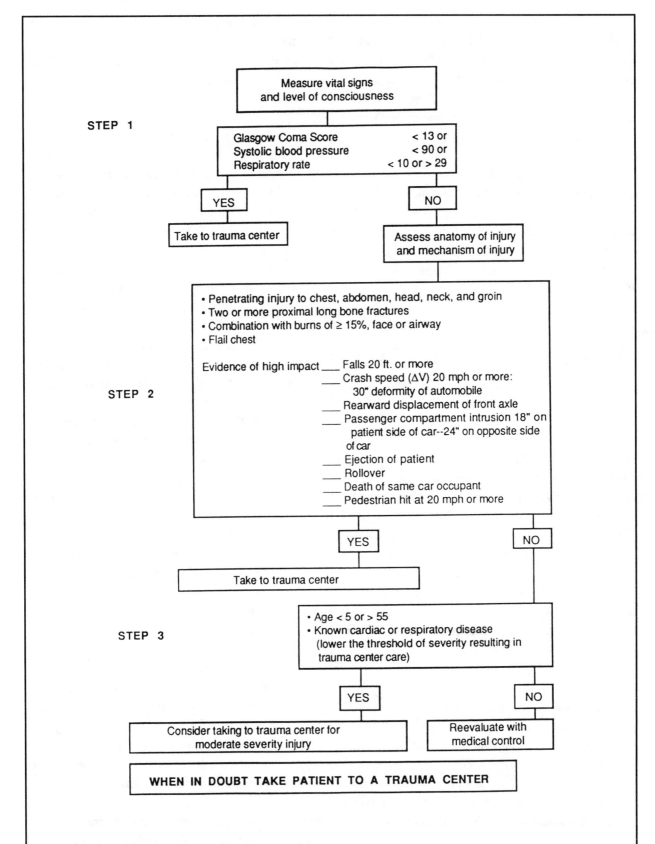

**Figure 1-1. Triage decision scheme.** Reprinted by permission from Cales, R. H., and Heilig, R.W., *Trauma care systems: A guide to planning, implementation, operation and evaluation.* Rockville, MD: Aspen, 1986.

ers and governmental agencies are already beginning to examine survival rates and patients' outcomes. Reimbursement funds may be channeled to those facilities with higher survival rates. Some facilities may be forced to close, and duplication of services may be reduced. Trauma patients may have to travel farther to receive specialized care, and intermediary facilities may assume more of the burden for initial stabilization and care of trauma patients.

Nurses can play a role in their facility's contribution to care, because nursing care, like other aspects of health care, is under scrutiny. This is the reason nursing diagnoses and specific interventions are included throughout this second edition of *Basic Trauma Nursing Skills.* By using nursing diagnoses and providing documentation of nursing care and its relation to patients' outcomes, nurses demonstrate and validate the value of nursing services.

# CRITICAL CONCEPTS

- Survival rates in trauma patients are influenced by rescue actions taken in the first hour after injury. This interval was termed the golden hour by R. Adams Cowley.

- Level 1 trauma centers are equipped and staffed 24 hr a day to meet the needs of trauma patients; these centers serve as outreach educators and resources for the entire trauma network.

- Accidents are the fourth leading cause of death in the United States, the leading cause of death in children, and the most common cause of death in the first 44 years of life.

- Drugs, alcohol, and firearms contribute significantly to the prevalence of accidental and intentional trauma in the United States.

# GLOSSARY

**Golden hour:** The first hour from the time trauma occurs; patients who receive skilled care in this hour have the best chance for recovery.

**Level 1 trauma center:** A regional trauma care center fully staffed and ready to provide complete trauma care to patients 24 hr a day.

**Level 2 trauma facility:** A hospital with selected professionals and services available at all times and other specialists available on short notice.

**Level 3 trauma facility:** A rural hospital with professionals on staff who are available to come in to examine and stabilize trauma patients before the patients are transferred to a higher level facility.

# EXAM QUESTIONS

## Chapter 1

## Questions 1 - 5

1. Which of the following is increasingly being characterized as the number one health problem in the United States?

   a. Driving under the influence of drugs
   b. Failure to take medication as prescribed
   c. Violent and abusive behavior
   d. Fractures in the elderly

2. Approximately how many teenagers are raped, robbed, or assaulted by their peers each year?

   a. 75,000
   b. 100,000
   c. 500,000
   d. 1,000,000

3. Who developed the concept of the golden hour in trauma?

   a. R. Adams Cowley
   b. A. Grace Noel
   c. James Comptom
   d. Ronald Wayne

4. Which level trauma center has facilities, surgeons, and specialists either immediately or rapidly available?

   a. Level 1
   b. Level 2
   c. Level 3
   d. Level 4

5. What is the second leading cause of fatal injury due to trauma?

   a. Gun shot wounds
   b. Motor vehicle accidents
   c. Drownings
   d. Bicycling accidents

# CHAPTER 2

# ASSESSING THE TRAUMA PATIENT

## CHAPTER OBJECTIVE

After completing this chapter, the reader should be able to evaluate a trauma scene, examine trauma patients, and formulate nursing diagnoses and plan nursing interventions for trauma patients.

## LEARNING OBJECTIVES

After studying this chapter, the reader should be able to

1. Assess a patient for trauma.

2. Suggest potential nursing diagnoses for trauma patients.

3. Relate signs and symptoms of trauma to the mechanism of injury.

4. Specify the five components of the nursing process and their potential uses in the assessment of trauma patients.

5. Specify adaptations in the nursing process that may be indicated because of the unique needs of trauma patients.

## INTRODUCTION

Accurate assessment is the key to caring for trauma patients. This chapter on basic trauma nursing skills forms the foundation for the rest of the book. It provides information on how to recognize the mechanism of injury, evaluate the trauma scene, examine trauma patients, and begin planning interventions and transport. It also reviews the nursing process and application of the process to the care of trauma patients. An understanding of basic cardiopulmonary resuscitation (CPR) is presumed.

## MECHANISM OF INJURY

Trauma results from absorption of energy generated by motion. When impact with an object occurs, the body must be able to absorb and redistribute that energy. If it cannot, it suffers disruption. Injury in the form of blunt or penetrating trauma is most often the result. The three basic mechanisms of motion injury are rapid forward deceleration, rapid vertical deceleration, and penetration by a projectile (Campbell, 1988).

### Blunt Trauma

Blunt trauma is caused by rapid deceleration. Deceleration is simply a decrease in speed. A person is traveling at a certain rate of speed when a sudden impact with another object halts his or her progress.

An example is the driver of a car that hits a tree: The car stops or decelerates suddenly, and so does the driver, but only after hitting structures within the car and consequently sustaining blunt trauma.

**Rapid forward deceleration.** When an object hurtling forward meets sudden resistance, rapid forward deceleration occurs. Rapid forward deceleration produces blunt trauma in a variety of areas, such as the head, neck, chest, abdomen, and extremities.

**Rapid vertical deceleration.** When an object traveling downward meets sudden resistance, rapid vertical deceleration occurs. A common example is a fall in which the victim slams against a surface and decelerates, or stops, sustaining trauma from the impact. Impact with the stationary surface will cause blunt trauma from the point of impact up and, occasionally, penetrating trauma, depending on the surface hit.

## Penetrating Trauma

When a missile traveling at high speed hits the body, piercing or penetration is likely to occur, leaving a path of destruction as the missile travels through the tissue. Most penetrating trauma is caused by guns or knives; however, any sharp object can penetrate the body and cause soft-tissue, visceral, or bony trauma.

## Typical Injuries

The types of injuries that occur in any trauma-causing event depend on the mechanism of injury. Thus, the typical injuries associated with a motor vehicle accident are different from those associated with an explosion or a fire. On the basis of the event that caused trauma, experienced trauma nurses can make rapid generalizations about potential injuries (Sheehy & Jimmerson, 1994). For example, the mechanism of injury in a fall is rapid vertical deceleration, which causes injury that must be absorbed from the site of impact. Thus, someone who has

fallen off a cliff is likely to have ankle or leg fractures, spinal fractures, or, possibly, internal injuries.

Most trauma patients are injured in accidents or assaults. Some trauma is self-inflicted, as in suicide attempts. Assaults produce both blunt and penetrating trauma. Accidental injuries most often occur in motor vehicle accidents, falls, water sports, occupational mishaps, and electrical accidents. Trauma caused by accidents generally includes fractures, dislocations, damage to internal organs, and soft-tissue injuries.

# ASSESSMENT OF TRAUMA PATIENTS

Seconds count in trauma care. R. Adams Cowley, associated with the renowned Shock Trauma Unit in Baltimore, Maryland, discovered the value of time in the treatment of traumatic injuries. He found that the highest rates of survival were influenced by rescue actions taken the first hour after the injury. You must act swiftly and accurately when presented with a trauma patient; precious minutes wasted never can be recaptured. The nursing goals are to assess and reassess accurately and to assist in resuscitation and stabilization. Ideally, these are accomplished in the first hour after injury.

An accurate assessment, including the patient's history and the mechanism of injury, is the key to a good outcome for trauma patients. The assessment described in this chapter is based on the principles proposed by the ACS Committee on Trauma (Trunkey, 1985) and includes the following four components:

1. Rapid and accurate assessment of the patient's condition.

2. Provision of resuscitation and stabilization on a priority basis.

3. Determination of whether a patient's needs likely will exceed local capability and arrangements for interhospital transfer if needed.

4. Assurance that optimal care is provided each step of the way.

In general, when confronted with a trauma patient, perform an initial rapid assessment (about 1–2 min) of the airway, breathing, and circulation and look for injuries that threaten life or limb. Once critical injuries are assessed, stabilized, or ruled out, you can do a more thorough secondary survey. For patients with severe trauma, the secondary survey takes place dur-

ing transport. Table 2-1 is a guide for setting priorities for injured patients.

Each trauma patient is unique, but generalizations can be made about many traumatic injuries. Knowledge of these injuries can facilitate assessment and intervention. The assessment plans presented in this chapter are general guidelines. They should be modified as indicated by the traumatic injuries and as nursing skills dictate. Points to remember include the following:

• Be aware that accurate assessment and compilation of an adequate history are crucial to survival and outcome for trauma patients.

---

**Table 2-1**

**Priority of Care:  Example of One Incident**

1. Determine responsiveness (LOC).
2. Maintain an open airway, protecting spine.
3. Make certain the patient is breathing or receiving rescue breathing (artificial ventilations).
4. Make certain circulation is present or CPR is provided.
5. Control severe, life-threatening bleeding.
6. Treat chest wounds that have opened the thoracic cavity and flail chest that compromises breathing.
7. Provide care for severe to moderate breathing distress.
8. Care for spinal injuries (cervical collar, etc.).
9. Treat severe, life-threatening shock.
10. Treat possible heart attack (patient unstable).
11. Determine severe head injuries and expedite transport.
12. Care for severe injuries of the chest, abdomen, and pelvis.
13. Treat severe medical problems or drug overdose.
14. Care for severe burns.
15. Control moderate bleeding.
16. Care for moderate medical problems.
17. Splint fractures.
18. Care for minor burns.
19. Care for minor cuts and bruises.

Note. LOC = level of consciousness, CPR = cardiopulmonary resuscitation.

Source: Grant, H. D., Murray, R. H., Jr., & Bergeron, J. D. (Eds.). *Brady emergency care* (5th ed.). Englewood Cliffs, NJ: Prentice-Hall, 1990.

- Familiarize yourself with your state's nursing practice regulations and professional licensing laws, and act within the scope of those boundaries.

- See Appendix A (Professional Resources list) for more information on organizations that can help nurses develop advanced trauma skills. This book is designed to develop knowledge of basic and fundamental trauma nursing skills.

## Initial Approach

When approaching the scene of an accident or assault where someone has been injured, scan the area to make certain that your own safety is not jeopardized by existing conditions: Stop, look, listen, and smell. Note downed power lines, fires, chemicals, and other environmental hazards that may threaten both rescuers and the injured person. If hazards exist, retreat to safety, and call for help.

If it appears safe, approach the injured person while continuing to survey the scene for clues to the accident or assault that caused the trauma. Table 2-2 gives more information on specific clues that can be gleaned from observation of the trauma scene. Note the position of the patient and the condition of the vehicle if a motor vehicle accident was involved and listen to bystanders' accounts. Check for major, obvious injuries first. Take in the scene and continue to gather information while assessing the patient. If possible, wear gloves, mask, and goggles for protection whenever examining and caring for a trauma patient.

Approach patients from the front if possible, so they will not have to turn their head to see you. Unless it is unsafe to approach the patient, do not wait until the patient is extricated from the scene of the accident to begin your assessment. If the patient is prone and unconscious, but you can determine clearly that air exchange is occurring (by the look-listen-and-feel assessment), wait for the arrival of additional rescuers to help logroll the patient onto a backboard.

State your name, and ask the patient what happened. A simple appropriate verbal response from the patient reveals valuable information: The patient is conscious (cerebral perfusion is adequate), and the airway is open (ventilation is occurring). Explain to the patient that you are there to help, and then ask permission to do so. Even though an emergency generally implies consent to nursing care, failure to obtain permission to touch the patient may be considered assault under some circumstances. Even if the patient appears to be unconscious, continue to speak as though he or she were conscious. Hearing is the last sense to be lost, and the patient who appears unconscious actually may be acutely aware of what is happening.

## Airway, Breathing, and Circulation

Begin the ABC plan of assessment: Evaluate the Airway, Breathing, and Circulation. Use this plan with every patient.

Ask all conscious patients their name and age, how the injury occurred, and where they think they are hurt. If the patient is a minor, ask someone else to try to locate a parent or guardian while emergency care is provided. Question patients about their medical history. Ask specifically if they are seeing a doctor, are taking any medication (prescription, over-the-counter, or illicit), are allergic to any medications, or have any medical conditions or physical limitations. Look for a medical identification tag if one can be found without moving the patient. Knowledge of existing medical problems can provide clues to the cause of an accident: An elderly woman who has fallen and fractured her hip, for example, may have had a syncopal episode caused by an arrhythmia.

Ask patients for permission to examine them, and warn them that they may feel pain. Protect patients' modesty when possible, but do a thorough examina-

## Table 2-2
## Assessment of the Trauma Scene

Accurate examination of the trauma scene can provide vital clues to the nature of the patient's injuries. The following are three common causes of trauma and specific information you should seek at the scene. This information will be valuable to you and the treating physician.

**Blunt trauma**

**Motor vehicle accidents**

Was the patient the driver or passenger?

Were seat belts in use?

What was the position of the patient in the car?

What was the point of impact of the patient with the car?

Was extrication necessary?

Were alcohol (drinking) or drugs involved?

What was the condition of the steering column and the windshield?

Was the patient ejected from the vehicle?

Was a fire or explosion involved?

Did the patient suffer loss of consciousness?

**Penetrating trauma**

**Gunshot wounds**

What type and caliber of weapon was used?

At what range or distance was the patient shot?

At what angle was the patient shot?

Where are the entrance and exit wounds?

What was the activity (lying down, running, walking) of the patient when he or she was shot?

**Knife or stab wounds**

What type of weapon was used (e.g., a butcher knife, scissors)?

What was the length of the blade?

What type of blade—was it curved, straight?

Was the attacker male or female? (Women usually stab down, at an angle; men tend to stab straight ahead.)

Compiled by Jon Carson, RN

tion. An examination cannot be complete when clothing covers the injuries or suspected site of trauma. Do not pull clothes off the patient; doing so could worsen injuries such as fractures. Cut clothing away with heavy scissors when necessary. Use a gentle touch; rushed and rough handling may aggravate injuries.

If the first contact establishes that the patient is unconscious, immediately further evaluate the airway, breathing, and circulation. If you cannot verify that a prone, unconscious patient is breathing, gently and carefully logroll the patient supine in order to evaluate the airway as described in the following list. Moving the patient may worsen injuries, but the alternative is certain death if the patient is not breathing. Presume that any unconscious trauma patient has spinal injuries until proved otherwise.

1. Kneel at the patient's head, and peering down at the chest, look, listen, and feel for breathing. Look for movement of the chest, listen for air moving in and out of the patient's nose and mouth, and feel for air exchange. If the patient is not breathing, take immediate action. Open the airway before doing anything else.

2. Clear any foreign matter from the patient's mouth. Do not move the patient's head or neck, as this may aggravate an injury to the cervical spine. If someone is available to help, have that person hold the patient's head and stabilize it to prevent any movement while you attempt to establish an airway. Open the airway by lifting the patient's chin with your index or middle fingers. This may be enough to lift the tongue from a position in the back of the throat, where it may be obstructing air flow. Another alternative is the jaw-thrust maneuver: Place your thumbs at the angles of the patient's jaw to lift the mandible and relieve any obstruction. Check for a pulse in the carotid artery while you are evaluating the breathing. Airway management techniques are discussed in greater detail in chapter 3.

3. If any obstruction of the airway is relieved and the patient still does not breathe spontaneously, begin CPR in accordance with current established guidelines.

4. If the patient is breathing, but respiration is noisy, an obstruction may still be present in the airway or the patient may have serious head, neck, or chest injuries. Remove clothing from the upper part of the patient's body (cut it off; do not pull it off), and again look, listen, and feel for trauma. Look for obvious deformities in, or trauma to, the neck and chest; feel for crepitus, escaping air, and variations in the chest structure; and listen

for sounds of breathing. This is a critical situation, and the patient should be transported immediately to the nearest hospital. Chest injuries are discussed in chapter 7; airway management, in chapter 3.

In summary, the first priority for trauma patients is to establish a patent airway and breathing. This is completed at the patient's head: The airway is opened, and ventilation is monitored or initiated. The next priority is to evaluate the circulation, as apnea and trauma can cause cardiac arrest from loss of circulating blood volume or hypoxia. If a pulse cannot be felt at the carotid artery next to the trachea, start CPR according to current established guidelines, and transport the patient as soon as possible. Frequent reassessment of the patient is essential.

## Secondary Survey

When the initial ABC survey is complete, the airway is secure, and the circulation is adequate, begin the secondary survey. The purpose of this assessment is to thoroughly evaluate the patient for further injury and begin recording findings as time permits. During the secondary survey, take time to stop any active bleeding and to determine other signs of trauma. Depending on the patient's condition, the secondary survey may take place at the scene or during transport.

General points to remember about the secondary survey include the following:

- Reassess the patient frequently; his or her condition can change at any time. Do not become fixated on a single injury and fail to note a decline in the patient's overall condition.

- Avoid palpating obvious injuries. Palpation causes the patient pain and may aggravate the injuries.

- Complete the secondary survey without visually examining the underside of the patient. Examination of the underside is done as the patient is moved onto the backboard or by the trauma team at a hospital, as spinal injury may be worsened by changing the patient's position.

- Expose the patient's body and examine it from head to toe. Cover the patient again as soon as the examination is completed. Ask someone to shield the patient from onlookers if necessary.

- Give the patient supplemental oxygen.

- Reassure the patient at regular intervals that you are doing everything possible to limit injuries and minimize discomfort. Explain your actions in simple terms.

- Do not give the patient anything by mouth in case surgery is necessary or in case the patient's level of consciousness decreases. Anything in the stomach could be inhaled into the lungs, causing a fatal pneumonia.

Specific aspects of the secondary survey include assessment of the following areas.

**Head.** Assume that a spinal injury exists until ruled out by objective testing and diagnosis by a physician at the hospital. All patients who have blunt trauma should be transported on a backboard with a rigid cervical Philadelphia collar in place. Do not move the patient's head. Look and feel over the head and scalp for lacerations, fractures, and contusions; ask the patient to report any tenderness or pain. Note drainage or bleeding from the ears, nose, eyes, or mouth. Do not attempt to remove an artificial hairpiece; it may be glued on permanently. Do not attempt to force open swollen or lacerated eyelids, as further damage may result. Do not apply pressure to lacerations of the eyelids; doing so may aggravate eye injuries. Chapter 11 reviews management of ocular

trauma; chapter 12 reviews management of maxillofacial trauma.

Although scalp lacerations are not always a serious injury, blood loss may exceed 0.5 L and appear quite dramatic. Hold a sterile gauze pad over any laceration, and continue with your assessment. Look in the patient's mouth for loose teeth, blood, and vomitus; all may obstruct the airway. Sniff the patient's breath for odors that may yield clues about the patient's history, such as the odor of ethanol from ingestion of alcohol, the fruity odor of diabetic ketoacidosis, or the odor of petroleum from ingestion of poison. Take just a moment to listen again to make certain the airway remains patent and air exchange is continuing.

Note the patient's level of consciousness. If behavior or speech is inappropriate or bizarre, consider this an indication of serious injury or of hypoxia. Chapter 5 reviews management of head trauma.

**Neck.** The trachea or windpipe should be midline. Note any swelling, discoloration, or tenderness of the neck. Check the strength of the bilateral carotid pulses again. Chapter 13 reviews management of maxillofacial and neck trauma.

**Chest.** If extraneous noise levels permit, use a stethoscope and listen to both sides of the chest in the midaxillary line; the breath sounds should be equal bilaterally. Note the symmetry of the chest as it rises and falls with inspiration and expiration; place your hands gently on each side of the chest and feel the expansion. Run your fingers over the ribs and palpate for possible fractures. Gently palpate the clavicles (collarbones) for possible fractures. Chapter 7 reviews management of thoracic trauma.

**Abdomen.** Look for discoloration, distortion, and distension of the abdomen. Palpate it gently for tenderness. If gentle pressure elicits pain, suspect internal injuries. An abdomen that is distended often is filled with blood, and shock is imminent. If either pain or distension is present, transport the patient immediately. Chapter 8 reviews management of abdominal trauma.

**Extremities.** Note any obvious deformities in the extremities that indicate a fracture. Do not attempt to straighten any fractures or move the limbs; doing so could make the injury worse. Palpate for a distal pulse in each extremity, and compare each extremity with its opposite; note the color and temperature of the skin. If the pulse is diminished or absent, or if the skin temperature or color of one extremity is different from that of the other extremity, the blood or nervous supply to one the extremities may be disrupted. Place a hand on each side of the pelvis and apply gentle pressure toward the midline. If this maneuver elicits pain, a pelvic fracture may be present. To evaluate for spinal cord injury in conscious patients, touch one of their fingers or toes and ask them to tell you where you are touching them. If no obvious injuries to the extremities are present, ask patients to move their fingers and toes and grasp your hand in order to check for neuromuscular injury. If a patient is conscious and alert but cannot move the arms or legs, suspect a serious spinal injury and be prepared for the onset of apnea at any time. Chapter 9 reviews management of orthopedic trauma; chapter 6 reviews management of spinal injury.

For more about evaluating trauma patients, see Figure 2-1 for the Champion Sacco Trauma Scale and Glasgow scoring systems used by trauma teams. Once the secondary survey is complete, record the findings and transport the patient to the appropriate facility if transport has not already been started. Remember: A rapid, accurate assessment and history are the keys to successful intervention for the trauma patient.

# TRANSPORT

Transport of the patient depends on the priorities determined in the assessment. As discussed previously, trauma patients whose condition is critical require immediate transport to the nearest hospital or level 1 trauma center. The decision to accept the patient at a level 1 facility is made by a physician at the facility; a helicopter and trauma team may be sent to the scene. Depending on the nature of the trauma and the assessment of the patient's condition, patients whose condition is less critical may travel by ambulance to a level 2 or level 3 facility.

Do not offer the trauma patient anything by mouth during transport, because immediate surgery may be necessary. Anything in the stomach will increase the risk of aspiration during anesthesia; a fatal pneumonia may result. The risk of aspiration is also high when the patient is semiconscious or unconscious. Report your findings to the team accepting your patient, and stay with the patient until the transfer is complete.

# THE NURSING PROCESS AND THE TRAUMA PATIENT

Many nurses remember tedious hours spent writing care plans when they were students, but they may give little more than cursory attention to such plans once they enter into practice. However, most accreditation standards require some type of care plan for each patient, and changes in the way health care is delivered in the United States call for accountability in health care practice. The nursing process is a reliable and uniform method of delivering and assessing the effectiveness of nursing care. It also provides docu-

# THE CHAMPION SACCO TRAUMA SCORE

The Trauma Score is used to give each injured patient a numerical score that can be used to estimate the severity of injury. The patient is graded in terms of cardiopulmonary and neurologic functions. Each category receives a numerical score. A high number indicates normal function, while a low number signifies impaired function. The numbers are totaled to give a Trauma Score. The lowest possible score is 1 (severe impairment). The highest possible score is 16 (normal for all categories).

The use of the Trauma Score can help to determine the order of care and transport, the level of care required, and if transport to a special facility is needed.

Each patient should be scored during the initial assessment and each time that vital signs are taken.

The following is based on the Trauma Score developed by Champion and Sacco. For additional information, see: Champion HR, Sacco WJ, Carnazzo AJ, et al: Trauma Score. *Critical Care Medicine* 9 (9): 672-676, 1981. Note that variations of this procedure have been adopted by some EMS Systems.

**WARNING:** Follow local guidelines if you are allowed to apply painful stimuli to a patient. Your local protocol should include what actions you may take when the mechanism of injury or state of consciousness indicates possible spinal injury.

## TRAUMA SCORE

| Respiratory Rate | 10-24/min | 4 | |
| | 24-35/min | 3 | |
| | 36/min or greater | 2 | |
| | 1-9/min | 1 | |
| | None | 0 | |
| Respiratory Expansion | Normal | 1 | |
| | Retractive | 0 | |
| Systolic Blood Pressure | 90 mmHg or greater | 4 | |
| | 70-89 mmHg | 3 | |
| | 50-69 mmHg | 2 | |
| | 0-49 mmHg | 1 | |
| | No Pulse | 0 | |
| Capillary Refill | Normal | 2 | |
| | Delayed | 1 | |
| | None | 0 | |
| Cardiopulmonary Assessment | | | |

## GLASGOW COMA SCALE

| Eye Opening | Spontaneous | 4 | |
| | To Voice | 3 | |
| | To Pain | 2 | |
| | None | 1 | |
| Verbal Response | Oriented | 5 | |
| | Confused | 4 | |
| | Inappropriate Words | 3 | |
| | Incomprehensible Words | 2 | |
| | None | 1 | |
| Motor Response | Obeys Command | 6 | |
| | Localizes Pain | 5 | |
| | Withdraw (pain) | 4 | |
| | Flexion (pain) | 3 | |
| | Extension (pain) | 2 | |
| | None | 1 | |
| Glasgow Coma Score Total | | | |

**TOTAL GLASGOW COMA SCALE POINTS**

| 14 – 15 = 5 | CONVERSION = |
| 11 – 13 = 4 | APPROXIMATELY |
| 8 – 10 = 3 | ONE-THIRD |
| 5 – 7 = 2 | TOTAL VALUE |
| 3 – 4 = 1 | |

| Neurologic Assessment | | |

**Total Trauma Score = Cardiopulmonary + Neurologic**

Figure 2-1. The Champion Sacco Trauma Scale.

# TRAUMA SCORE CONTINUED

## SCORING THE PATIENT

There are four elements to the cardiopulmonary assessment. The numerical values are added together to produce a cardiopulmonary score.

There are three elements to the neurological assessment. These are derived from the Glasgow Coma Score. Each category of the Glasgow Coma Score is given a numerical value. These numerical values are added together to produce a subtotal. This number is then reduced by approximately one-third its value to produce the neurologic assessment score.

The cardiopulmonary assessment and the neurologic assessment scores are added together to give the Trauma Score.

For example, a patient has a respiratory rate of 30 breaths per minute (3), retractive chest movements (0), a systolic blood pressure of 80 mmHg (3), and delayed capillary refill (1). The total score for cardiopulmonary function is 3+0+3+1=7.

This same patient shows no eye opening (1), no verbal response (1), and an extension reaction to pain (2). Added together, the total is 4. Approximately one-third of this number is 1. The cardiopulmonary and neurologic scores are added together (7+1) to give a Trauma Score of 8.

## TRAUMA SCORE DEFINITIONS

**RESPIRATION RATE**
The number of respirations (1 inspiration and 1 expiration) in 30 seconds, multiplied by two.

**RESPIRATION EXPANSION**
NORMAL — clearly visible chest wall movements that are associated with breathing.
RETRACTIVE — the use of accessory muscles (neck and abdominal muscles) to assist with breathing.

**SYSTOLIC BLOOD PRESSURE**
The systolic pressure recorded by auscultation or palpation (see pages 60-61).

**CAPILLARY REFILL**
This is determined by pressing a nail bed, the skin on the forehead, or the lining of the mouth (oral mucosa) until there is a loss of normal color (blanching or turning white). The pressure is released and the time for color return is measured. Normal return of color will take place in approximately two seconds (about the time it takes to say to yourself, "capillary refill").
NORMAL REFILL — the color returns within two seconds.
DELAYED REFILL — the color returns sometime after two seconds.
NONE — there is no indication of capillary refill.

## GLASGOW COMA SCALE DEFINITIONS

**EYE OPENING**
This test is valid only if there is no injury or swelling that prevents the patient from opening the eyes.
SPONTANEOUS — the patient opens his or her eyes without any stimulation.
TO VOICE — the patient will open his or her eyes in response to your request. Say, "Open your eyes." If the patient's eyes remain unopened, shout the command.
TO PAIN — if the patient does not open his or her eyes in response to your voice command, pinch the back of his or her hand or the skin at the ankles (apply the stimulus to an uninjured limb).

**VERBAL RESPONSE**
ORIENTED — an aroused patient should be able to tell you his or her name, where he or she is, and the date in terms of the year and month.
CONFUSED — the patient cannot give accurate responses, but he or she is able to say phrases or sentences and perhaps take part in a conversation.
INAPPROPRIATE WORDS — the patient says one or several inappropriate words, usually in response to a physical stimulus. Often, the patient will curse or call for a specific person. This may happen without any stimulus.
INCOMPREHENSIBLE SOUNDS — the patient mumbles, groans, or moans in response to stimuli.
NO VERBAL RESPONSE — repeated stimulation will not cause the patient to make any sounds.

**MOTOR RESPONSE**
OBEYS COMMANDS — this is limited by the apparent nature of the patient's injuries and the injuries that can be associated with the mechanism of injury. The patient is asked to perform a simple task such as moving a specific finger or holding up two fingers.

If the patient does not carry out the command, painful stimuli can be utilized by applying firm pressure to an uninjured nail bed for five seconds or pinching the skin on the back of an uninjured hand or at an uninjured ankle.
LOCALIZES PAIN — the patient reaches to the source of the pain. Often, the patient will try to remove your hand from the pain site.
WITHDRAWS — the patient moves the limb rapidly away from the source of the pain. The arm may be moved away from the trunk.
FLEXION — the patient slowly bends the joint (elbow or knee) in an attempt to move away from the pain. The forearm and hand may be held against the trunk.
EXTENSION — the patient will straighten a limb in an effort to escape the pain. The movement appears slow and "stiff." There may be an internal rotation of the shoulder and forearm.
NONE — the patient does not respond to the repeated application of the stimulus.

NOTE: A special thanks is given to the people at Emergency Health Services, Department of Health, Commonwealth of Pennsylvania for their help in supplying information for this figure.

**Figure 2-1. The Champion Sacco Trauma Scale (cont.)**

Reprinted by permission from Grant, H. D., Murray, R. H., Jr., & Bergeron, J. D. (Eds.). *Brady emergency care* (5th ed.). Englewood Cliffs, NJ: Prentice-Hall, 1990.

mentation of the value of that care. When nurses supply written evidence of the care they provide, their contribution to the patient's health care and their impact on the patient's outcome are clear. Professional respect and autonomy should be enhanced.

Using the nursing process to plan care is not simply an academic exercise. In trauma care, the nursing process facilitates professional care and decision making amid often chaotic circumstances. It helps nurses get organized and determine priorities. With practice, applying the nursing process can enhance your ability to deliver consistent quality care and ensure continuity of care. The process provides a guide to care, so that each patient is not treated as a jumbled and pressing assortment of needs.

Efficient use of time and setting of priorities are essential characteristics of trauma nurses because of the urgent needs of trauma patients, which are often followed by long-term needs, including rehabilitation.

The nursing process has five steps: assessment, diagnosis, planning, implementation, and evaluation. Diagnosis was added as a component in recent years. Although the nursing diagnosis and the medical diagnosis may overlap, the nursing diagnosis generally reflects the nursing needs of the patient. The nursing diagnosis specifies actual or potential health problems that nurses can determine and that nursing care can resolve (Sparks & Taylor, 1991). All five steps of the nursing process are reviewed here to show how the process can be adapted for trauma care. The discussion is not comprehensive, because details can be found in textbooks on the subject.

## Assessment

Gathering information about the patient and the injury is the first step in the nursing process. An accurate assessment is the key to effective nursing care and a good outcome for the patient.

## Diagnosis

As defined by the North American Nursing Diagnosis Association (NANDA, cited in Sparks & Taylor, 1991), the nursing diagnosis is a "clinical judgement about individual, family, or community responses to actual or potential health problems or to life processes. Nursing diagnosis provides the basis for selection of nursing interventions to achieve outcomes for which the nurse is accountable." A nursing diagnosis includes problems the nurse can act on independently, without a physician's order. This second step uses all a nurse's skills and enhances professional autonomy. In addition, formulating a nursing diagnosis helps because it requires focusing not just on the disease but on the patient's whole being: mind, body, and spirit. The nursing diagnosis also helps determine potential concerns before they become major problems. Subsequent chapters list common nursing diagnoses for specific trauma specialties.

## Planning

According to Sparks and Taylor (1991), planning involves four stages:

1.  Assigning priorities: In any patient, assessment of airway, breathing, and circulation is the first priority.

2.  Establishing expected outcomes: Setting goals helps determine where you hope your patient will be when nursing care ceases. This stage also forms the basis for evaluating progress and accepting accountability for nursing care.

3.  Selecting nursing actions: The nursing diagnosis and expected outcomes lead you to select nursing actions from a common pool of nursing interventions.

4. Providing documentation of care: This phase includes recording your care and the patient's response. Obviously, in trauma care, documentation is often delayed until the patient is stabilized. Nevertheless, accurate and clear documentation is essential. Appendix B, Trauma Assessment Nurses' Notes and Shock Trauma Flowsheet, are examples of records for rapid and uniform documentation of trauma nursing care. Accurate documentation may reduce liability in the event of litigation.

## Implementation

Implementation is nursing in action. Specific nursing actions described in each of the following chapters are based on patients' needs as determined for the specific type of trauma.

## Evaluation

The final step of the nursing process, evaluation, guides you to cease or continue the intervention or move to another action if the initial intervention is ineffective.

## Using the Nursing Process in Trauma Care

Familiarity with nursing diagnoses and the associated characteristics leads to a set of expected outcomes and the interventions proposed to achieve these outcomes. Evaluation and documentation logically follow. The nursing process therefore generates a plan of care for the general injuries the patient has sustained. This plan then only needs to be individualized to the patient's unique needs.

Consider this brief sketch in trauma nursing: Alice was a trauma nurse working in a level 1 facility when a car roared up to the entrance. Two men rushed in dragging a third man who had been shot three times in the chest. On the basis of her understanding of penetrating chest trauma, Alice mentally formulated several potential nursing diagnoses as she helped place the unconscious patient on a stretcher. As she worked, she began her assessment and planned and then implemented nursing actions. Documentation would be completed when the patient's condition permitted. She constantly reassessed the patient as she worked and adjusted her care accordingly. (In some settings, a person may be designated to record events during the resuscitative effort.) The possible nursing diagnoses for this patient included the following:

- Airway clearance, ineffective; breathing pattern, ineffective; gas exchange, impaired. Alice anticipated that endotracheal intubation and artificial ventilation would be necessary, so she made certain the instruments and supplies were available at the bedside. Securing the airway is the first priority, and in this case, endotracheal intubation was established promptly because the patient was not breathing. Artificial ventilation with a bag-valve device was begun.

- Cardiac output, decreased; fluid volume deficit. With the patient's systolic blood pressure at 60 mm Hg and his heart rate at 140 beats per minute, Alice knew the trauma team would begin fluid resuscitation. She inserted two large-bore intravenous catheters and began infusing crystalloids. She also asked the clerk to secure emergency blood supplies in the event blood was needed. Preparations were made to transfer the patient to the operating suite.

- Coping, ineffective individual; grieving, anticipatory. After they were notified by the police, the patient's family arrived at the hospital distraught and anxious, so Alice notified the hospital chaplain. She accompanied the family to a private consultation room and spent some time allowing them to process the news and express concerns. Care of the patient's family is an important aspect of the patient's care. Indeed, the trauma nurse has acquired additional patients when the patient's family arrives.

# SUMMARY

Because accurate assessment and continuing reassessment are the keys to caring for trauma patients, this chapter on basic trauma nursing skills forms the foundation for all subsequent chapters. Nursing intervention at the scene of an accident can be crucial to the trauma patient's optimal outcome. Swift prioritization and immediate intervention are necessary when trauma threatens life or limb. At the same time, rescuers must consider their own safety at the accident scene. A secondary survey after management of critical injuries allows the nurse to plan further intervention and prepare for transport of the patient.

# CRITICAL CONCEPTS

- Establish a patent airway and adequate circulation before doing anything else.

- Divide your assessment of the patient into two phases: a rapid initial survey and a more detailed secondary survey.

- A key to successful nursing care of the trauma patient is an accurate assessment and continuing reassessment.

- The nursing process is a systematic method of planning and delivering nursing care. The five steps in the process are assessment, diagnosis, planning, implementation, and evaluation.

- Presume that spinal injury exists in all unconscious trauma patients until proved otherwise.

- Act to preserve life and limb and prevent further injury.

# GLOSSARY

**Blunt trauma:** Motion energy that disrupts body tissue with a blow that does not penetrate.

**Nursing diagnosis:** A clinical judgment about individual, family, or community responses to actual or potential health problems or to life processes. Nursing diagnoses provide the basis for selection of nursing interventions to achieve outcomes for which the nurse is accountable.

**Penetrating trauma:** Motion energy that disrupts body tissue with penetrating force.

# EXAM QUESTIONS

## Chapter 2

## Questions 6 - 10

6. Trauma patients should not be given anything to eat or drink until it has been determined that they are stable and that surgery will not be needed because anything in the stomach increases the risk of:

   a. Unconsciousness
   b. Nausea
   c. Aspiration
   d. Diarrhea

7. Which step in the nursing process includes assigning priorities, establishing expected outcomes, selecting appropriate nursing actions, and providing documentation of the process?

   a. Assessment
   b. Implementation
   c. Planning
   d. Evaluation

8. Knowledge of which of the following helps trauma nurses anticipate potential injuries in a trauma patient?

   a. How the patient got to the trauma unit
   b. The mechanism of injury
   c. How long the patient has been without food or drink
   d. The patient's occupation

9. Which of the following is NOT a likely initial nursing diagnosis for a trauma patient?

   a. Adjustment impairment
   b. Airway clearance, ineffective
   c. Breathing pattern, ineffective
   d. Fluid volume deficit

10. During the assessment of a trauma patient, what method should be used to expose the patient's body completely and rapidly?

    a. Pulling off all clothing
    b. Cutting away clothing that cannot be removed except by pulling
    c. Pushing clothing out of the way but not removing it
    d. Stripping clothing off the extremities

# CHAPTER 3

# AIRWAY MANAGEMENT

## CHAPTER OBJECTIVE

After completing this chapter, the reader should be able to relate the importance of maintaining a patent (open) airway, list specific techniques for opening and securing the airway, and describe nursing strategies in airway management.

## LEARNING OBJECTIVES

After studying this chapter, the reader should be able to

1. Recognize normal airway anatomy and physiology.

2. Describe assessment of the airway in a trauma patient.

3. Recognize signs of airway obstruction.

4. List basic techniques for opening and securing the airway.

5. Differentiate among equipment used to open and secure the airway.

6. Select nursing diagnoses for a patient whose airway is compromised.

## INTRODUCTION

Establishing a patent airway with adequate ventilation is the first priority in every trauma patient; without adequate ventilation, severe brain damage and death are inevitable. With each trauma patient, the first concerns are to establish an open or patent airway, ensure that the airway remains open (secure), and confirm that adequate air exchange (ventilation) occurs.

This chapter reviews basic normal anatomy and physiology of the air passages in the human body. It discusses the causes of airway obstruction and gives instructions on how to assess the airway in trauma patients. It also describes the techniques and equipment used in airway management and reviews nursing considerations.

## BASIC ANATOMY AND PHYSIOLOGY OF THE NORMAL AIRWAY

The function of the airway or air passages is to direct oxygen to the lungs, where it is exchanged for carbon dioxide, the by-product of metabolism. Oxygen is critical to survival. Without it, brain cells begin to die within minutes.

## Anatomy

The air passages of the human body begin at the nose and lips and end in the alveoli. The upper part of the airway consists of the air passages from the nose and lips to the epiglottis. The nose contains projections called turbinates that may impede insertion of nasal airways. The tongue is a muscle attached to the hyoid bone located just under the chin. The epiglottis, a floppy piece of cartilage covered by mucosa, is located at the top of the trachea. Both the tongue and the epiglottis are attached to the hyoid bone; both can obstruct the flow of air through the passage. Some of the landmarks of the human airway include the following structures:

**Hyoid bone.** The hyoid bone is a U-shaped bone attached to the tongue. It does not touch any other bone in the body. The hyoid may play a role in airway obstruction because it is attached to the tongue.

**Pharynx.** A muscular structure commonly referred to as the throat, the pharynx begins at the base of the skull. The airway may become obstructed if food, blood, or foreign bodies lodge in the pharynx. Opening into the esophagus and larynx, the pharynx also plays a role in speech.

**Larynx.** The larynx is composed of a series of cartilages and muscles that assist in speech. However, its most critical function is as an air passage.

**Epiglottis.** A floppy mucosa-covered cartilage, the epiglottis is attached to the thyroid cartilage, which commonly is referred to as the Adam's apple, and is part of the larynx. In unconscious or trauma patients, the epiglottis may flop over the opening to the trachea and obstruct the flow of air.

**Trachea.** Serving as the passageway for air from the upper part of the airway to the main bronchi that branch out into the lungs, the trachea is composed of C-shaped rings of cartilage joined by tough membranes. If the upper part of the airway is obstructed, skilled professionals may cut between the rings of the trachea to open an air passage. The trachea branches into the left and right main bronchi, and from there air flows to the bronchioles.

**Vocal cords.** The vocal cords are found at the opening of the trachea. They may obstruct the airway by closing spasmodically. If you have ever choked on a liquid that "went down the wrong way," you have experienced a laryngospasm, which is a labored inspiration accompanied by a crowing sound and some reflex coughing.

## Physiology

Because the brain controls breathing automatically, apnea or absence of respirations may indicate severe head trauma, shock, or cardiac arrest. Inspiration is initiated by the downward movement of the diaphragm, the muscle separating the thoracic cavity from the abdominal cavity. The muscles surrounding the ribs also aid inspiration. These actions cause the lungs to expand, generating negative pressure within them. This is different from most types of artificial ventilation, which generally use positive pressure to force air into the lungs. Air passively flows back out of the lungs during expiration.

# MECHANISM OF INJURY IN AIRWAY OBSTRUCTION

As discussed in chapter 2, trauma results from absorption of energy generated by motion, and takes two forms, blunt and penetrating. Either type may disrupt the air passages. Patients with obstructing trauma to the airway require immediate intervention; otherwise, they may die within minutes. Specific types of maxillofacial and neck trauma that obstruct the airway are discussed in chapter 13.

The most common cause of airway obstruction in an unconscious or semiconscious trauma patient is the tongue falling back into the throat to block air flow through the pharynx. This usually occurs because of a decrease in the level of consciousness and is similar to the airway obstruction characterized by snoring in persons who are in deep slumber. Other causes include the epiglottis falling back to occlude the trachea; blood, vomit, teeth, or foreign bodies obstructing the airway; and trauma to the head and neck.

The human body has reflexes to protect the airway: Gagging and coughing often expel foreign substances that threaten the patency of the trachea. However, in an unconscious patient, reflexes may be dulled, and foreign substances such as blood, teeth, or food may enter the lungs. Further obstruction or a serious life-threatening pneumonia usually results.

# ASSESSMENT OF THE AIRWAY

Accurate assessment of the airway plays a key role in the patient's survival. However, remember that an unconscious trauma patient is assumed to have spinal injuries until proved otherwise. Movement of the patient's head and neck could aggravate any spinal injury and cause permanent disability. Whenever possible, have a second rescuer immobilize the patient's head while you assess the airway. The three steps in the assessment are as follows:

1. **Look.** Quickly scan the entire patient. Look for obvious trauma and note skin color and affect; patients with inadequate oxygen in their blood will become restless and agitated. Stand or kneel at the patient's head, peer down at the chest, and look for movement. The patient's rib cage should rise and fall with each breath. Both sides of the chest should move together with equal expansion. If the movement is not equal, cut away (do not pull off) clothing to expose the chest; serious trauma may be present.

2. **Listen.** Lean close to the patient's head and listen for the sound of air passing in and out of the patient's nose or mouth. Snoring or gurgling sounds may indicate the airway is partially obstructed. If the patient is hoarse, suspect damage to the laryngeal structures.

3. **Feel.** Hold the palm of your hand near the patient's nose and lips; feel for the flow of air. Place your palms lightly on each side of the patient's chest over the ribs; feel for both sides of the chest rising equally. Take a moment to evaluate the integrity of the rib cage, and gently feel for fractures or distorted areas.

# AIRWAY MANAGEMENT TECHNIQUES

This section describes both basic and advanced techniques for airway management; advanced techniques are presented for your information only. It is not recommended that you attempt to use the advanced techniques unless you have special training in them and their use is accepted within your hospital's standard of practice.

The first goal with any trauma patient is to ensure a patent airway. Even if the initial evaluation determines that the airway is open, reassess the patient often to be certain that a patent and secure airway is maintained. If the patient cannot maintain a patent airway spontaneously, secure it artificially.

If the look-listen-and-feel assessment determines that the patient's air flow is minimal, try to improve the flow. Sometimes simply lifting and holding the patient's tongue off the back of the throat by using the jaw thrust or chin lift will enhance air flow markedly. Placement of an artificial airway may be necessary to keep the airway open if the patient is unconscious or semiconscious. Positive pressure with oxygen from a bag-valve device may be necessary to help the patient breathe.

If your assessment indicates that air exchange is not occurring, open the airway by using the techniques outlined here. Remember that unconscious trauma patients are presumed to have cervical spine injury until proved otherwise. Moving the patient could worsen the injury, but if the patient is not breathing, death is certain. Logroll the patient as a unit when turning him or her supine.

The most common cause of airway obstruction is the tongue falling back in the throat, often the result of a decrease in the patient's level of consciousness. If no spontaneous respiratory effort occurs after you open the airway, begin artificial respirations and secure the airway. To reduce the possibility of transmission of body fluids, use a barrier device whenever you perform mouth-to-mouth breathing. Give the patient oxygen at the earliest possible moment. If oxygen is available at the scene but cannot be delivered to a nonbreathing patient because only nasal prongs are available, then the person performing mouth-to-mouth breathing should wear the oxygen as supplied. This increases the amount of oxygen delivered to the patient.

Techniques to open and secure the airway range from simple maneuvers performed at the scene of the trauma to sophisticated invasive procedures that only skilled professionals should attempt. Equipment used in these techniques is described briefly in the next section.

## Basic Techniques

The patient should be supine for the following simple techniques. Another rescuer should stabilize the patient's head, and a rigid cervical collar (Philadelphia collar) should be placed to prevent movement of the head and neck that might aggravate a spinal injury. Wear gloves, if possible, and use your fingers to sweep out the patient's mouth before beginning; blood, teeth, or foreign objects may be present. Be alert, and withdraw your fingers if necessary; the patient may bite down if you stimulate the gag reflex. If suction is available, use a rigid "tonsil" suction. Flexible suction catheters may enter the cranial vault if a skull fracture is present.

To open the airway, begin with the simplest maneuver and progress until the airway is secure or your skills are exhausted. First, attempt to lift the tongue off the back of the throat. If this is not successful, attempt to raise the epiglottis from the position where it may be obstructing the trachea. Use the jaw thrust or chin lift to accomplish either of these goals.

**Jaw thrust.** The jaw thrust (Figure 3-1) involves sliding the mandible (lower jaw) up. Because the tongue is connected to the mandible, this simple maneuver may be all that is needed to open the airway. To perform the jaw thrust, kneel or stand at the patient's head, facing his or her feet. Stabilize the patient's head between your wrists as necessary, and place your thumbs at the angle of the patient's jaw near the ears. Push up. You should feel the mandible slide up; the tongue will be lifted off the back of the throat, and air flow should resume.

**Chin lift.** As an alternative to the jaw thrust, you may be able to use the chin lift (Figure 3-2). Grasp the patient's mandible itself and pull gently up, thereby lifting the tongue from the back of the throat. You may see this maneuver accompanied by the head tilt, but this is not recommended in trauma patients unless cervical injury has been ruled out.

**Insertion of an oral or a nasal airway.** An artificial airway may be all that is needed to maintain a patent airway in the unconscious or semiconscious patient. However, nurses should be trained in the placement of these airways before attempting to insert one. Placed to keep the tongue from occluding the airway, an oral airway actually can worsen obstruction if it is not inserted properly, and one should not be used on a conscious patient, because it will stimulate gagging and retching. Nasal airways sometimes get hung up on the turbinates and may trigger serious nose bleeds. Worse yet, the tube may enter the cranial vault if a skull or mid-face fracture is present.

## Advanced Techniques

**Oral or nasal endotracheal intubation.** Endotracheal intubation is placement of a breathing tube into the trachea or windpipe via the nose or the mouth (Figure 3-3). A trauma patient who is unconscious should have the airway secured by an endotracheal tube as

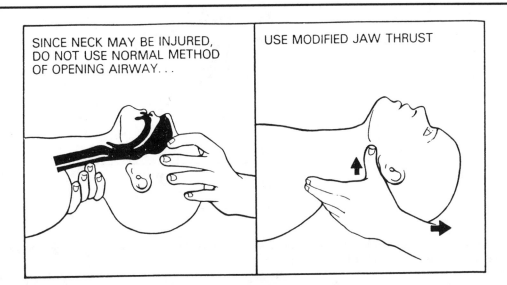

**Figure 3-1. Modified jaw thrust.** Reprinted by permission from Campbell, J. *Basic trauma life support: Advanced prehospital care* (2nd ed.). Englewood Cliffs, NJ: Prentice-Hall, 1988.

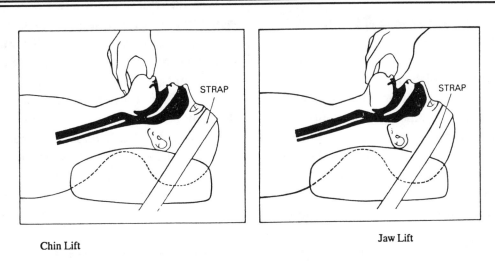

**Figure 3-2. Chin and jaw lift**. Reprinted by permission from Campbell, J. *Basic trauma life support: Advanced prehospital care* (2nd ed.). Englewood Cliffs, NJ: Prentice-Hall, 1988.

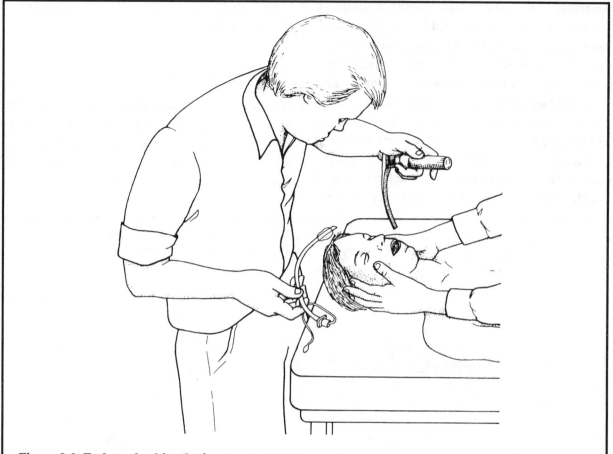

**Figure 3-3. Endotracheal intubation.** Reprinted by permission from Kitt, S., & Kaiser, J. *Emergency nursing: A physiologic and clinical perspective.* Philadelphia: Saunders, 1990.

soon as possible. Common indications for this procedure in trauma patients are as follows (Miller, 1990):

- Head injury and score of 9 or less on Glasgow Coma Scale
- Shock
- Airway obstruction
- Combative patient requiring sedation
- Chest trauma with hypoventilation
- Cardiac arrest

Only those trained in endotracheal intubation should attempt this procedure. Intubation can be performed under direct vision with the aid of a laryngoscope, or it can be performed blindly. Several different techniques are used. These include guiding the tube into the trachea by listening for the breath sounds, grasping the epiglottis between the fingers and sliding the tube past it into the trachea (digital intubation), and even threading the tube over a catheter inserted through the trachea and directed back up into the mouth (retrograde intubation). Although a nasal endotracheal tube is less uncomfortable for the patient, nasal intubation should be avoided in the initial management of head injuries because the tube may enter the cranial vault if a fracture is present at the base of the skull. In order to protect the lungs from gastric secretions and foreign bodies such as teeth, a balloon (cuff) near the end of the tube can be inflated. Complications from endotracheal intubation range from damage to the teeth and lips to death from unrecognized esophageal intubation that leads to hypoxia.

**Surgical airways.** Severe head or maxillofacial trauma may make it impossible to secure the airway via the mouth or nose. When intubation of the trachea via the nose or mouth is impossible or contraindicated, air flow may be established by penetrating the trachea, an invasive technique that is undertaken only by those trained to perform it. In needle cricothyroidotomy, a large-bore (12- to 14-gauge) over-the-needle catheter (such as that used for establishing an intravenous line) is speared through the membrane between the cricoid and the thyroid cartilages. The needle is removed, and the catheter is left in place. The catheter is then connected to a jet ventilation device (Figure 3-4). In surgical cricothyroidotomy, an incision is made, and a small endotracheal tube or tracheostomy tube is guided through the opening (Figure 3-5).

# AIRWAY MANAGEMENT EQUIPMENT

Establishing a patent airway may require no more equipment than your hands. However, the equipment used in the preceding techniques is briefly described here. Training in their use is required with all these devices.

**Oral airways.** Oral airways are curved pieces of plastic that are slipped into the mouth to hold the tongue off the back of the throat. They are available in a variety of sizes. They are not tolerated by conscious patients because they stimulate gagging.

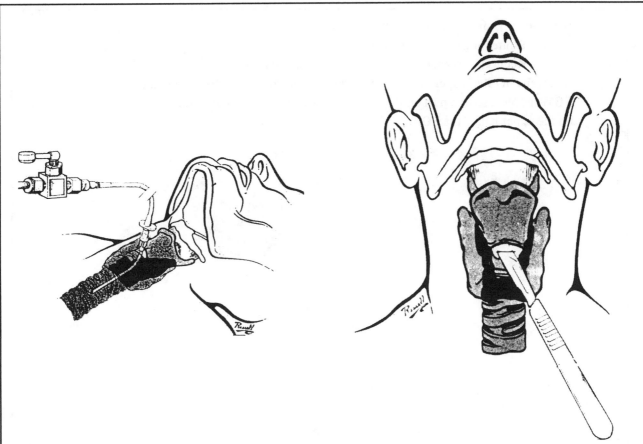

**Figure 3-4.** Attachment of a transtracheal ventilation system to an intratracheal catheter.

**Figure 3-5.** Cricothyroidotomy performed with scalpel.

Both figures reproduced with permission. *Textbook of advanced cardiac life support*, 1994. Copyright American Heart Association.

**Nasal airways.** Nasal airways are trumpet-shaped, soft, pliable rubber tubes that are slid down through a nostril to keep the tongue off the back of the throat and thus ensure flow of air. Nasal airways are better tolerated by conscious or semiconscious patients because they do not stimulate the gag reflex as vigorously as oral airways do.

**Bag-valve device.** Known to most nurses as an "ambu bag," the bag-valve device is a manual ventilating bag that can be connected to a mask, endotracheal or tracheostomy tube, or other airway. The bag-valve device generates positive pressure and should force air into the lungs. For apneic patients, mouth-to-mouth or mouth-to-mask breathing can also be used.

**Esophageal obturator airway.** Designed for use by those without skills in endotracheal intubation or whenever endotracheal intubation is difficult, the esophageal obturator airway (EOA) consists of a tube and a mask. The tube is inserted into the esophagus, where the cuff or balloon is inflated to seal off the stomach from the lungs. Then the mask is connected to a bag-valve device. Presumably, positive pressure on the bag via the mask will force air into the lungs. Use of the EOA is limited to unconscious patients only, and it should not be used in patients with trauma to the face or the upper part of the airway. However, it eliminates the need for extending the patient's head and neck and does not require visualization of the trachea. Unintentional intratracheal placement of an EOA can be fatal to the patient, because inflating the cuff when it is in the trachea could rupture the trachea. Another version of the EOA includes a gastric tube that is used for aspiration and decompression of the stomach (Figure 3-6).

1.  Improved version of the EOA
    - Route for gastric decompression added
    - Reduces the chance for regurgitation and aspiration
2.  Distal end of tube is open, allowing passage of a tube for gastric decompression
3.  EGTA added a second port on the mask for ventilation and removed the small holes that are present on the upper half of the EOA

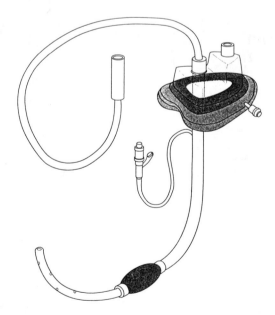

**Figure 3-6. Esophageal gastric tube airway.**

Reprinted by permission from Aehlert, B., *ACLS quick review study guide.* St. Louis: Mosby–Year Book, 1992.

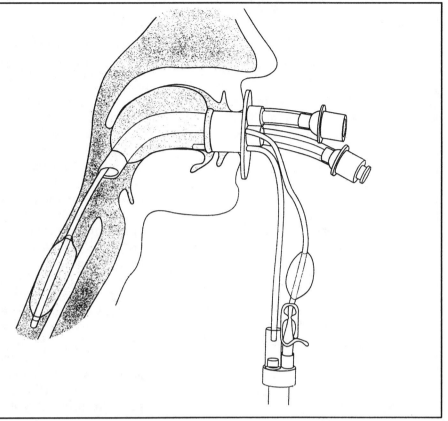

**Figure 3-7. Pharyngotrachael lumen airway in position.**

Reprinted by permission from Aehlert, B., *ACLS quick review study guide.* St. Louis: Mosby–Year Book, 1992.

**Pharyngotracheal lumen airway.** The pharyngotracheal lumen airway (PTL) consists of two tubes, one short and one long. Inserted blindly like the EOA, the PTL should provide ventilation of the lungs regardless of whether the long tube enters the esophagus or the trachea. The short tube contains a cuff that seals the pharynx (Figure 3-7). The longer tube then either functions as an endotracheal tube, or if it is in the esophagus, the balloon can be inflated and air directed to the lungs. Elimination of the need to maintain a good mask seal is one of the primary advantages of the PTL over the EOA.

**Laryngoscope.** The laryngoscope is a lighted instrument that consists of (1) a handle containing the batteries and (2) a detachable blade. The blade is placed in the mouth to displace the tongue and illuminate the epiglottis and the glottic opening to the trachea. The blades come in different sizes and styles.

**Endotracheal tubes.** Endotracheal tubes are plastic tubes that are introduced through the mouth, throat, or nose or directly into the trachea to maintain air flow. They come in a variety of sizes and styles. A cuff or balloon near the tip of the tube is inflated to seal off and protect the lungs from the contents of the stomach or throat.

# NURSING STRATEGIES IN PATIENTS WITH AIRWAY COMPROMISE

Nursing care of patients with airway compromise focuses on opening and maintaining the airway within the limits of your skills and training. Table 3-1 gives common nursing diagnoses and interventions for trauma patients with airway compromise. The following nursing strategies may also be relevant.

## Table 3-1
## Potential Nursing Diagnoses and Interventions
## for Trauma Patients with Airway Compromise

| Diagnosis | Interventions |
| --- | --- |
| Airway clearance, ineffective, r/t presence of tracheobronchial obstruction or secretions such as blood | Look, listen, and feel to assess air exchange. Presume that any unconscious trauma patient has spinal injury until proved otherwise. If air exchange is adequate, do not manipulate the airway or the head or neck, but continue to monitor the patency of the airway, as this status may change rapidly. If air exchange is inadequate, logroll the patient supine while maintaining cervical alignment. Wear gloves when possible; sweep debris and foreign objects or teeth out of mouth. Relieve the obstruction if possible. Have other rescuers (if available) stabilize the head and neck, and then attempt the jaw thrust, chin lift, and jaw lift to open the airway. Prepare to assist with intubation or establishment of a surgical airway if the patient's condition indicates. |
| Breathing pattern, ineffective, r/t trauma | Monitor respiratory status and be prepared to start artificial respiration as necessary. Use a barrier method to prevent transmission of body fluids. Prepare for needle aspiration or insertion of a chest tube if indicated by the patient's condition. Monitor vital signs, and report changes. |
| Gas exchange impairment r/t altered oxygen supply or decreased blood pressure | When available, supply oxygen to the patient. Rescuer can wear oxygen nasal cannula until a more suitable source arrives. Perform CPR as indicated and according to standards. Monitor and record vital signs, when possible, and report changes. Assist in fluid resuscitation when appropriate; monitor intake and output. |
| Anxiety r/t situational crisis and hypoventilation | Reassure the patient as you work, even if you are not certain he or she is conscious. Because inability to breathe or restricted breathing is a terrifying experience, explain to the patient what you are doing and how you are working to improve his or her breathing. Hypoventilation can lead to hypoxia, which often leads the patient to become increasingly restless, anxious, and even combative as it progresses. |
| Aspiration, potential, r/t decreased level of consciousness, blunted reflexes | Do not give the patient anything by mouth until he or she has been examined by a physician and the potential for surgery has been ruled out. Assist with placement of endotracheal tube and inflation of cuff to seal lungs off from stomach; apply pressure over the cricoid cartilage in the trachea if requested. |

Note.—This is a sample of potential nursing diagnoses. It is not presented as or intended to be a complete care plan for a trauma patient. More complete information can be found in a medical-surgical nursing course and textbook. r/t = related to.
Adapted from Sparks, S., and Taylor, C. M. *Nursing diagnosis reference manual*, Springhouse, PA: Springhouse Corp., 1991, and Chitwood, L., *Ambulatory patient care*, San Diego: Western Schools, 1994.

Your intervention should be within the scope of your professional license; commensurate with your skills and training; consistent with your state's nurse practice act; and when performed in a health care institution, adherent to that facility's standard of practice.

- Maintain basic cardiopulmonary life support skills consistent with current professional practice. Consider completing training in advanced cardiac life support and basic trauma life support.

- Familiarize yourself with the types and uses of various equipment for airway management so that you can recognize the devices quickly and use them properly in an emergency situation.

# SUMMARY

Establishing a patent airway with adequate ventilation is the first priority in every trauma patient, because without adequate ventilation, severe brain damage and death are inevitable. With every trauma patient, the first concerns must be to establish an open or patent airway, ensure that the airway remains open (secure), and confirm that adequate air exchange (ventilation) is started or continues. The trauma patient's outcome is directly related to the ability to open and maintain the airway.

# CRITICAL CONCEPTS

- Establishing a patent airway and adequate ventilation is the first priority in every trauma patient.

- Presume that every unconscious patient has a cervical spinal injury until proved otherwise.

- Look, listen, and feel to assess the airway.

- Actions taken to establish and maintain a patent airway can mean life or death for a trauma patient.

- The most common cause of airway obstruction is the tongue falling back into the throat because of a decreased level of consciousness.

- Use the jaw thrust or chin lift initially to open the airway.

# GLOSSARY

**Bag-valve device:** A pliable reservoir connected to a source of oxygen; squeezing it generates positive pressure and delivers a breath to the patient; often referred to as an "ambu bag."

**Endotracheal intubation:** Placement of a tube into the trachea; usually accomplished by passing a tube through the mouth, nose, or throat; past the epiglottis; and into the trachea.

**Epiglottis:** Floppy mucosa-covered cartilage located at the opening to the trachea.

**Esophageal obturator airway (EOA):** An artificial airway device that consists of a tube and a mask. The tube is inserted into the esophagus, where the cuff or balloon is inflated to seal off the stomach from the lungs. Then the mask is connected to a bag-valve device, and the device is used to force air into the lungs.

**Pharyngotracheal lumen airway (PTL):** An artificial airway device that consists of two tubes, one short and one long. Inserted blindly like the EOA, the PTL should provide ventilation of the lungs regardless of whether the long tube enters the esophagus or the trachea.

# EXAM QUESTIONS

## Chapter 3

### Questions 11 - 16

11. One sign of partial obstruction of the airway is:

    a. Apnea
    b. Snoring
    c. Retching
    d. Coughing

12. A potential nursing diagnosis for a trauma patient with airway compromise is:

    a. Fluid volume deficit
    b. Altered protection
    c. Sensory or perceptual alteration
    d. Anxiety

13. Which of the following is done initially to assess the status of the airway in a trauma patient?

    a. Use a stethoscope to auscultate breath sounds in all fields.
    b. Look, listen, and feel for respirations.
    c. Flip the patient onto his or her back and feel for air exchange
    d. Percuss all quadrants of the thorax.

14. What is the first step in attempting to open an obstructed airway in a trauma patient?

    a. Use the jaw thrust or chin lift to lift the tongue off the back of the throat.
    b. Insert an oral or a nasal airway.
    c. Using a barrier method, inflate the lungs with four quick breaths.
    d. Pierce the cricothyroid membrane and start jet ventilation.

15. An airway maintenance device that can lead to tracheal rupture if it is improperly placed is the:

    a. Oral airway
    b. Esophageal obturator airway
    c. Jet ventilator
    d. Endotraeheal tube

16. In humans, the upper part of the airway begins at the lips and nose and ends at the:

    a. Epiglottis
    b. Carina
    c. Pharynx
    d. Hyoid bone

# CHAPTER 4

# SHOCK AND CARDIAC ARREST

## CHAPTER OBJECTIVE

After completing this chapter, the reader should be able to name the different types of shock, list common causes of shock in trauma patients, differentiate between common causes of cardiac arrest in trauma patients, and describe nursing care for trauma patients in shock.

## LEARNING OBJECTIVES

After studying this chapter, the reader should be able to

1. Identify the five basic types of shock.

2. Describe the physiologic response to shock.

3. Indicate the mechanism of shock in trauma patients.

4. Estimate blood pressure on the basis of palpated pulse.

5. Select common nursing diagnoses for patients in shock.

## INTRODUCTION

Shock is failure of the body to maintain adequate organ perfusion. The American Heart Association (AHA) defines shock as "syndrome of diverse causes characterized by variable presentations. The common denominator for all shock states is inadequate cellular perfusion and inadequate oxygen delivery for existing metabolic demands" (Cummins, 1994). Shock can be fatal within minutes. Cardiac arrest associated with trauma may be due to several causes (Table 4-1), and, in general, treatment in these instances is different from that used when cardiac arrest is the primary event.

This chapter reviews normal cardiovascular anatomy and physiology and the mechanism of injury that results in shock or cardiac arrest. It also describes assessment of a trauma patient for shock, discusses common causes of shock and of cardiac arrest related to trauma, and reviews nursing strategies for the care of patients in shock.

## BASIC NORMAL CARDIOVASCULAR ANATOMY AND PHYSIOLOGY

The following is a basic review of the cardiovascular system.

## Table 4-1
## Causes of Cardiac Arrest Associated with Trauma

- Severe central neurologic injury with secondary cardiovascular collapse.

- Hypoxia resulting from neurologic injury, airway obstruction, large open pneumothorax, or severe tracheobronchial laceration or crush.

- Direct and severe injury to vital structures such as the heart or aorta.

- Underlying medical problems that led to the injury, such as sudden ventricular fibrillation.

- Severely diminished cardiac output due to tension pneumothorax or pericardial tamponade.

- Exsanguination leading to hypovolemia and severely diminished delivery of oxygen.

- Injuries in a cold environment (e.g., fractured leg) complicated by severe hypothermia.

Adapted from Cummins, R. O. (Ed.) *Textbook of advanced cardiac life support*, Dallas: American Heart Association, 1994.

## The Heart

The heart (Figure 4-1) is a muscular, four-chambered organ that acts as a pump to deliver blood to the body through two circuits, the systemic and pulmonary circulation. The heart receives its blood supply from the coronary arteries; perfusion of the heart occurs during diastole when the heart is relaxed.

## The Vessels

Arteries carry freshly oxygenated blood from the heart to the body. Veins carry blood that has given up its oxygen to the tissues back to the heart for circula-tion to the lungs, where the oxygen will be replenished and the carbon dioxide released for excretion. Oxygen gives arterial blood its bright red color; arterial pulsations coincide with the pumping action of the heart. The arteries become progressively smaller and finally branch into thin, microscopic capillaries. Oxygen is given up to the tissue at this level, and the waste products of metabolism are picked up for transport. The veins carry the dark-red or maroon deoxygenated blood back to the heart, where the process begins again. The muscular linings of the blood vessels have nerve endings that can change the diameter of the vessels by causing constriction or dilation. Major arteries in the body include the following:

Aorta. The aorta is referred to as a great vessel; it exits from the left ventricle of the heart, arches up and then back down through the chest, runs the length of the torso as the descending aorta, and subdivides at the legs. Three vessels exit from the arch of the aorta to supply the upper extremities and the head.

**Pulmonary artery.** The pulmonary artery exits from the right ventricle of the heart and directs blood returning from the body to the lungs.

**Vena cava.** The vena cava empties into the right atrium. The superior vena cava drains blood from the head and upper extremities; the inferior vena cava collects blood from the trunk and legs.

## The Lungs

The lungs receive blood from the right ventricle via the pulmonary artery, which subdivides into progressively smaller vessels that eventually interface with the alveoli in the lungs. It is in these microscopic structures that gas exchange occurs: Carbon dioxide is removed from the blood, and oxygen is replenished. The freshly oxygenated blood returns to the left upper chamber of the heart via the pulmonary veins.

## The Blood

A fluid that circulates throughout the body, blood is composed of plasma, a straw-colored liquid that makes up more than half its volume, and the formed elements: red blood cells, white blood cells, and platelets (Grant et al., 1990). See Table 4-2 for more information on blood volume and critical losses. Some of the functions of blood include transporting gases, waste products of metabolism, nutrients, and hormones and fighting disease. The average adult male has 5-6 L of blood.

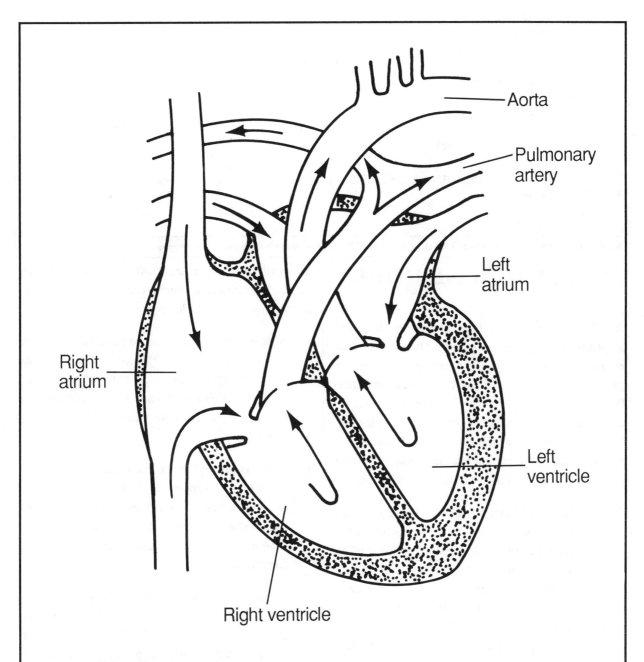

**Figure 4-1. Circulation through the heart.** Reprinted by permission from Miller, B.F., and Keane, C.B. *Encyclopedia and dictionary of medicine and nursing.* Philadelphia: Saunders, 1972.

**Table 4-2**
**Blood Volumes**

| Subject | Total Blood Volume | Lethal Blood Loss If Not Replaced (Rapid) |
|---|---|---|
| Adult male (154 lb, 70 kg) | 5.0–6.6 L | 2.0 L |
| Adolescent (105 lb, 4.8 kg) | 3.3–4.5 L | 1.3 L |
| Child (early to late childhood; depends on size) | 1.5–2.0 L | 0.5–0.7 L |
| Infant (newborn, normal weight range) | 300+ ml | 30–50 ml |

Reprinted by permission from, Grant, H. D., Murray, R. H., Jr., & Bergeron, J. D. (Eds.). *Brady emergency care* (5th ed.). Englewood Cliffs, NJ: Prentice-Hall, 1990.

Note.—One liter equals about 2 pints. One milliliter is about the same as 20 drops from a medicine dropper.

# MECHANISM OF INJURY

As discussed in chapter 2, trauma results from absorption of energy generated by motion. When that energy strikes the body, it causes either blunt or penetrating trauma and disrupts the body's integrity. Blunt or penetrating trauma to soft tissue, organs, or bones may result in shock. According to Grant et al. (1990), "Regardless of the mechanism, shock results in the failure of the cardiovascular system to provide sufficient blood to all the vital tissues of the body."

Trauma can cause hemorrhagic shock due to blood loss. That loss may be obvious on inspection, or it may be occult. Blood loss from blunt trauma is often slower than that seen with penetrating trauma. Blunt trauma often causes internal hemorrhage; penetrating trauma that fractures bones or lacerates internal organs may also cause internal hemorrhage. A contusion or bruise on the shin after a bump into a table is associated with minor internal hemorrhage. In trauma patients, however, internal hemorrhage may be massive and cause death within minutes, so early detection is critical. Common causes of internal hemorrhage include the following:

- **Abdominal trauma:** Blunt or penetrating trauma may rupture the liver, spleen, or other intraabdominal organs. As blood fills the abdominal cavity, the abdomen becomes distended and tender. Blood loss may be minor, life-threatening, or fatal.

- **Aortic rupture:** Blunt or penetrating trauma can cause tearing, rupture, or dissection of the aorta; shock will result. Death usually occurs within minutes; a few patients survive the initial injury long enough to get to a hospital for definitive treatment.

- **Cardiac tamponade:** Blunt or penetrating trauma may cause bleeding into the inelastic sac surrounding the heart. This constricts the heart and results in cardiac tamponade, which can result in flow obstruction shock.

- **Myocardial contusion:** Blunt trauma may bruise the heart to the point that it cannot contract effectively. This can result in pump failure and shock.

- **Bone fracture:** The femur, humerus, and pelvis lose substantial amounts of blood into the site of injury when fractured. For example, bleeding from a fractured femur can reach 1 L, even in a closed fracture in which the skin remains intact over the break. Concurrent fracture of both femurs can result in life-threatening blood loss.

# PHYSIOLOGIC RESPONSE TO SHOCK

Although the body has superb compensatory mechanisms to cope with blood loss, this capacity is not infinite. The ability to compensate also depends on the condition of the patient before the injury. When the healthy body sustains trauma, the fight-or-flight stress response is initiated. This response from the sympathetic nervous system generates the release of catecholamines, hormones that stimulate the heart and constrict the blood vessels, among other actions.

The goal of the compensatory drive is to maintain perfusion and therefore oxygenation of the vital organs: the brain, the heart, and the kidneys. The compensatory mechanisms triggered by the stress response include the following:

- **Tachycardia:** The heart pumps progressively faster through all levels of shock in an effort to meet the body's oxygen and perfusion needs. However, as severe shock progresses and hypoxia develops, the heart rate will begin to slow and eventually stop. Bradycardia in a hypoxic shock patient is therefore an ominous sign.

- **Vasoconstriction:** The vessels supplying blood to the skin, muscles, and internal organs begin to constrict or narrow their diameter to increase and divert blood flow to the vital organs: the heart, brain, and kidneys.

- **Changes in cardiac output:** Although it may rise at first because of the stimulation from stress, cardiac output inevitably falls as blood volume falls.

- **Narrowing of pulse pressure:** The pulse pressure is the difference between the diastolic pressure and the systolic pressure. For a blood pressure of 120/80 mm Hg, for example, the pulse pressure is 40. During mild hemorrhage, the pulse pressure may widen slightly. As blood loss continues, the pulse pressure narrows as the body attempts to maintain organ perfusion by increasing the diastolic pressure.

- **Hypotension:** Compensatory mechanisms maintain a normal blood pressure during mild hemorrhage, but the blood pressure will inevitably decrease as blood loss increases.

- **Tachypnea:** If the airway is patent, and other injuries have not caused changes in the respiratory drive that originates in the brain, the respiratory rate will increase as the body tries to increase intake of oxygen.

- **Oliguria:** Output of urine remains stable in mild shock but then begins to fall as shock progresses and the kidneys succumb to inadequate perfusion.

- **Altered mental status:** The stress response releases catecholamines that heighten awareness in the patient who has mild hemorrhaging. However, because of inadequate perfusion of the brain, mental status deteriorates as shock progresses: The patient becomes restless, confused, and sometimes even combative.

- **Metabolic changes:** Cells that do not receive enough oxygen shift to anaerobic metabolism; this increases the production of lactic acid and can lead to metabolic acidosis. Human cells function only within a narrow pH range, and irreversible damage progressing to death will occur if acidosis is not corrected.

# ASSESSMENT OF THE PATIENT IN SHOCK

When approaching the scene of an accident or assault, stop, look, listen, and smell to make certain that your own safety is not jeopardized. If it appears safe to approach the trauma patient, do so cautiously but quickly while noting the position of the patient and any obvious deformities, major injuries, or bleeding. Remember that any unconscious trauma patient is presumed to have a spinal injury until it is proved otherwise.

Approach patients from the front if possible so they will not have to turn to see you. State your name, tell the patient that you are there to help, and ask what happened. A simple appropriate verbal response yields valuable information: The patient is conscious (perfusion to the brain is adequate at this point), and the airway is patent. The next step is to stop any major bleeding and then evaluate the adequacy of the circulation.

If the patient does not respond, begin to evaluate and secure the airway, establish respiratory exchange, and check for a pulse. Quickly palpate the pulse at the carotid artery. If no pulse is felt, begin CPR according to accepted guidelines. If a pulse is present, evaluate the adequacy of the circulation by observing these signs:

- **Skin color:** Cyanosis indicates that ventilation and perfusion are inadequate. Cyanosis is a late and ominous sign of hypoxia; death is imminent. Make certain that the patient's airway is patent and that adequate supplemental oxygen is being inspired. If these are confirmed, presume that circulation is inadequate and that cardiac arrest is imminent. A pale skin tone indicates that perfusion is less than adequate.

- **Skin temperature:** The skin of a patient in shock is generally cool to the touch, because blood is shunted away from the skin to the vital organs: the heart, brain, and kidneys. One exception is septic shock, in which the skin is warm, pink, and sometimes mottled.

- **Capillary refill:** The skin color should return to pink within 2 sec of the release of pressure that blanches the skin. Perform the capillary refill test by pressing on and then releasing the patient's skin at the base of the fingernail. The skin should become pink again within 2 sec if capillary refill is adequate. A slow return to pink means that perfusion or circulating blood volume or both are low.

- **Vital signs:** The blood pressure begins to fall in proportion to the amount of blood loss: the greater the hemorrhage, the greater the drop in blood pressure. It is helpful to know what the baseline blood pressure is for the patient, but when this information is unavailable, a patient is considered to have hypotension when the systolic blood pressure is less than 90 mm Hg. The heart rate increases as the heart attempts to maintain cardiac output by pumping a diminished stroke volume more often. Unless affected by a head injury or other trauma, the patient's respiratory rate generally will increase as the blood pressure falls in the body's effort to acquire adequate oxygen and excrete carbon dioxide.

# TYPES OF SHOCK

When a patient is in shock, the second priority (after establishing the airway) is to determine the cause of shock and attempt to reverse the process. The five categories of shock are hypovolemic, cardiogenic, distributive, flow obstruction, and anaphylactic (Cummins, 1994). Try to determine the cause of shock so effective interventions can be started. In trauma, shock is often due to hemorrhage or loss of circulating volume. However, shock in the trauma patient may also be neurogenic related to a spinal injury, or it may be related to flow obstruction, such as cardiac tamponade. Also, in some patients, the trauma occurs after the initial injury. An example is a man who has a heart attack while driving and then has an accident that results in trauma.

The AHA (Cummins, 1994) recommends that providers seeking the cause of shock consider the "cardiovascular triad" (Table 4-3) and try to determine if shock is due to a rate problem, a pump problem, or a volume problem. An important concept is that no part of the circulatory system exists in isolation, so each part influences the other: When one system fails, others may follow. Figure 4-2 is an algorithm for assessment and treatment of hypotension and shock.

## Hypovolemic Shock

Hemorrhagic or hypovolemic shock is the most common type of shock in trauma patients. Volume replacement is the treatment of choice for hemorrhagic and hypovolemic shock (Cummins, 1994). The ACS committee on trauma recognizes four types of hypovolemic shock (Trunkey, 1985):

1. Class I hemorrhage is a loss of up to 15% of the blood volume, or about 750 ml. Most patients can lose this amount of blood with-

---

### Table 4-3
### The Cardiovascular Triad

| Rate Problems | Pump Problems | Volume (Includes Vascular Resistance) Problems |
|---|---|---|
| *Too slow* | *Primary* | *Volume loss* |
| • Sinus bradycardia | • Myocardial infraction | • Hemorrhage |
| • Type I and II second-degree heart block | • Cardiomyopathies | • Gastrointestinal loss |
| • Third-degree heart block | • Myocarditis | • Renal losses |
| • Pacemaker failures | • Ruptured chordae | • Insensible losses |
| | • Acute papillary muscle dysfunction | • Adrenal insufficiency (aldosterone) |
| | • Acute aortic insufficiency | |
| | • Prosthetic valve dysfunction | |
| | • Ruptured intraventricular septum | |
| *Too fast* | *Secondary* | *Vascular resistance* |
| • Sinus tachycardia | • Drugs that alter function | (Vasodilatation or redistribution): |
| • Atrial flutter | • Cardiac tamponade | • Central nervous system injury |
| • Atrial fibrillation | • Pulmonary embolus | • Spinal injury |
| • PSVT | • Atrial myxomata | • Third space loss |
| • Ventricular tachycardia | • Superior vena cava syndrome | • Adrenal insufficiency (cortisol) |
| | | • Sepsis |
| | | • Drugs that alter tone |

Reproduced with permission. *Advanced cardiac life support*, 1994. Copyright American Heart Association.

---

out exhibiting signs or symptoms because of the body's compensatory mechanisms.

2. Class II hemorrhage is a 15-30% loss of the body's blood volume, or up to 1500 ml. Signs and symptoms include increased heart and respiratory rates, narrowed pulse pressure, anxiety, pale cool skin, and slow capillary refill.

3. Class III hemorrhage is a 30-40% loss of blood volume, or up to 2 L in an adult male. Signs of inadequate perfusion appear, including hypotension, tachycardia, tachypnea, and a decline in mental acuity.

4. Class IV hemorrhage is a loss of more than 40% of the blood volume. This is a critical situation, and death may be imminent. The pulse is fast and shallow as are respirations; the skin is cold and clammy; urine output

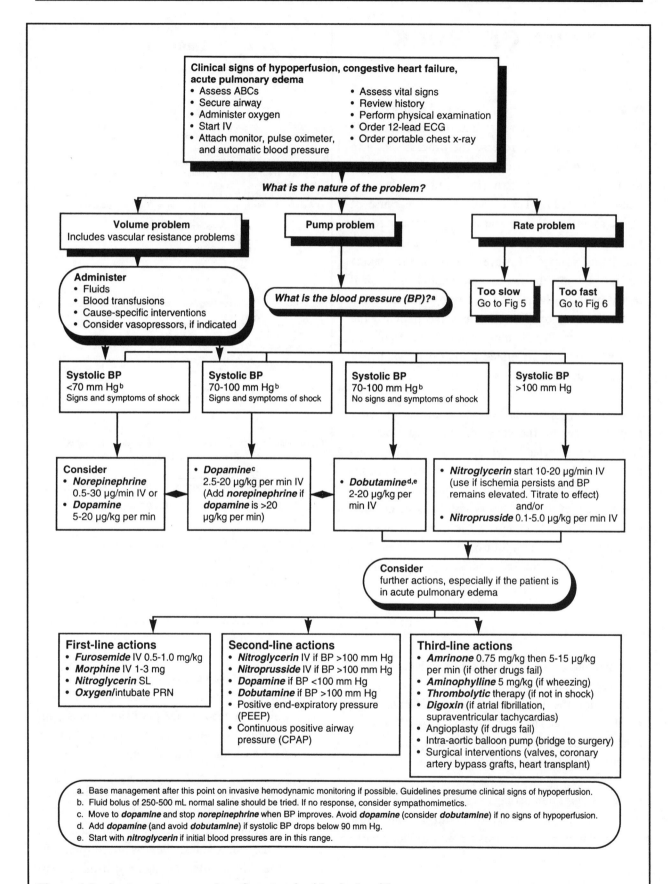

**Figure 4-2. Acute pulmonary edema/hypotension/shock algorithm.** Reproduced with permission. *Advanced cardiac life support*, 1994. Copyright American Heart Association.

dwindles or stops; the patient may lapse into a coma. As death looms, the heart slows and finally stops.

## Cardiogenic Shock

Shock also may be due to failure of the heart as a pump. Although cardiogenic shock is not as common as hypovolemic shock in trauma patients, it must be considered when no evidence of blood loss is present, but the patient has signs and symptoms of shock. Cardiogenic shock may originate with trauma to the heart, as in a motor vehicle accident or a myocardial infarction triggered by the stress of the accident or assault.

## Distributive Shock

When the circulating volume is adequate but the distribution of it is impaired, distributive shock has developed. The AHA (Cummins, 1994) identifies two types of distributive shock:

1. **Septic shock:** The patient often shows the signs of infection: The skin may be warm, pink, or ruddy rather than cool and clammy. The pulse pressure is widened rather than narrowed in septic shock. Unless treatment of the patient was delayed, or trauma has caused contamination of the abdominal cavity from disruption of the gastrointestinal system, septic shock is seldom a concern in the initial management of trauma patients.

2. **Neurogenic shock:** Although a single head injury seldom produces shock, serious injury to the spinal cord can cause shock. Neurogenic shock is a complex phenomenon in which the nerve pathways controlling the diameter of the vessels are interrupted and hypotension results. Suspect neurogenic shock in any trauma patient who has paralysis and whose hypotension is not accompanied by tachycardia. Indeed, if the cardioaccelerator

nerves T1-T4 are blocked by spinal injury, the patient may be severely bradycardic.

## Flow Obstruction Shock

When the ejection of blood from the heart is impeded, flow obstruction shock can develop. This may be the result of pathologic changes such as an embolism or heart disease. In trauma patients, flow obstruction shock is most often caused by injuries such as cardiac tamponade.

## Anaphylactic Shock

Anaphylactic shock develops in response to the administration of a substance to which the patient is allergic. Cardiovascular collapse may be sudden and severe. Anaphylactic shock is seldom an issue in trauma patients.

# CONSIDERATIONS IN RESUSCITATION

Health professionals who routinely provide care to trauma patients outside the hospital generally practice under guidelines for the care of such seriously or gravely injured patients. However, a nurse who happens on a trauma scene or who is asked to help may not have the benefit of such specialized education. The AHA (Cummins, 1994) offers the following information on resuscitation of a trauma patient in cardiac arrest:

- Start resuscitative efforts when the patient appears to have a chance for survival.

- Do not attempt resuscitation of (1) patients in cardiac arrest who have total body burns, hemicorporectomy, or decapitation or (2) other patients with obvious severe trauma who have no vital signs, no pupillary response, and no shockable electrical cardiac rhythm.

- Patients with deep penetrating cranial injuries and patients with penetrating cranial or truncal wounds associated with asystole and a transport time of more than 15 min to a definitive care facility are unlikely to benefit from resuscitative efforts.

- Make rapid extrication to and notification of a trauma facility of paramount importance if resuscitation is attempted.

- Chances of survival are inversely proportional to the period of pulselessness and time required for basic CPR.

- Administration of cardiac medications and chest compressions in trauma patients with cardiac arrest are of uncertain value. Control of the airway should be obtained first, and then defibrillation, if possible.

- Minimize delays in getting the patient to a hospital with a fully equipped resuscitation team.

Obviously the outlook can be bleak when trauma causes cardiac arrest. Those who do survive are generally young, in good health, and have been rapidly transported to a trauma facility. Figure 4-3 outlines emergency cardiac care for adults.

In rare instances, efforts to resuscitate a trauma patient may go beyond advanced cardiac life support; cardiopulmonary bypass may even be used. The purpose is to oxygenate and circulate the blood to the pulseless patient while the source of shock is eliminated. This obviously requires tremendous expertise and immediate availability of all personnel to perform the procedure.

# NURSING STRATEGIES FOR THE CARE OF PATIENTS IN SHOCK

Care of a trauma patient in shock presents the challenge of determining the cause of shock, halting the blood loss, and supporting the cardiovascular system until circulating volume can be replenished. That means replacing lost volume and aiding the pumping action of the heart. The ultimate goal is to return enough oxygenated blood to the circulation so the heart can maintain adequate organ perfusion. Supplying oxygen, administering fluids or blood transfusions, and compressing the chest to continue circulation if cardiac arrest develops are common methods to maintain perfusion and ventilation.

Table 4-4 gives potential nursing diagnoses and interventions for the care of patients in shock. The following nursing strategies may also be useful. It is presumed with each that the patient's airway, breathing, and circulation have been established and that the patient is being transported to the hospital without delay. Also, every trauma patient is presumed to have a spinal injury until it is proved otherwise. Your interventions should be within the scope of your professional license; commensurate with your skills and training; consistent with your state's nurse practice act; and when performed in a health care institution, adherent to that facility's standards of practice.

- Apply direct pressure to a bleeding wound to slow the outflow of blood and encourage clotting. Wear gloves and place a sterile dry dressing over the wound. In general, do not remove a dressing once it has been placed; renewed bleeding or exacerbation of the injury could occur. Do not apply direct pressure to bleeding from an injured eye, because this could cause loss of vision and loss of the eye itself.

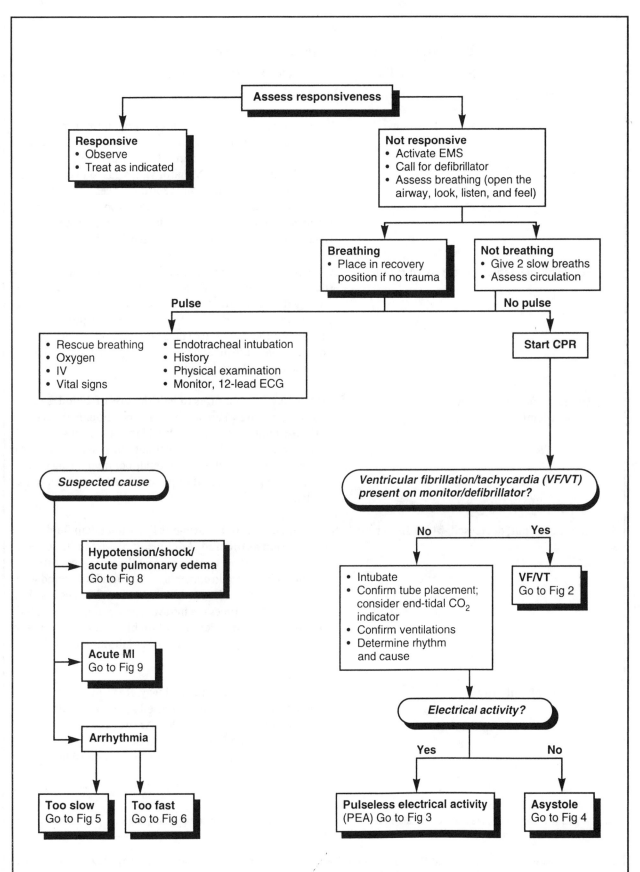

**Figure 4-3. Universal algorithm for adult emergency cardiac care.** Reproduced with permission. *Advanced cardiac life support*, 1994. Copyright American Heart Association.

## Table 4-4

## Potential Nursing Diagnoses and Interventions
## for Trauma Patients in Shock or Cardiac Arrest

| Diagnosis | Interventions |
|---|---|
| Fluid volume deficit, actual, r/t trauma | Secure intravenous access with two large-bore intravenous lines and begin volume replacement as ordered, because rapid deterioration may occur. Place the patient in the Trendelenburg position. Monitor vital signs, skin color, and temperature as indicated, and report changes or trends. Administer crystalloids, colloids (plasma volume expanders), blood, and blood products as ordered, according to policy. Hypertonic saline infusions may be used. Monitor urine output. |
| Fluid volume deficit, potential, r/t trauma | Apply pressure to bleeding sites to reduce or halt blood loss (do not apply pressure when tissue at the site may be further damaged by pressure, as in an open eye injury). Transport patient to a definitive care facility as soon as possible. Prepare for the insertion of invasive monitoring devices. Do not allow patients to sit or stand if they are hypotensive; syncope or a fall may result. |
| Tissue perfusion alteration r/t hypovolemia | Perform nursing measures to halt the loss of blood, such as applying pressure where appropriate, positioning the patient or the extremity to minimize blood loss, or assisting in invasive procedures. Keep the patient warm to increase tissue perfusion; when possible, warm fluids before infusing them. Assist with application of pneumatic antishock garment as needed. |
| Cardiac output, decreased, r/t cardiac arrest | Start two large-bore intravenous lines and begin fluid resuscitation as ordered. Administer oxygen to increase oxygenation of blood. Remember that the emergency drugs atropine, lidocaine, and epinephrine can be administered via an endotracheal tube if venous access has not been established; the dose is 2.0–2.5 times the intravenous amount. Administer inotropic agents if ordered. Obtain blood for determination of arterial blood gases and for other laboratory studies as ordered. |
| Fear r/t unfamiliarity | Explain what you are doing and why. Reassurance and explanations can prevent increased stress of the already stressed patient (Russell, 1994). Answer the patient's questions when possible; when possible, allow a family member or a friend of the patient to be at bedside. |

Note.—This is a sample of potential nursing diagnoses. It is not presented as or intended to be a complete care plan for the trauma patient. More complete information can be found in a medical-surgical nursing course and textbook. r/t = related to.

Adapted from Sparks, S. and. Taylor, C. M *Nursing diagnosis reference manual*, Springhouse, PA: Springhouse Corp., 1991, and Chitwood, . L, *Ambulatory patient care*, San Diego: Western Schools, 1994.

- Elevate the injured part to reduce blood flow if that extremity has no fractures and spinal injury has been ruled out.

- Note that agitation, restlessness, and combativeness may indicate that hypoxia and inadequate perfusion of the brain are developing.

- Know the patient's baseline vital signs and health status whenever possible so you can treat the patient, not the numbers. For example, you might encounter two trauma victims, each with a blood pressure of 90/50 mm Hg. One is a healthy young woman whose blood pressure is generally in this range; the other is her obese 65-year-old father with poorly controlled chronic hypertension who usually has a blood pressure of 140/90 mm Hg. In the first patient, a blood pressure of 90/60 mm Hg generally would require only continued observation; in the second, a blood pressure of 90/60 would require aggressive intervention, especially when correlated with other signs and symptoms of shock.

- Apply a tourniquet only if you are skilled in its use and understand the hazards associated with it, such as loss of the limb. A tourniquet is a last resort and is seldom appropriate. In rare cases, such as traumatic amputation, a tourniquet may be considered. Do not apply a tourniquet on or below the elbow or knee (Grant et al., 1990).

- Note that if you can palpate a carotid pulse, the systolic blood pressure is presumed to be at least 60 mm Hg; the femoral pulse, 80 mm Hg; the radial pulse, 90-100 mm Hg.

- Infuse fluids under pressure when possible and as directed for any patient who is exsanguinating. Pressure infusing equipment can inject intravenous fluids at flow rates far faster than gravity drip sets. Some facilities are able to warm fluids during infusion, and this reduces the hazards of hypothermia and chilling.

- Administer oxygen to every seriously injured trauma patient to reduce the potential for development of hypoxia.

- Begin fluid resuscitation with crystalloids (e.g., a clear intravenous fluid, such as lactated Ringer's solution, capable of passing through a semipermeable membrane), colloids (e.g., a plasma expander), or donated blood. Fluid resuscitation increases the circulating volume and enhances perfusion. Although blood should be transfused only when the indications to do so are clear, do not hesitate to administer blood to a critically injured trauma patient who is in shock. Even a transfusion of "red-tag" blood (donated blood that is type specific but has not been fully cross-matched with the patient's blood) is preferable to watching a patient hemorrhage to death. McAlary (1994) states that reactions to this type of blood are rare and generally easily treated, and the alternative of waiting for cross-matched blood could result in the patient's death.

- Avoid hypotension in any patient who has been resuscitated; it can impair recovery of cerebral function (Cummins, 1994).

- Assume that internal hemorrhage has occurred whenever a trauma patient has a distended or tender abdomen, fractured long bones in the arm or thigh, bleeding from body orifices, penetrating trauma of the torso, or hematemesis.

- Assist with application of a pneumatic antishock garment if such a procedure is not contraindicated by the patient's injuries and if a trauma professional skilled in the garment's use can apply it. The garment must be not be used by anyone who is not a member of the trauma team or specially trained in its application. The garment consists of trousers that are wrapped around the patient's legs and abdomen and inflated to compress the vasculature and raise blood pressure.

The compression also may reduce further bleeding and serve as a splint for fractures.

- For trauma patients with hemorrhagic shock, aggressive fluid resuscitation and rapid transport to a hospital with immediate operative facilities are generally essential to a good outcome.

# SUMMARY

Shock is failure of the body to maintain adequate organ perfusion. The common denominator for all shock states is inadequate cellular perfusion and inadequate oxygen delivery for existing metabolic demands. Cardiac arrest associated with trauma may be due to several causes, and, in general, treatment is different than that used when cardiac arrest is the primary event. The ultimate goal is to return enough oxygenated blood to the circulation so the heart can maintain adequate organ perfusion. Usually caused by loss of blood volume in trauma victims, shock can be fatal if appropriate intervention is not begun.

# CRITICAL CONCEPTS

- Establish a patent airway first.

- Return enough oxygenated blood to the circulation so the heart can maintain adequate organ perfusion; this is the goal of shock management.

- Transport all patients who are in shock to the hospital without delay.

- Administer oxygen to all trauma patients who are in shock.

- Presume that any trauma patient who has an increased heart rate and cold pale skin is in shock until it is proved otherwise.

# GLOSSARY

**Cardiogenic shock:** Failure of the heart as a pump; not as common as hypovolemic shock in trauma patients.

**Catecholamines:** Hormones such as epinephrine released by the adrenal glands in response to stress. These hormones raise blood pressure, increase the heart rate and breathing, speed up clotting, release sugar into the bloodstream, and initiate the fight-or-flight response.

**Hypovolemic shock:** Failure of the body to maintain adequate organ perfusion because of inadequate blood volume; the most common type of shock in trauma patients.

**Neurogenic shock:** A complex phenomenon in which nerve pathways controlling vessels are interrupted and hypotension results. Tachycardia does not develop during neurogenic shock.

# EXAM QUESTIONS

## Chapter 4

## Questions 17 - 21

17. A 155-lb (70 kg) man has received multiple injuries in a motor vehicle accident. His blood pressure is 70/40 mm Hg, his heart rate is 138 beats per minute, and his respiration is 36 breaths/min. He is confused. You estimate a blood loss of 30–40% of his total blood volume. What type of shock is likely in this patient?

    a.  Cardiogenic shock
    b.  Hypovolemic shock, class III
    c.  Neurogenic shock
    d.  Septic shock, class IV

18. Hormones that stimulate the heart and constrict blood vessels in response to shock are called:

    a.  Endorphins
    b.  Catecholamines
    c.  Serotonergics
    d.  Pitocins

19. A common potential nursing diagnosis for a trauma patient in hypovolemic shock might be:

    a.  Fluid volume deficit
    b.  Hyperthermia
    c.  Disuse syndrome
    d.  Mobility impairment

20. An intoxicated driver runs his car into a telephone pole in front of your house. He gets out of the car but then collapses on the pavement. You cannot palpate a radial or femoral pulse, but you can feel a carotid pulse. You estimate that his systolic blood pressure is:

    a.  120 mm Hg
    b.  90 mm Hg
    c.  70–80 mm Hg
    d.  60 mm Hg

21. Pericardial tamponade can result in which type of shock?

    a.  Septic
    b.  Flow obstruction
    c.  Distributive
    d.  Neurogenic

# CHAPTER 5

# HEAD INJURY

## CHAPTER OBJECTIVE

After completing this chapter, the reader should be able to differentiate between the basic structures and functions of the head, recognize common causes of head trauma, and initiate appropriate intervention for patients with head injuries.

## LEARNING OBJECTIVES

After studying this chapter, the reader should be able to

1. Recognize signs and symptoms of a head injury.

2. Select methods to stabilize a patient who has a head injury.

3. List common types of head injuries.

4. Choose nursing strategies useful in caring for patients who have a head injury.

5. Indicate common nursing diagnoses and interventions for patients with a head injury.

## INTRODUCTION

Trauma patients with head injuries have a death rate twice as high (35% vs. 17%) as that of victims without central nervous system injuries (Campbell, 1988). Prevention is crucial, but when head injuries do occur, prompt recognition and swift interventions are the keys to the best possible outcome for the patient. Although the brain can sustain minor trauma without serious sequelae, severe head and brain injuries can result in death or culminate in difficult quality-of-life issues.

This chapter reviews normal anatomy and physiology of the head and brain and the pathologic changes associated with common head injuries. It also discusses assessment and management of these injuries and reviews nursing strategies for the care of patients with head injuries.

## BASIC ANATOMY AND PHYSIOLOGY OF THE HEAD AND BRAIN

Knowledge of the basic anatomy and physiology of the head and brain is essential to assessment and management of the patient who has head trauma. See Figure 5-1 for a cross-sectional view of the tissues in the head.

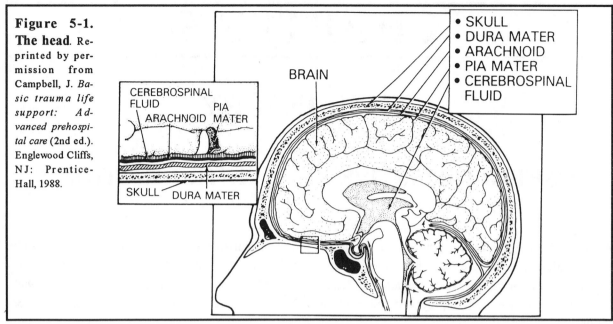

**Figure 5-1. The head**. Reprinted by permission from Campbell, J. *Basic trauma life support: Advanced prehospital care* (2nd ed.). Englewood Cliffs, NJ: Prentice-Hall, 1988.

## Scalp

The scalp is a thick layer of skin and hair covering the skull. It is highly vascular, and it bleeds freely. Although quite dramatic, scalp wounds are not usually severe enough to lead to hypotension, but blood loss may exceed 1 L.

## Skull

The skull is a rigid box: It is not flexible, and it holds a fixed amount of material. The brain, covered by the thin membranous meninges, is protected by the skull. Because the skull is rigid, any increase in the volume it holds can be disastrous. Figure 5-2 shows the major bones that form the skull.

## Brain

Formed from billions of nerve cells, the brain weighs about 3 lb (1.4 kg). The cerebrum composes the main part of the brain and is divided into two hemispheres. Unfortunately, just as a slightly swollen area or bruise will form on the shin in response to a bump, so will the brain swell in response to trauma. However, because the brain is enclosed in the rigid skull, swelling can cause death in minutes. Like other tissues,

the brain requires oxygen. It is generally accepted that the brain can go no longer than 4–6 min without oxygen before irreversible damage occurs. This is not a firm rule; victims of hypothermia are often an exception.

## Meninges

The three meninges (Figure 5-3) are fibrous membranes that cover the brain and spinal cord:

1. **Dura mater:** The dura mater is the toughest and outermost of the meninges; it covers the brain. A head injury can cause bleeding between the dura mater and the arachnoid mater. The resulting pressure can cause brain injury.

2. **Arachnoid mater:** The arachnoid mater is the thinner membrane that lies under the dura mater.

3. **Pia mater:** Adherent to the brain, the pia mater is the innermost of the three meninges.

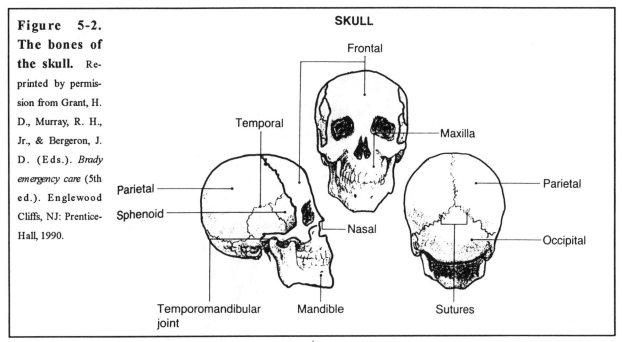

**Figure 5-2. The bones of the skull.** Reprinted by permission from Grant, H. D., Murray, R. H., Jr., & Bergeron, J. D. (Eds.). *Brady emergency care* (5th ed.). Englewood Cliffs, NJ: Prentice-Hall, 1990.

## Cerebrospinal Fluid

About 150 ml of cerebrospinal fluid (CSF) bathes the brain and spinal cord. The CSF provides a cushion of support and protects against some harmful substances by acting as the blood-brain barrier.

## Cranial Nerves

Twelve pairs of cranial nerves arise from the underside of the brain. The most frequently injured cranial nerve is the third one, the oculomotor nerve (Strange, 1987). The major functions of this nerve include regulation of eye movements and pupil size. The first two cranial nerves, the olfactory and optic nerves, are also subject to injury.

# MECHANISM OF INJURY

Trauma results from absorption of energy generated by motion. When impact with an object occurs, the body must be able to absorb and redistribute that energy, or its integrity is disrupted. A head injury may be the result of blunt or penetrating trauma. Head injuries also are classified as open (the brain is exposed) or closed (the skull is intact, although the scalp may be disrupted).

Because the brain is protected by the skull, most brain injuries are caused by blunt trauma to the head. Just as the occupants of motor vehicles continue forward and crash into the interior of the vehicle when it hits a stationary object or another vehicle, so does the brain continue forward when the skull hits an object. This causes a deceleration injury to the brain as it hits the skull, absorbs energy, and rebounds to the opposite side of the skull. The first collision of the brain with the skull is the *coup;* the second collision, with the opposite side, is the *contrecoup.* This movement of the brain in the skull can tear blood vessels and damage structures in the brain, leading to collections of blood that occupy space or to swelling of the brain.

Blunt or penetrating trauma can cause the brain to swell, just as any other soft tissue swells as a result of leaking capillaries and the body's inflammatory response to injury. Trauma also may cause bleeding in the cranium, and the blood from the hemorrhage must occupy space. The intracranial pressure (ICP) will increase because the skull is rigid and inelastic.

**Figure 5-3. Epidural and subdural hematomas.** Reprinted by permission from Sherman, D. N. *Nursing 90, 20*(4), 47–51, 1990.

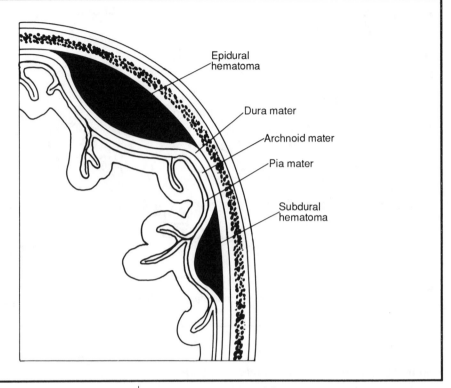

Epidural hematoma

Dura mater

Archnoid mater

Pia mater

Subdural hematoma

Increased ICP is a serious event. As the ICP rises, so does the blood pressure, as the body attempts to continue to perfuse the brain. In later stages, the heart rate slows by reflex, the body decompensates, and death results. Increased ICP may also force the brain down through the foramen magnum and herniate the brainstem, another grave event.

Projectiles such as bullets or knives may enter the brain. A projectile that penetrates the brain must enter through the skull, so bone fragments may be driven into the wound along with the foreign object, causing additional injury to the brain. Intracranial bleeding and structural damage may result. Penetrating trauma usually fractures the skull, and the projectile may be retained in the brain. Figure 5-4 shows examples of skull fractures.

# ASSESSMENT OF THE PATIENT WITH HEAD INJURIES

Whenever a patient has a head injury, follow the standard ABC assessment plan. Assume that the patient also has injury to the cervical spine, and immobilize the head and the neck. If necessary, a second rescuer can stabilize the patient's head and neck until a team arrives with a rigid Philadelphia cervical collar.

One of the most important tasks in assessing and managing patients with head injuries is continual monitoring of the patient's condition. This monitoring is essential; it enables you to recognize variations from the baseline that indicate pathologic changes (Trunkey, 1985). Determine a baseline of the patient's condition, and then act on any deviation from that baseline. The condition of a patient who has a head injury can change radically within minutes.

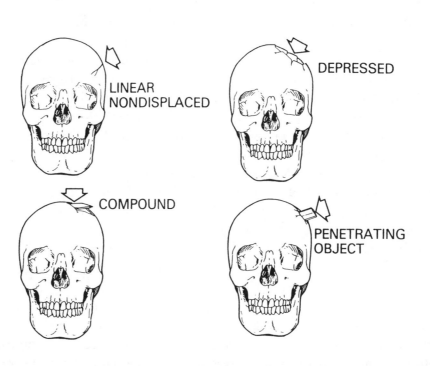

**Figure 5-4. Types of skull fractures.** Reprinted by permission from Campbell, J. *Basic trauma life support: Advanced prehospital care* (2nd ed.). Englewood Cliffs, NJ: Prentice-Hall, 1988.

LINEAR NONDISPLACED

DEPRESSED

COMPOUND

PENETRATING OBJECT

If the patient is unconscious, consider all potential causes, including head injury, that might account for the loss of consciousness. Sheehy and Jimmerson (1994) propose the following mnemonic for ruling out potential causes of loss of consciousness:

A = Alcohol (acute or chronic)
E = Epilepsy
I = Insulin (too much or too little)
O = Overdose (or underdose)
U = Uremia (or other toxic problems)
T = Trauma/tumors
I = Infections
P = Psychiatric
S = Stroke

Assessment proceeds as with any patient: Observe the accident scene, and obtain a history of the injury while evaluating the patient. Ask bystanders about the patient's actions and level of consciousness before the trauma occurred. This can provide information for the baseline assessment and clues about the nature of the injury. Note that alcohol and substance abuse frequently are factors in assaults and accidents that result in head injury. Knowing what the patient's mental status was before the accident is helpful in evaluating the patient after the accident. Many trauma professionals think that the level of consciousness and any change in it are the most important indicators of head injury, so monitor this parameter closely. Do this by talking with the conscious patient while you work so that you will be immediately aware of any deterioration in the level of consciousness or any slurred or inappropriate speech.

Head injury is highly likely if any of the following occurs:

• The patient had a blow to the head.

• The patient complains of a headache.

• Deformity or fracture of the skull, face, or jaw is obvious.

• Blood or clear fluid that may be CSF leaks from the patient's nose or ears.

- The blood pressure is elevated, but the pulse rate is slow (this is an ominous and late sign of increased ICP).

- The pupils are unequal, dilated, or unresponsive to light, or the patient reports visual disturbances or a reduction in visual acuity. Do not force open injured eyelids to assess the pupils; doing so may aggravate an eye injury. Also, be aware that some drugs, such as narcotics, can alter the size and reactivity of the pupils.

- The patient is unconscious or lost consciousness after the trauma.

- The patient shows alterations in the level of consciousness such as drowsiness, hyperactivity, or irrational behavior. Do not assume that the trauma patient who slurs words or staggers is intoxicated or a substance abuser. Head injury can cause confusion, slurred speech, and problems with comprehension. Conversely, do not assume that the obviously intoxicated patient's slurred speech or staggering gait is the result of alcohol ingestion rather than a head injury.

- The patient has paralysis or motor weakness, especially on just one side of the body.

- The patient has abnormal posturing and rigidity of the extremities.

- Bruising appears over the mastoid process behind the ears (Battle's sign) or underneath the eyes (raccoon eyes); it may take several hours for this discoloration to appear.

- The patient has or had a seizure.

- The patient has any changes in the level of consciousness as evidenced by orientation to time, place, and person.

Assessment of the patient who has head injury also requires a brief neurologic examination to evaluate the patient's eye opening, verbal response, and motor responses. Do this assessment, which follows the design of the Glasgow Coma Scale (Figure 2-1), when you begin the secondary survey. Much of the value of noting and recording this information is that it helps form a baseline reference for the patient and aids in early recognition of any changes. It also supports continuity of care. The assessment is easily duplicated, and changes in the patient's condition can be documented reliably.

When assessing a child with head injuries, view both the injury and the trauma scene with suspicion unless the injury was clearly the result of an motor vehicle accident or other accident. If you suspect a child's injuries may have been inflicted intentionally, ask a second rescuer to notify the police, and ask the police to investigate. See chapter 16 for more on trauma in children and child abuse.

# COMMON HEAD INJURIES

## Scalp Laceration

The scalp is vascular and bleeds freely. The blood loss is seldom life-threatening, however, except in children, who have a lower blood volume than adults.

## Skull Fracture

A skull fracture may be obvious because it deforms the skull, or it may not be diagnosed until a radiograph of the head is obtained. Suspect a skull fracture in any patient who is unconscious or who has penetrating head injury, unequal or unreactive pupils, blood or CSF flowing from the nose or ears, or bruises under the eyes or behind the ears. The base of the skull is a common fracture site, and basilar skull fractures can provide an opening between the nasal air passages and the brain. Consequently, attempts to insert a nasogastric tube or nasal airway can result in the tube entering the brain.

## Concussion

A concussion is a mild closed head injury without detectable damage to the brain (Grant et al., 1990). Blunt trauma to the head, as in a fall or a sports accident, can cause a concussion; consciousness may be lost briefly. Some amnesia is common, and the patient often complains of a headache. Although this injury generally is not considered serious, any patient who has lost consciousness should be transported to a hospital for examination. If the loss of consciousness exceeds 5 min, the patient may be hospitalized for further observation.

## Cerebral Contusion

A cerebral contusion is another closed head injury caused by blunt trauma to the head. Bruising of the brain results because of bleeding from blood vessels in the cranium that are torn on impact. Loss of consciousness occurs, usually for a prolonged period. The patient should be transported to a hospital for examination. Because it is difficult to determine the degree of cerebral contusion in the prehospital setting, be on guard for any deterioration or change in the patient's condition.

## Hematoma

Trauma to the brain may cause hematoma. Surgery often is necessary to evacuate the mass. Any patient with a possible hematoma should be transported to a hospital. Figure 5-3 shows the two common types of hematoma caused by head injury.

**Subdural hematoma.** A collection of blood under the dura, a subdural hematoma may develop over a period of hours or days or weeks after the injury, because bleeding is often from a venous source. A patient who has a subdural hematoma may complain of headache and have alterations in neurologic status, such as changes in the level of consciousness or slurred speech. The outcome is improved by early recognition and intervention.

**Epidural hematoma.** A collection of blood above the dura, an epidural hematoma is caused by arterial bleeding, so the signs and symptoms appear sooner than those of a subdural hematoma. Typically, loss of consciousness occurs. This is followed by a brief period when the patient is conscious and lucid, but then the patient again lapses into unconsciousness and evidence of neurologic injury becomes apparent, especially paralysis on one side of the body. Immediate surgery is required to evacuate the hematoma, otherwise the prognosis can be poor.

## Intracerebral Hemorrhage

Penetrating head injury, and sometimes blunt trauma, can cause bleeding into the brain similar to that associated with a stroke. The ICP increases, and death may occur. Any patient with possible intracerebral hemorrhage should be transported to a hospital. Frequent monitoring of the patient during transport is essential.

## Impalement

Any object lodged in the head should be left in place. Removing it could make the injury worse. The object should be stabilized, and the patient should be transported to a hospital immediately.

## Table 5-1
### Potential Nursing Diagnoses and Interventions for Patients with Head Injuries

| Diagnosis | Interventions |
|---|---|
| Airway clearance, ineffective, r/t decreased level of consciousness | Maintain a patent airway. Presume that a spinal cord injury due to head injury exists in patients with head injuries until it is proved otherwise at a hospital. Do not manipulate the patient's head or neck; stabilize it in a rigid Philadelphia collar. Until a basilar skull fracture has been ruled out, do not insert anything into the nose (e.g., airways, endotracheal tubes, gastric tubes, suction catheters) because the device could enter the brain. |
| Breathing pattern, ineffective, r/t trauma | Monitor level of consciousness and respiration constantly and be prepared to start artificial ventilation as necessary. Monitor and record vital signs and level of consciousness; report changes immediately. |
| Gas exchange impairment r/t altered oxygen supply or ineffective respiration | Supply oxygen to the patient when possible; follow physician's orders about hyperventilation to decrease $CO_2$. Increases in $pCO_2$ in the blood due to ineffective breathing will dilate the blood vessels and increase intracranial pressure; hyperventilation will reduce $pCO_2$ and may reduce this swelling. |
| Anxiety r/t head injury and potential for impairment | Head injuries especially distress patients and families, who fear brain damage and limited recovery, so reassure them that everything possible is being done for the patient. Explain that bleeding scalp wounds look quite dramatic but are seldom life threatening if not associated with a skull or brain injury. Reassure the patient as you work, because hearing may be present even in an apparently unconscious patient. |
| Injury, potential for, r/t possible seizure activity | Be careful when you put your fingers into a trauma patient's mouth, because a seizure may develop quickly. Do not restrain the patient if a seizure occurs, but keep patients from hurting themselves or others during the seizure. |
| Aspiration, potential, r/t decreased level of consciousness, blunted reflexes | Do not give the trauma patient anything by mouth until he or she has been examined by a physician and the potential for surgery is ruled out. Vomiting frequently accompanies head injury; have suction available and take steps to prevent aspiration. |

Note.—This is a sample of potential nursing diagnoses. It is not presented as or intended to be a complete care plan for the trauma patient. More complete information can be found in a medical-surgical nursing course and textbook. r/t = related to.

Adapted from Sparks, S. and Taylor, C. M. *Nursing diagnosis reference manual*, Springhouse, PA: Springhouse Corp., 1991, and Chitwood,, L. *Ambulatory patient care*, San Diego: Western Schools, 1994.

# NURSING STRATEGIES FOR PATIENTS WITH HEAD INJURIES

Head injuries are potentially serious, are associated with significant morbidity and mortality, and may affect a patient's quality of life. The first minutes of the golden hour can have a critical impact on the outcome of patients who have head injury. The goal of trauma care is to return the patient to his or her pretrauma stage of functioning, and when that is not possible, to help the patient achieve the best possible outcome with minimal limitations.

Table 5-1 gives potential nursing diagnoses and interventions for the care of patients with head injuries. The following common nursing strategies may also be useful. It is presumed with each that airway, breathing, and circulation are already established. Your intervention should be within the scope of your professional license; commensurate with your skills and training; consistent with your state's nurse practice act; and when performed in a health care institution, adherent to that facility's standards of practice.

- Monitor arterial blood gases as ordered and notify physician or respiratory therapist of abnormal values so that adjustments and interventions can be planned.

- Determine the size and reactivity of the pupils at regular intervals; immediately report any changes.

- Administer intravenous fluids as indicated to combat shock, but be aware that excessive fluid administration can contribute to increased ICP.

- Remember that head injury is seldom a cause of hypotension. Hypotension most likely is caused by hemorrhage in another area of the body. In a patient with a normal pulse rate and without pallor, hypotension may indicate neurogenic shock associated with a spinal injury.

- Do not probe through a scalp laceration to determine its depth. Simply apply gentle pressure with a sterile dressing to reduce blood flow, and transport the patient to a hospital. Do not apply pressure over an obvious deformity of the skull. The deformity could be a fracture, and pressure on it could injure the brain further.

# SUMMARY

Because patients with head injuries have a death rate twice as high (35% vs. 17%) as that of trauma patients who do not have injuries to the central nervous system, prompt recognition and swift intervention are the keys to the best possible outcome. Although the brain can sustain minor trauma without serious complications, severe head and brain injuries result in death or disability.

# CRITICAL CONCEPTS

- Assume that all patients who have a head injury also have injury to the cervical spine until proved otherwise.

- Note that most head injuries are not the result of direct force to the brain but rather are due to the movement of the brain inside the rigid skull.

- Continually monitor the patient's level of consciousness. It can deteriorate rapidly, and immediate intervention may be necessary.

- Do not insert any tubes through the nose of a patient with a head injury until the possibility of a basilar skull fracture has been ruled out. The tube could penetrate the brain through this fracture.

# GLOSSARY

**Cerebral contusion:** A closed head injury caused by blunt trauma. Bruising of the brain results because of bleeding from blood vessels in the cranium that are torn on impact. Loss of consciousness is common and may be prolonged. Hospitalization and further evaluation are necessary.

**Concussion:** A mild closed head injury without detectable damage to the brain; may or may not involve brief loss of consciousness. The patient generally makes a complete recovery.

**Cranial nerves:** Twelve pairs of nerves that arise from the underside of the brain and perform specific functions. The most commonly injured cranial nerve is the oculomotor, or third cranial nerve.

**Epidural hematoma:** A collection of blood above the dura; caused by arterial bleeding, so the signs and symptoms appear sooner than those of a subdural hematoma. Immediate surgery is often required, or the prognosis may be poor.

**Subdural hematoma:** A collection of blood under the dura; may develop over a period of hours or days or weeks after injury, because bleeding is often from a venous source. This is a serious injury.

# EXAM QUESTIONS

## Chapter 5

### Questions 22 - 26

22. You are working in the emergency department when a patient arrives complaining of a headache, nausea, and vomiting. He mentions that he was involved in a motor vehicle accident 3 weeks ago in which he hit his head on the steering wheel but had only brief loss of consciousness. What is a likely head injury in this patient?

    a. Subdural hematoma
    b. Cerebral contusion
    c. Scalp laceration
    d. Epidural hematoma

23. Lowering the pco2 in a patient with head injury does which of the following?

    a. Increases oxygenation in the cerebral arteries through vasodilation
    b. Lowers intracranial pressure by increasing vasoconstriction
    c. Blocks increases in intracranial pressure by reducing sodium transport in the brain
    d. Reduces intracranial hemorrhage

24. Insertion of tubes into the nose should be avoided in patients with head injuries until which of the following has been ruled out?

    a. Tentorium tear
    b. Basilar skull fracture
    c. Cerebral contusion
    d. Optic nerve damage

25. Sudden deceleration of the brain within the cranium is what type of injury?

    a. Cranial neuropathy
    b. Cerebral hematoma
    c. Coup-contrecoup
    d. Intracranial hemangioma

26. A common initial nursing diagnosis for a patient with head trauma is:

    a. Oral mucous membrane alteration, related to head trauma
    b. Injury, potential for, related to possible seizure activity
    c. Sleep pattern disturbance, related to increased intracranial pressure
    d. Incontinence, stress, related to trauma

# CHAPTER 6

# SPINAL INJURY

## CHAPTER OBJECTIVE

After completing this chapter, the reader should be able to differentiate between the basic structures and functions of the spinal cord and spinal column, recognize common causes of spinal trauma, and describe care of patients with spinal injury.

## LEARNING OBJECTIVES

After studying this chapter, the reader should be able to

1. Recognize the signs and symptoms of spinal injury.

2. List common types of spinal injuries.

3. Name drugs used to treat patients with spinal injury.

4. Select common nursing diagnoses and interventions for patients with spinal injury.

## INTRODUCTION

Feared by many because of the potential for permanent paralysis, spinal injury is one of the most distressing and devastating of all injuries. Patients who a

have spinal injury require careful handling, "packaging," transportation, and swift emergency intervention. Nearly 13,000 new spinal cord injuries occur each year, and estimates indicate that 4,860 of these patients die before reaching a hospital (National Spinal Cord Injury Association [NSCIA], 1988). Injuries to the spinal cord are one of the few in which early interventions have such a profound influence on the outcome of the trauma. Although the mechanics of the primary spinal injury cannot be undone, the rescuers can alter the effects of hemorrhage, hypotension, and hypoxia that cause secondary trauma to the spinal cord and thus limit further damage (Campbell, 1988).

This chapter reviews normal anatomy and physiology of the spinal cord and spinal column and the pathologic changes associated with common spinal injuries. It also describes assessment and management of these injuries and presents potential nursing diagnoses and strategies.

## BASIC ANATOMY AND PHYSIOLOGY OF THE SPINAL CORD AND SPINAL COLUMN

Knowledge of the basic structures and functions of the spinal cord and spinal column is essential to assessment and management of a patient who has a spinal injury.

## Spinal Cord

The spinal cord is a soft tissue that is housed in the spinal column. The foramen magnum is the opening in the base of the skull through which the brainstem merges with the spinal cord. The three meninges that cover the brain also encircle the spinal cord, a structure about 1 cm in diameter. Cerebrospinal fluid bathes and cushions the spinal cord just as it does the brain. Nerve tissue in the spinal cord is bundled together in tracts. The spinal cord receives sensory input from ascending tracts, and the brain commands the body's motor functions by sending messages through the descending tracts. Thirty-one pairs of nerves branch out from the spinal cord.

The body has one nervous system with several subdivisions. The brain and the spinal cord compose the central nervous system. The peripheral nervous system consists of the other nerves that exist outside the brain and spinal cord. The autonomic nervous system has two branches: the sympathetic and the parasympathetic. The sympathetic nervous system initiates the body's fight-or-flight stress response; the parasympathetic system acts to mediate or counter those responses.

Acting as the control center, the brain receives signals through the neural network and reacts if necessary by sending a message to the body. For example, if you are driving and another motorist pulls out in front of you, you react by depressing the brake pedal, a motor response. Your heart rate and blood pressure also may increase in response to the perception of danger, a sympathetic response.

In a spinal cord injury, this message-sending network is disrupted or even eradicated, so the body cannot react and respond as it did before the injury. Depending on the point of disruption, a person with a spinal cord injury may have paralysis, lose control of body functions, or even stop breathing. Because the spinal cord is quite delicate, relatively limited trauma can result in major malfunctioning. Occasionally, swelling from trauma around the spinal cord can cause temporary compression of the cord and the disruption of transmissions through the cord, resulting in paralysis. As the swelling subsides, function may return. In most instances though, damage to the spinal cord is permanent, because the spinal cord, like the brain, has little healing capacity.

## Spinal Column

The spinal column protects the spinal cord and gives humans the ability to walk upright. Figure 6-1 is a diagram of the 33 vertebrae that form the spine: 7 cervical, 12 thoracic, 5 lumbar, 5 sacral (fused), and 4 (fused) that form the coccyx. Each vertebra forms a protective ring; the spinal cord runs through the spinal canal, which is the protective housing formed from these rings. Cartilaginous disks are sandwiched between the vertebrae to cushion the spine.

The vertebrae of the cervical spine are quite flexible; this flexibility allows humans to monitor their surroundings but also makes the neck prone to injury in trauma, because the head is relatively heavy. The thoracic vertebrae receive additional stability from the attached ribs, but the flexible junction with the lumbar vertebrae is another potential site of injury.

# MECHANISM OF INJURY

The spinal cord or spinal column may be injured by blunt or penetrating trauma. Most spinal injuries are closed and not visible to the rescuer. The spinal column can be damaged without harming the spinal cord, and the spinal cord can be damaged without evidence of damage to the spinal column.

Rapid vertical deceleration from a fall and rapid forward deceleration during a motor vehicle accident are the two primary causes of spinal injury. Motor vehicle accidents account for 48% of spinal cord injuries; falls, for 20%; and sports accidents, for 15%

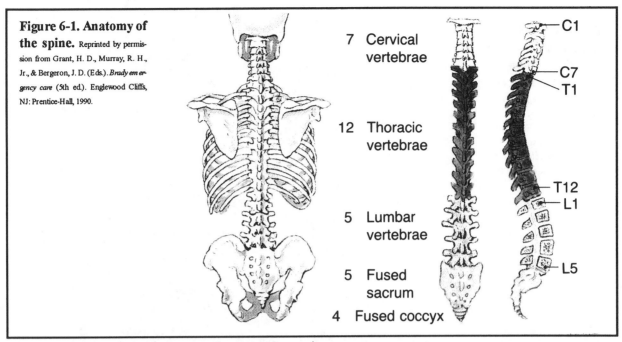

**Figure 6-1. Anatomy of the spine.** Reprinted by permission from Grant, H. D., Murray, R. H., Jr., & Bergeron, J. D. (Eds.). *Brady emergency care* (5th ed.). Englewood Cliffs, NJ: Prentice-Hall, 1990.

7 Cervical vertebrae

12 Thoracic vertebrae

5 Lumbar vertebrae

5 Fused sacrum

4 Fused coccyx

C1

C7
T1

T12
L1

L5

(two-thirds of these sports injuries are from diving). In patients more than 45 years old, falls overtake motor vehicle accidents as the leading cause of spinal cord injury (NSCIA, 1988). As Figures 6-2 and 6-3 show, rupture of ligaments stabilizing the vertebrae allows individual vertebrae to dislocate and press on the spinal cord. Flexion of the head (chin to chest) is a major mechanism of injury in most spinal trauma. Compression and rotational injuries can shatter vertebrae and force bone fragments into the cord (Figure 6-4).

According to Shea (1985), the mechanism of injury is important in determining the type of injury. Hyperflexion injuries have a mortality rate of 45 per 10,000, and hyperextension injuries have a mortality rate of 3 per 10,000. Rear-end collisions usually cause hyperextension; head-on collisions cause hyperflexion.

In addition to dislocation of the vertebrae and the resulting compression of the spinal cord, foreign bodies may lodge in the cord and directly disrupt its structure and function. Projectiles such as bullets or knives are the most frequent objects involved in penetrating spinal cord injury. A projectile that penetrates the cord may drive bone fragments into the cord along with the foreign object, inflicting fur-

ther injury. Bleeding or hematomas at the trauma site can compress the cord; loss of blood supply to the cord can cause irreversible damage.

Because of the flexibility of the spine in the cervical and lumbar regions, injury often occurs at these sites. The most common site of spinal cord injury is between the cervical vertebrae C5 and C6; the second most common site is between T12 and L1. When the spinal cord is injured, the patient has partial or complete loss of function and sensation in certain parts of the body. The loss begins at the site of the lesion or injury and continues downward. Spinal cord injuries are classified as complete when the loss of sensation and function is total and as incomplete when the loss is partial. Slightly more than one-half of all spinal cord injuries result in quadriplegia, or loss of sensation and function from the shoulders down. Patients with paraplegia are affected from about the waist down (NSCIA, 1988).

Spinal cord injuries not only can cause permanent paralysis but also can be life threatening. If the spinal cord is disrupted, the body cannot signal vital organs: Breathing may stop, the pulse rate may become dangerously slow, and blood pressure can fall. Death may occur if interventions are not swift.

**Figure 6-2. Posterior ligament rupture caused by forward dislocation of the vertebrae.** Reprinted by permission from Kitt, S., & Kaiser, J. *Emergency nursing: A physiologic and clinical perspective.* Philadelphia: Saunders, 1990.

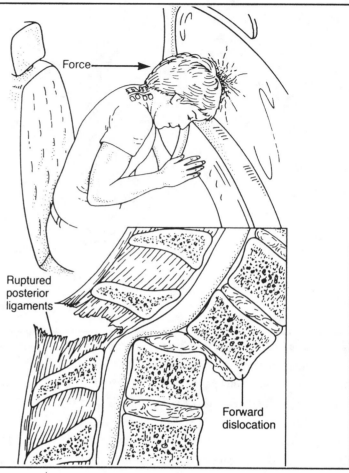

Force

Ruptured posterior ligaments

Forward dislocation

# ASSESSMENT OF PATIENTS WITH SPINAL INJURY

Whenever a patient has a spinal injury, follow the ABCs and assessment described in chapter 2: Evaluate the airway, breathing, and circulation. Because any movement of a patient with a spinal injury can make the injury worse, and because a spinal injury is frequently not obvious or visible, act as if all trauma patients have spinal injury. In general, assume that a spinal injury exists if the patient has any of the following:

• Unconsciousness.

• Trauma to the head, neck, or upper part of the chest.

• Paralysis or loss of sensation in any part of the body.

• Difficulty breathing despite no obvious thoracic trauma.

• Involuntary loss of control of bowel and bladder.

• Priapism.

• Signs of spinal shock: hypotension with warm skin and slow pulse rate.

Assessment of a patient who has a spinal injury proceeds as with any other patient. Observe the accident scene and elicit a history of the injury while assessing the patient. Ask bystanders about the accident or as-

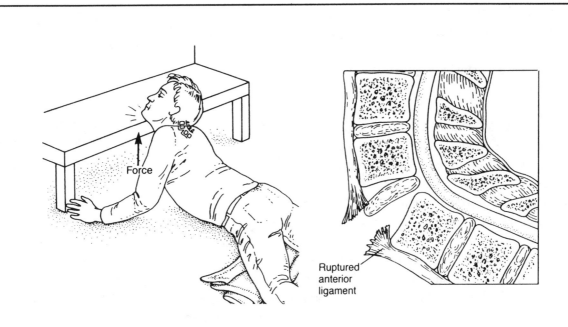

**Figure 6-3. Anterior ligament rupture caused by hyperextension and posterior dislocation of the vertebrae.** Reprinted by permission from Kitt, S., & Kaiser, J. *Emergency nursing: A physiologic and clinical perspective.* Philadelphia: Saunders, 1990.

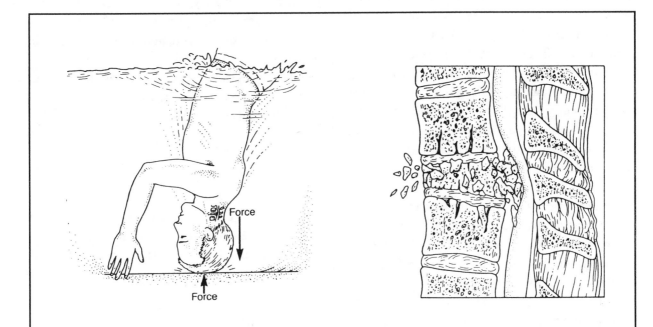

**Figure 6-4. Compression force causing wedging and crush-type injury of the vertebrae.** Reprinted by permission from Kitt, S., & Kaiser, J. *Emergency nursing: A physiologic and clinical perspective.* Philadelphia: Saunders, 1990.

sault; this can provide information for a baseline assessment and clues about the mechanism of injury.

When assessing a patient for a spinal injury be aware of the following:

- The prevalence of spinal cord injury is high in motor vehicle accidents when the occupants are unrestrained; 13% of occupants thrown from a vehicle have neck fractures (Shea, 1985). Occupants who use restraints are much less likely to have spinal cord injury.

- Most patients with spinal cord injury are 16-30 years old. Men are injured more often than women (82% vs. 18%). Most of the patients are single.

- Diving accidents are associated with a high prevalence of spinal cord injury. The prevalence is higher in the summer.

Assessment of a conscious patient who has a spinal injury also requires a brief neurologic examination during the secondary survey to evaluate the patient's motor and sensory function. Ask patients to wiggle their toes and fingers, squeeze your hand, and determine which of their toes or fingers you are touching. Figure 6-5 is a summary of the assessment and possible conclusions. Shea (1985) recommends investigating the "*P's*"øpain, position, paralysis, paresthesias, ptosis, and priapismøin any patient with suspected spinal cord injury.

If patients can wiggle their fingers and toes, their motor function may be intact; if they can feel your touch, sensory function may be intact. However, do not decide, on the basis of these signs, that a patient does not have spinal injury. Spinal injury is confirmed or ruled out in a hospital setting, and you should assume that it exists until it is proved otherwise.

# COMMON SPINAL INJURIES

Sheehy and Jimmerson (1994) classify the three major types of spinal injuries as injury to the cord itself, fracture of the vertebrae, and injury to the spinal nerves.

## Cervical Injury

Most patients with a complete spinal cord injury at C3 die before receiving medical attention because respirations cease (NSCIA, 1988). Others may experience respiratory distress or require artificial ventilation for the rest of their lives. Also, 27% of patients with cervical spine injuries have concomitant head injuries (Sheehy & Jimmerson, 1994).

## Thoracic Injury

Because of its stability, the thoracic spine is not injured as often as other parts of the spine. Nevertheless, the neck of any patient who has a suspected injury of the thoracic spine should be immobilized, and the patient should be transported to the hospital on a long spine board. Thoracic trauma can impair ventilation and circulation.

## Lumbar Injury

The lumbar vertebrae join the thoracic vertebrae at a flexible joint. Unfortunately, this flexibility also makes the T12-L1 area the second most common site of spinal injury. This injury is common in patients who cannot move their legs.

## Impalement

Any object that lodges in the spinal column should be left in place. Removing in could make the injury worse.

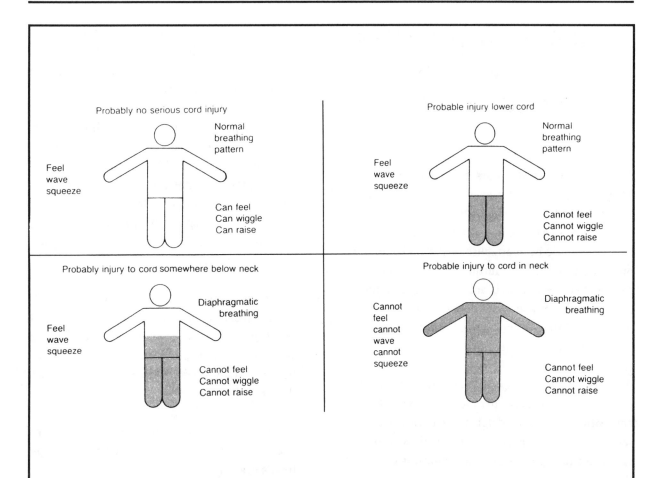

Probably no serious cord injury

Normal breathing pattern

Feel wave squeeze

Can feel
Can wiggle
Can raise

Probable injury lower cord

Normal breathing pattern

Feel wave squeeze

Cannot feel
Cannot wiggle
Cannot raise

Probably injury to cord somewhere below neck

Diaphragmatic breathing

Feel wave squeeze

Cannot feel
Cannot wiggle
Cannot raise

Probable injury to cord in neck

Diaphragmatic breathing

Cannot feel
cannot wave
cannot squeeze

Cannot feel
Cannot wiggle
Cannot raise

Warning: If the patient is unconscious or the mechanism of injury indicates possible spinal injury, assume that spinal injury is present.

**Figure 6-5. Summary of observations and possible conclusions in assessment of a conscious patient with suspected spinal cord injury.** Reprinted by permission from Grant, H. D., Murray, R. H., Jr., & Bergeron, J. D. (Eds.). *Brady emergency care* (5th ed.). Englewood Cliffs, NJ: Prentice-Hall, 1990.

## Spinal Shock

Spinal shock, or neurogenic shock, is a condition associated with spinal injury. Normally, the nervous system controls the blood pressure by constricting or dilating vessels in response to signals from the body. When the flow of information through the spinal cord is impaired, control over the vessels is lost, and they dilate, causing a drop in blood pressure; pooling of the blood may make the skin feel warm and pink. The sympathetic system generally stimulates an increase in pulse rate to compensate for any decrease in

blood pressure, but this impulse is impaired in spinal cord injury. The pulse rate may not increase; in fact, it may fall to dangerously low levels if the cardiac accelerator nerves in the thoracic vertebrae are blocked. The emergency team may apply a pneumatic antishock garment to help support the blood pressure by compressing the lower extremities; fluids may help somewhat, but inotropic agents are often necessary to sustain life.

# NURSING STRATEGIES FOR PATIENTS WITH SPINAL INJURY

Spinal injuries must always be considered serious. They are associated with high rates of morbidity and mortality, and they significantly affect the patient's quality of life. After a patent airway, breathing, and circulation have been established, the goal of prehospital care is to limit any further damage to the spinal cord and column. This is accomplished by immobilizing the patient and maintaining perfusion and oxygenation of the nervous system while transporting the patient to a hospital.

Patients who have a spinal injury are always transported on a long spine board to hold the whole body and with a rigid Philadelphia collar in place. This series of steps is called packaging the patient. In general, leave the application of immobilizing devices to the emergency team called to the trauma scene. Also note that specialists may recommend intravenous administration of methylprednisolone to reduce the severity of a spinal cord injury or enhance recovery. This protocol generally must be started within a few hours of the trauma if it is to be effective (Sheehy & Jimmerson, 1994).

Table 6-1 gives potential nursing diagnoses and interventions for patients with spinal injury. The following strategies may also be useful. It is presumed with each that the airway, breathing, and circulation have been established. Your intervention should be within the scope of your professional license; commensurate with your skills and training; consistent with your state's nurse practice act; and when performed in a health care setting, adherent to that facility's standards of practice.

- Do not move the patient if he or she is conscious, is breathing adequately, and has a pulse and you see no immediate threats to the patient's life or to your own safety. Continue monitoring and be prepared to act; the patient's condition may deteriorate suddenly.

- Move the patient by yourself only if the patient or you are in immediate danger (e.g., the patient is prone and not breathing, you are by yourself, or an explosion or fire at the trauma scene seems imminent). Do your best to keep the patient's head, neck, and spine in alignment when you move him or her. Never drag or pull the patient by the head or neck.

- Leave application of the Philadelphia collar to the emergency team unless you are familiar with the device and have developed the skills necessary for correct application. Continue to stabilize the patient's head and neck with your hands (Figure 6-6).

- Use the jaw thrust to open the patient's airway if necessary while preventing movement of the patient's head and neck.

- Do not attempt to remove a helmet from the victim of a motorcycle or sports accident unless necessary to access the patient's airway, sustain respirations, or control life-threatening hemorrhage.

- Use appropriate rescue techniques (Figure 6-7) for patients injured in a water accident.

- Expect at least four trained professionals to place the patient on a spine board unless the patient's condition is so critical that the need to transport is immediate. Logroll the patient as a unit, keeping the head in alignment with the body.

- Quickly scan the patient's back for obvious injuries before the patient is rolled onto the spine board.

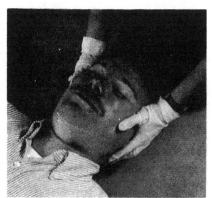

Properly position both hands.

Do not apply traction to the head and neck, or pull and twist the head. You are trying to stabilize the head and neck.

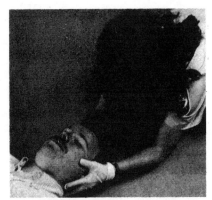

Maintain stabilization - keep head in neutral alignment.

**Figure 6-6. Applying manual stabilization.** Reprinted by permission from Grant, H. D., Murray, R. H., Jr., & Bergeron, J. D. (Eds.). *Brady emergency care* (5th ed.). Englewood Cliffs, NJ: Prentice-Hall, 1990.

- A Philadelphia collar does not adequately prevent lateral or side-to-side movement of the patient's head, so the emergency team often adds additional support with rolled towels or intravenous bags placed on each side of the patient's head. The head is then taped in place to the back board to further restrict movement.

- Remember that the patient with a spinal cord injury often can no longer perceive pain from other injuries because of the disruption of the spinal cord's messenger functions. Be certain to evaluate the chest, abdomen, and lower extremities, and continue to monitor the status of these structures.

- Note that a full bladder may burst if the patient has a spinal cord injury that prevents the sensation of fullness from being transmitted to the brain. Catheterization is often indicated, but not until the potential for urethral damage due to a pelvic fracture has been ruled out, because catheterization may cause further urethral damage.

- Do not allow the patient to eat or drink until he or she is seen by a neurosurgeon. Immediate surgical intervention may be indicated for some spinal injuries, and oral intake will increase the risk of a fatal aspiration during the perioperative period. Also, the patient's condition may deteriorate, and vomiting or aspiration may occur.

# SUMMARY

Spinal injuries can be devastating and deadly. Nursing interventions play a key role in the outcome of the injury; the NSCIA (1988) reports that 86% of patients with spinal cord injury who survive the first 24 hr will still be alive 10 years later.

# CRITICAL CONCEPTS

- Assume that all unconscious trauma patients have a spinal injury until proved otherwise; immobilize the head and neck in a straight line with the body.

- Intravenous methylprednisolone may help reduce the severity of a spinal cord injury, but this drug must be administered within hours of the

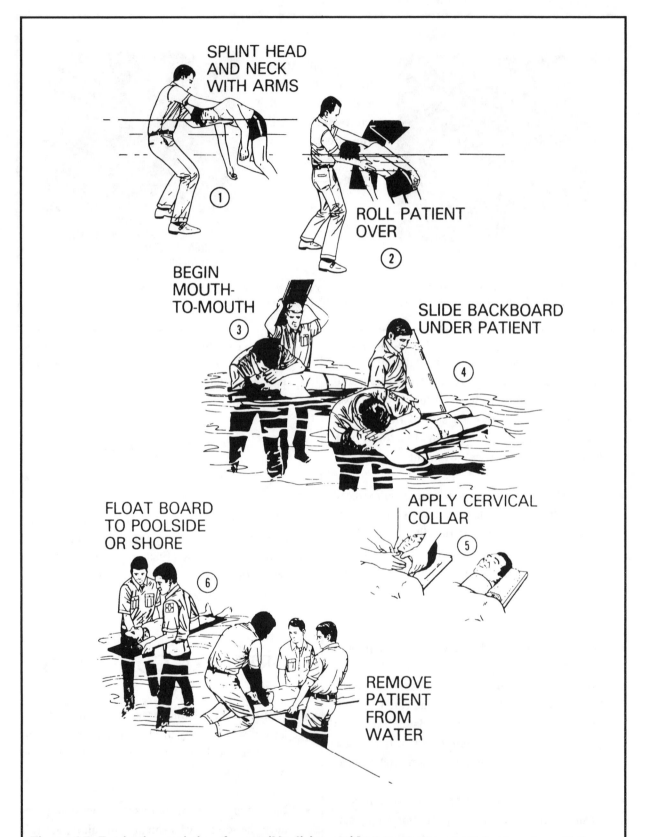

**Figure 6-7. Extricating a victim of a possible diving accident.** Reprinted by permission from Grant, H. D., Murray, R. H., Jr., & Bergeron, J. D. (Eds.). *Brady emergency care* (5th ed.). Englewood Cliffs, NJ: Prentice-Hall, 1990.

## Table 6-1
## Potential Nursing Diagnoses and Interventions for Patients with Spinal Injury

| Diagnosis | Interventions |
|---|---|
| Airway clearance, ineffective, r/t spinal injury | Maintain a patent airway. Use the jaw thrust to open the airway while preventing movement of the patient's head and neck; stabilize the head between your wrists until a Philadelphia cervical collar can be applied; use your hands and knees to maintain the head in alignment. |
| Breathing pattern, ineffective, r/t spinal injury | Maintain a patent airway. Be prepared to assist respirations or provide artificial ventilation if the patient cannot breathe. Administer oxygen as soon as possible to enhance oxygenation of all body structures, including the spinal cord. |
| Fluid volume deficit, potential, r/t spinal shock | Secure venous access and administer intravenous fluids, plasma expanders, and inotropic agents as ordered to support the blood pressure. Anticipate possible application of pneumatic antishock garment. |
| Fear r/t unfamiliarity with spinal injury | Reassure the patient frequently that you are doing everything possible to help him or her; offer calm simple explanations. Even the apparently unconscious patient may benefit from voice contact. |
| Injury, potential for, r/t loss of sensation | Monitor the condition and placement of extremities and body parts. Patients with spinal cord injury may not be able to tell you when something hurts, for example, a stretcher rail pinching the leg. |
| Adjustment impairment r/t spinal injury | Encourage the patient to express feelings by providing a safe and nonthreatening environment. Reassure the patient that his or her feelings are normal after trauma including spinal injury. Suggest consultation with mental health professional, social worker, or chaplain. |

Note.—This is a sample of potential nursing diagnoses. It is not presented as or intended to be a complete care plan for the trauma patient. More complete information can be found in a medical-surgical nursing course and textbook. r/t = related to.

Adapted from Sparks, S. and Taylor, C. M. *Nursing Diagnosis reference manual,* Springhouse, PA: Springhouse Corp., 1991, and Chitwood, *L. Ambulatory patient care,* San Diego: Western Schools, 1994.

trauma to be effective and is only given on a physician's order.

- Most spinal injury due to blunt trauma is sustained in automobile or sports accidents and falls. Most spinal injuries due to penetrating trauma are caused by guns or knives.

- Administer oxygen to all patients who have suspected a suspected spinal injury to increase oxygen supply to the spinal cord.

# GLOSSARY

**Compression injury:** Compaction of vertebrae caused by application of opposing forces through the spinal column; may shatter vertebrae and drive bone fragments into the spinal cord.

**Hyperextension injury:** Force applied to the head that snaps it back, causing the occiput to lurch back against the thoracic spine; common cause is rear-end motor vehicle accidents.

**Hyperflexion injury:** Sudden forcing downward and forward of the head (chin to chest) that may cause dislocation of vertebrae and spinal cord injury; common cause is head-on motor vehicle accidents.

**Spinal shock:** A type of neurogenic shock characterized by warm pink skin, hypotension, and bradycardia. Spinal shock is due to impaired sympathetic vasomotor control secondary to spinal cord injury.

# EXAM QUESTIONS

## Chapter 6

### Questions 27 - 31

27. Which type of injury of the cervical spinal cord is likely in a patient involved in a head-on motor vehicle accident?

    a. Rotational
    b. Hyperflexion
    c. Hyperextension
    d. Compression

28. What drug may be administered soon after a spinal cord injury to reduce the severity of the injury?

    a. Dexamethasone
    b. Captopril
    c. Methylprednisolone
    d. Diazepam

29. A common potential nursing diagnosis for a patient with spinal cord injury is:

    a. Diarrhea
    b. Nutrition, altered
    c. Fatigue
    d. Fluid volume deficit, potential

30. During your assessment of a patient who has a spinal injury you note the onset of hypotension and bradycardia. The patient's skin feels warm. Which of the following conditions is most likely?

    a. Pump failure
    b. Spinal shock
    c. Neurogenic bladder
    d. Cardiogenic shock

31. Treatment of spinal shock may include administration of which of the following drugs?

    a. Antibiotics
    b. Antiinflammatory agents
    c. Inotropic agents
    d. Corticosteroids

# CHAPTER 7

# THORACIC TRAUMA

## CHAPTER OBJECTIVE

After completing this chapter, the reader should be able to differentiate between the organs found in the thoracic cavity, describe their basic structures and functions, list common types of thoracic trauma, and select nursing interventions for patients with thoracic trauma.

## LEARNING OBJECTIVES

After studying this chapter, the reader should be able to

1. Recognize signs and symptoms of thoracic trauma.

2. List common types of thoracic trauma.

3. Differentiate among interventions in the care of patients with thoracic trauma.

4. Specify common potential nursing diagnoses for patients with thoracic trauma.

## INTRODUCTION

Henderson et al. (1994) report that the first surgical intervention in a penetrating cardiac injury occurred in 1893. The patient survived the surgery to repair the pericardium and close the stab wound that penetrated the right ventricle. Less than 15% of thoracic injuries today require the skills of a thoracic surgeon, so responsibility for the management of most patients with chest injuries falls to health care professionals who can intervene swiftly with relatively simple but life-saving procedures (Trunkey, 1985) In many cases, specially trained nurses and paramedics perform these procedures at the trauma scene or during transport.

Thoracic trauma is entirely responsible for 25% of all trauma deaths; injuries to the chest are the most frequently missed injuries in the first hour of care (Sheehy & Jimmerson, 1994). Half of the patients who have multiple trauma have thoracic trauma; two thirds of those with fatal thoracic trauma live to reach the hospital (Campbell, 1988).

This chapter reviews basic anatomy and physiology of the thoracic cavity and the organs contained within it and describes common mechanisms of injury that produce blunt and penetrating thoracic trauma. It also describes assessment of patients with thoracic trauma, discusses common thoracic trauma, and presents nursing strategies and interventions for care of patients with thoracic trauma.

# BASIC THORACIC ANATOMY AND PHYSIOLOGY

The chest or thoracic cavity is the area between the diaphragm and the neck. The primary structures in the chest cavity are the trachea, the lungs, and the heart. The diaphragm separates the thoracic cavity from the abdominal cavity and aids in inspiration. Surrounded by the bony cage formed by the ribs, some of the abdominal structures such as the liver and spleen lie in an area called the thoracic abdomen. Knowledge of the location and an understanding of the structure and function of these thoracic organs provide the foundation for assessment and management of patients who have thoracic trauma. Figure 7-1 shows the structures of the thoracic cavity.

## Rib Cage

Twelve pairs of ribs form the rib cage. Although fracture of a single rib often is not a serious injury, fractures of multiple ribs can produce an unstable segment of the rib cage that may impair respiration. Rib fractures may also penetrate, lacerate, or otherwise damage underlying structures.

## Sternum

The sternum offers additional protection to the heart and lungs and consists of three parts: the manubrium at the top (nearest the head), the body or midsection, and the smaller xiphoid process at the bottom. Blunt trauma from impact of the thorax against the steering wheel is a major cause of a fractured sternum and myocardial contusion in motor vehicle accidents.

## Trachea

The trachea divides into the right and left main bronchi and then divides further still into the bronchioles, which eventually lead to the alveoli, which mediate the exchange of oxygen and carbon dioxide between the air and the blood. Trauma may crush or penetrate the trachea, which obviously has a vital role as the airway.

## Lungs

Although the body can function with just one lung, the lungs are the major organs of respiration and are essential to life. Penetrating trauma from stab and gunshot wounds may deflate one or both of the lungs and lead to hypoxia. The lungs naturally operate with *negative* pressure, which pulls air into the lungs. The diaphragm descends, and air is sucked into the lungs, or inhaled. Current technology for artificial respiration uses *positive* pressure. Positive pressure pushes air into the lungs: Oxygen is blown down the trachea to cause inflation of the lungs. This fundamental difference in the way the lungs are inflated is significant in patients who have thoracic trauma.

## Pleura

The pleura is the serous membrane that covers the lungs (the pulmonary pleura) and lines the inside of the rib cage (the parietal pleura).

## Pleural Cavity

As a potential space between the parietal pleura lining the rib cage and the pulmonary pleura, the pleural cavity can fill with blood or air as a result of trauma.

## Diaphragm

Attached to the ribs, sternum, and spine, the diaphragm contracts, generating a negative pressure gradient that pulls air down the trachea to inflate the

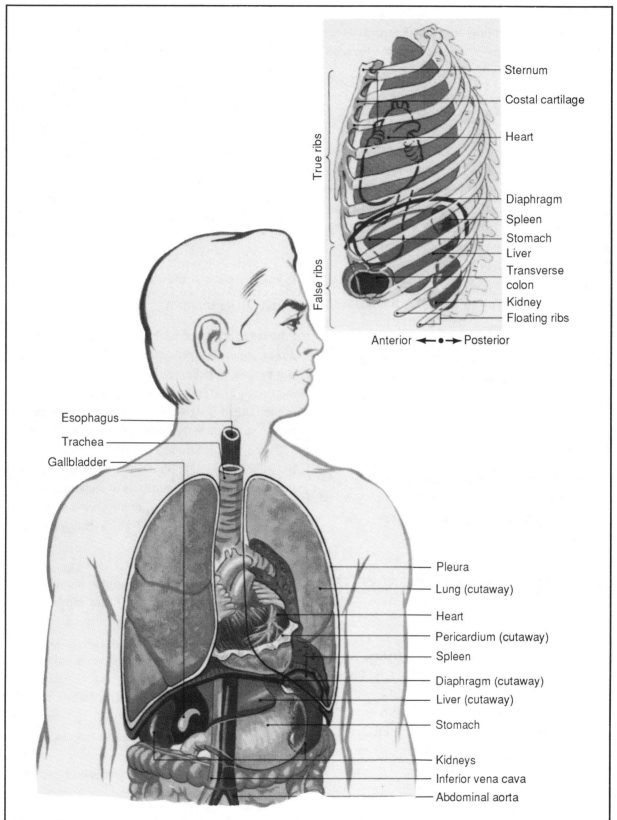

**Figure 7-1. Anatomy of the chest and upper part of the abdomen**. Reprinted by permission from Grant, H. D., Murray, R. H., Jr., & Bergeron, J. D. (Eds.). *Brady emergency care* (5th ed.). Englewood Cliffs, NJ: Prentice-Hall, 1990.

lungs. Both blunt and penetrating trauma can tear the diaphragm and allow abdominal organs to slip into the thoracic cavity. The presence of the organs in the cavity can impair respiration.

## Heart and Great Vessels

Protected by the sternum and ribs, about two thirds of the heart lie to the left of the body's center or midline. Arising from the left ventricle of the heart, the aorta carries freshly oxygenated blood to the body. The vena cava collects blood from the body and returns it to the right upper chamber of the heart. The pulmonary artery transports blood from the right lower chamber of the heart to the lungs, where oxygen content is replenished. Blunt trauma to the thorax can rupture the aorta and other great vessels or even tear the valves within the heart. Objects that penetrate the thorax can pierce the heart, coronary arteries, and great vessels, leading to rapidly fatal exsanguination.

## Esophagus

The esophagus is a muscular tube, about 10 in. (25.4 cm) long, that lies behind the trachea. It also can be torn or penetrated during thoracic trauma.

# MECHANISM OF INJURY

The mechanism of injury in thoracic trauma may be either blunt or penetrating trauma. Falls, motor vehicle accidents, gunshot and stab wounds, and crush injuries are common causes of thoracic trauma. The resulting trauma can range from a fractured rib to a fatal heart injury. The addition of air bags to motor vehicles has decreased the prevalence and severity of trauma to the head, neck, and chest caused by motor vehicle accidents.

## Blunt trauma

Blunt trauma causes most chest injuries (Sheehy & Jimmerson, 1994). Most blunt thoracic trauma is caused by rapid deceleration. Falls, motor vehicle accidents, assaults, and sporting accidents account for much of blunt thoracic trauma. Energy from blunt trauma reverberates through the thorax, so crushing of soft tissues against the rigid spine and rupture of the thoracic organs may occur. Rapid vertical deceleration, as in a fall, can shear the aorta and great vessels from the heart. Blunt trauma of force sufficient to fracture the rib cage often is associated with bruising of the heart and lungs.

## Penetrating trauma

Projectiles are responsible for most penetrating thoracic trauma. The projectile can be a knife or a missile such as a bullet, although gunshot wounds are increasing in prevalence. There are 200 million guns in the United States. Since 1933, firearms have been the cause of 500,000 deaths in the United States, and 732 shootings occur each day (Ordog, Wasserberger, Balasubramanium, & Shoemaker, 1994). Penetrating thoracic trauma from gunshots or stabbings can lead to impalement, laceration, or rupture and puncture of the thoracic organs, all of which can cause loss of both structure and function.

Stab wounds to the chest may appear innocuous, but they are associated with significant morbidity and mortality because of injuries to intrathoracic structures, including the heart, major vessels, lungs, tracheobronchial tree, esophagus, and spinal cord (Ordog, Balasubramanium, Wasserberger, Kram, Bishop, & Shoemaker, 1994). In contrast to bullet wounds, which often leave a well-defined wound track and an end point of either a bullet or an exit wound, stab wounds cannot be visualized, and estimation of the depth of the wound is based solely on the patient's signs and symptoms.

# ASSESSMENT OF PATIENTS WITH THORACIC TRAUMA

For any patient with thoracic trauma, follow the standard ABC assessment plan: Evaluate the airway, breathing, and circulation. Be aware that thoracic trauma is not usually the sole injury. Observe the trauma scene and elicit a history of the injury while examining the patient. Try to determine the object that caused the injury, the speed of force of the object, and the area of the thorax hit by the object (Kitt & Kaiser, 1990). Work quickly. Early detection, intervention, and transport are critical to the patient's survival. Lerer and Knottenbelt (1994) report that the key to improved outcome after survivable sharp penetrating chest trauma is rapid transportation by the quickest available means to adequate emergency care.

Remember that any patient who has multiple trauma is presumed to have a spinal injury until proved otherwise. Do not move the patient's head or neck; apply a rigid Philadelphia collar as described in chapter 6, or have a second rescuer stabilize the patient's head.

Signs and symptoms of thoracic trauma include the following:

- Dyspnea.

- Obvious deformity of the chest wall, trachea, rib cage, or neck.

- Shock.

- Hypoxia and cyanosis.

- Deviation of the trachea from the midline of the body (a late and ominous sign in most thoracic trauma).

- Unequal expansion or excursions of the chest.

- Hemoptysis.

- Subcutaneous emphysema.

- Pain with breathing or at the site of thoracic injury.

- Impalement of an object in the thorax.

- Sucking, bubbling, or gurgling sounds from the thorax.

# TYPES OF THORACIC TRAUMA

Thoracic trauma is generally serious and requires prompt skilled interventions. Trauma specialists (Campbell, 1988; Trunkey, 1985) have identified 12 common thoracic injuries found in patients who have multiple trauma (Table 7-1). Six are considered immediately life-threatening and are the top priority at the trauma scene. The other 6 are considered potentially life-threatening and require attention when you begin the secondary survey.

## Pneumothorax

When a lung is punctured, air inspired through that lung rushes out into the pleural cavity. As the air fills the pleural space, the space expands. The expanding pleural cavity impairs normal expansion of the affected lung; hypoxia may occur, depending on the degree of impairment or pulmonary deflation. The body is often able to seal small defects made in the chest wall by a penetrating object. The types of pneumothorax (Figure 7-2) include open pneumothorax and tension pneumothorax.

**Table 7-1**
**Priorities in Thoracic Trauma**

| Immediately Life-Threatening, Top-Priority Trauma | Potentially Life-Threatening Thoracic Trauma; Managed During the Secondary Survey |
| --- | --- |
| • Airway obstruction<br>• Open pneumothorax<br>• Tension pneumothorax<br>• Massive hemothorax<br>• Flail chest<br>• Cardiac tamponade | • Pulmonary contusion<br>• Aortic disruption<br>• Tracheobronchial disruption<br>• Esophageal disruption<br>• Traumatic diaphragmatic hernia<br>• Myocardial contusion |

Source: Campbell, J., *Basic Trauma life support*, Advanced prehospital care, Englewood Cliffs, NJ: Prentice-Hall, 1988, and Trunkey, D. D., *Advanced trauma life support course for physicians*, Chicago: American College of Surgeons, Committee on Trauma, 1985.

**Open pneumothorax.** Referred to as a sucking chest wound, an open pneumothorax is caused by trauma that pierces the chest wall and leaves a pathway from the thorax to the outside environment that the body cannot seal off. Air may be drawn in and out through the defect with attempts at respiration, but because the air does not enter the lungs and the blood does not exchange gases, dyspnea and hypoxia occur. Signs and symptoms of open pneumothorax include obvious open defects in the chest wall, dyspnea, tachycardia, shock, and cyanosis.

**Tension pneumothorax.** When the chest wall remains closed, but the lung is injured and air escapes from the lung, this air accumulates in the thorax. Pressure from the accumulating air compresses the lung and intrathoracic structures, impairing the functioning of the heart and lungs. This can shift the heart and other structures of the chest from their normal position and further impair functioning, creating a life-threatening situation. This is a tension pneumothorax. A tension pneumothorax also can be caused by a rescuer who applies excessive positive pressure to a manual ventilating device and subsequently ruptures a lung. It can also occur when the occlusive dressing applied to seal an open pneumothorax does not allow adequate escape of air. Tension pneumothorax is a life-threatening situation, and death may be imminent. The patient is dyspneic, and the neck veins may

be distended; few or no breath sounds can be heard on the affected side, and shock ensues.

## Massive Hemothorax

Penetrating thoracic trauma most commonly pierces the organs contained in the chest; blunt trauma may tear vessels. Either can result in the loss of 1.5 L or more of blood into the pleural cavity; each pleural cavity can contain up to 3.0 L of blood (Campbell, 1988). A hemothorax (Figure 7-2) also can be associated with a pneumothorax. Suspect massive hemothorax when a patient with thoracic trauma is in shock and has no breath sounds or diminished breath sounds. This is a serious and life-threatening emergency that generally requires an emergency thoracotomy.

## Flail Chest

When three or more consecutive ribs are fractured in two places, a segment of chest wall is separated from the thorax. This condition is known as a flail chest (Figure 7-3). Because of the force required to fracture multiple ribs, the lung lying under the flail segment often is injured, and a pneumothorax may exist concurrently. Flail chest often is diagnosed on the basis of its paradoxical movement: The affected ribs move in an uncoordinated fashion that is opposite from movements of the rib cage. The flail segment

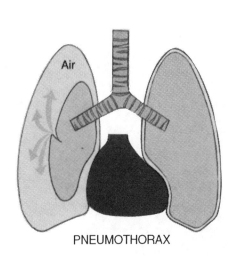

PNEUMOTHORAX

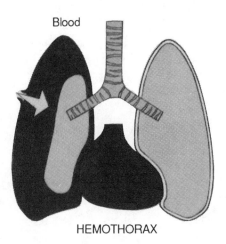

HEMOTHORAX

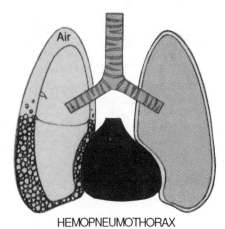

HEMOPNEUMOTHORAX

**Figure 7-2. Conditions produced by chest injuries.** Reprinted by permission from Grant, H. D., Murray, R. H., Jr., & Bergeron, J. D. (Eds.). *Brady emergency care* (5th ed.). Englewood Cliffs, NJ: Prentice-Hall, 1990.

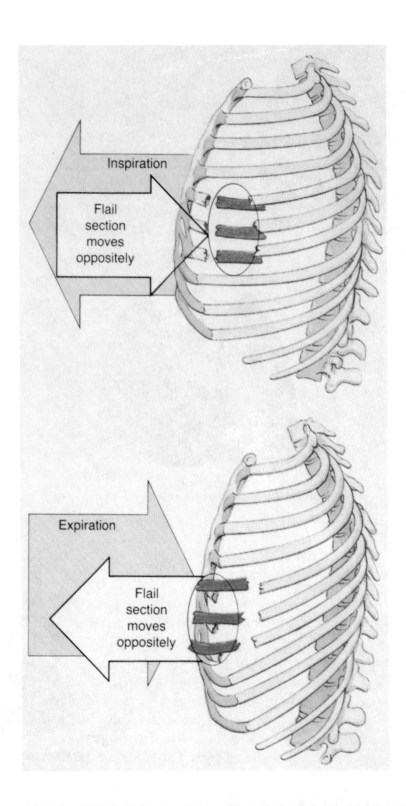

**Figure 7-3. Paradoxical motion in flail chest.** Reprinted by permission from Grant, H. D., Murray, R. H., Jr., & Bergeron, J. D. (Eds.). *Brady emergency care* (5th ed.). Englewood Cliffs, NJ: Prentice-Hall, 1990.

may be overtly visible, or it may be palpated during assessment.

## Cardiac Tamponade

When penetrating trauma causes blood to leak out of the heart and into the inelastic sac surrounding the heart (pericardium), a condition known as cardiac tamponade develops. The pressure builds around the heart because the pericardium does not stretch, and the heart's pumping action is hampered. A triad of signs aids in the diagnosis of cardiac tamponade: hypotension, distended neck veins, and muffled heart sounds (Campbell, 1988). Unfortunately, noise at the trauma scene may make it difficult to ascertain any decrease in heart sounds, and the other two signs are also consistent with tension pneumothorax, so diagnosis often requires advanced skills and knowledge.

## Pulmonary Contusion

Pulmonary contusion, or bruising of the lung, occurs with blunt trauma. It may cause immediate, life-threatening hypoxia or develop into respiratory distress later. Suspect a pulmonary contusion if a patient has rib fractures or bruising of the chest.

## Tracheobronchial Disruption

Both blunt and penetrating trauma can disrupt the trachea or bronchi or fracture the larynx. Massive crepitus is often noted from the level of the nipples up, and frothy or bloody sputum is present in the airway. Gaining control of the airway in this situation can be challenging; refer to chapter 3 for more on airway management. Bleeding is often profuse in neck injuries; associated injuries of the upper part of the airway may make opening the airway at the trachea the only option, and even that can be difficult.

## Esophageal Disruption

Although most esophageal injuries are caused by penetrating trauma, the esophagus can also be torn by blunt trauma. Esophageal trauma usually is diagnosed in the hospital during posttrauma assessment and evaluation. Management of esophageal trauma is usually not as pressing as the other injuries described here; treatment usually takes place in a hospital.

## Myocardial Contusion

Bruising of the heart muscle is caused by blunt trauma to the anterior part of the chest. Whenever a patient has blunt trauma to this part of the chest, assume that a myocardial contusion exists. This damage to the heart muscle is similar to that sustained in a myocardial infarction; chest pain, dysrhythmia, and cardiogenic shock may occur (Campbell, 1988).

## Aortic Rupture

The aorta can be injured by either blunt or penetrating trauma. Sudden decelerative forces may tear the artery, compression against the spine as when a driver hits the steering wheel may rupture it, and bullets may lacerate it. Rapid exsanguination and death are the result; 90% of patients who have aortic rupture die. Most have been involved in motor vehicle accidents or falls. Aortic rupture is not listed as a first-priority thoracic injury because of this fatality rate. Patients who survive the initial trauma have a second chance if you can get them to the hospital quickly. If conscious, the patient may complain of pain between the scapulae (shoulder blades) and dyspnea.

## Traumatic Diaphragmatic Hernia

When the diaphragm is disrupted, the thoracic contents may slip up into the chest cavity and impair breathing. Sometimes, however, the injury is not even noted until the thorax is explored surgically. Breath sounds may be decreased on one side of the chest, or the heart sounds may be shifted, because the lung and heart are displaced further into the abdomen by the thoracic organs. The patient may complain of dyspnea, and cyanosis may be evident because the lungs no longer can function efficiently. More often though, diaphragmatic injury is diagnosed at the hospital on the basis of radiographic findings.

## Lacerations and Contusions of the Thorax

Thoracic lacerations and contusions cause pain, discoloration, and obvious or occult bleeding. Be aware of the potential for damage to organs and structures underlying the injury.

## Rib Fracture

The ribs most often fractured in blunt trauma are the 5th through the 10th. The upper ribs are protected by the shoulders, and the loner ribs float and are thus more flexible (Grant et al., 1990). Fractures of the upper three ribs, which are quite strong, indicate a significant blow to the upper part of the chest and may indicate serious head and neck trauma. Suspect injury to the subclavian vessel or even the aorta if the first, second, or third rib is fractured; arteriograms are usually obtained in the hospital to rule out such injuries. In general, when a patient has an injury at the clavicle or above, assume that he or she has three injuries: closed-head injury, neck injury, and facial fractures (McAlary, 1994) until it is proved otherwise. Fracture of a single rib, although painful, is seldom serious. Patients often splint the injury themselves by favoring the affected side and limiting movement of the arm. Respiration may be impaired by pain in patients who are conscious.

## Impalement

An object impaled in the thorax should be left in place. The pressure exerted by the object acts to tamponade, or compress, damaged vessels and thus reduce bleeding. Pulling the object out could trigger massive hemorrhage. Removal of the object must be done in the hospital.

## Traumatic Asphyxia

When a patient has a severe crush injury to the chest, as in a motor vehicle accident, or compression of the chest, the motion energy may squeeze blood out of the heart and into the head and neck. The patient's head and neck swell, and cyanosis of the face and lips occurs (Figure 7-4). Although the skin below the level of the injury is pink, suspect other injuries in a patient who has traumatic asphyxia (Campbell, 1988).

## Fractured Sternum

The sternum may be fractured in blunt trauma to the anterior part of the chest. The fracture sometimes can be palpated or may be obvious to inspection. A fractured sternum causes severe chest pain and sometimes dyspnea. Suspect a myocardial contusion if a patient has a fractured sternum, and be alert for evidence of hypoxia, hypotension, arrhythmias, or other indications of further thoracic trauma. Sternal fractures may not be quite as serious as once thought. Roy-Shapira, Levi, and Khoda (1994) write that these fractures are generally benign and do not require special treatments or an expensive workup. They propose that patients with sternal fracture who are not dyspneic, have normal findings on electrocardiograms, and are hemodynamically stable can be safely discharged early.

* Distended neck veins.
* Head, neck and shoulders appear dark blue or purple.
* Eyes may be blood-shot and bulging.
* Tongue and lips may appear swollen and cyanotic.
* Chest deformity may be present.

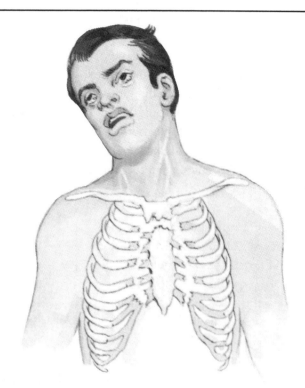
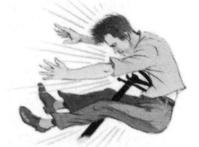

**Figure 7-4. Signs of traumatic asphyxia.** Reprinted by permission from Grant, H. D., Murray, R. H., Jr., & Bergeron, J. D. (Eds.). *Brady emergency care* (5th ed.). Englewood Cliffs, NJ: Prentice-Hall, 1990.

# NURSING STRATEGIES FOR THE CARE OF PATIENTS WITH THORACIC TRAUMA

Table 7-2 gives potential nursing diagnoses and interventions for patients with thoracic trauma. The following nursing strategies may also be useful. It is presumed that the patient's airway, breathing, and circulation have been established and that the patient is being transported to the hospital without delay. Your interventions should be within the scope of your professional license; commensurate with your skills and training; consistent with your state's nurse practice act; and when performed in a health care institution, adherent to that facility's standards of practice.

* Completely expose seriously injured patients who have multiple trauma. Cut off clothing; pulling it off could aggravate injuries. Examine the patient for trauma. Observe and palpate the neck veins; they may become distended in serious chest trauma. Evaluate the trachea for a normal midline position. Protect the patient's privacy and warmth and recover him or her as soon as possible to prevent heat loss and embarrassment.

* Begin administration of supplemental oxygen; thoracic trauma may cause hypoxia.

* Monitor the patient's electrocardiogram (heart rhythm). Serious arrhythmias may result from myocardial and vascular damage sustained during thoracic trauma.

* Place the stethoscope in the midaxillary line to compare the equality of breath sounds. Breath sounds detected by auscultation directly off each

side of the sternum may include sounds referred from the opposite side of the chest.

- Monitor vital signs closely and as indicated by the patient's condition and suspected injuries in order to note changes and trends in the patient's condition. Remember that the numbers (e.g., blood pressure, heart rate) are not as important as the patient's clinical condition and the trends involved.

- Help relieve the pressure of a tension pneumothorax when necessary. In this procedure, the tension pneumothorax may be converted to an open pneumothorax by inserting a large-bore needle into the chest wall to release the trapped air and decompress the chest. This should be done only by those with special training and skills. Nursing care includes monitoring the patient's condition and vital signs, offering explanations to the conscious patient, keeping the patient warm, and ensuring the flow of oxygen and intravenous fluids to the patient during the procedure.

- Make preparations for an emergency thoracotomy in the trauma suite or emergency department if the patient is critically injured and his or her condition is unstable. Table 7-3 gives the indications for emergency thoracotomy.

- Cover an open pneumothorax wound with any available material, including a rubber glove or plastic dressing. Many trauma teams now use a special taping method (Figure 7-5) that allows air to escape from the chest but prevents entry of additional air: An occlusive dressing is taped on three sides. The dressing is pulled over the wound with inhalation, but air escapes during exhalation through the loose border of the dressing. This one-way flutter-valve effect prevents accumulation of air in the chest cavity. If the patient's condition worsens after application of this dressing, reopen the seal; it may be aggravating the condition.

- Stabilize an object impaled in the chest by putting bandages around it (Figure 7-6). Secure venous access, administer oxygen, monitor the electrocardiogram and vital signs, and transport the patient to the hospital. The impaled object may be compressing internal structures and preventing hemorrhage, so it should be removed only under controlled circumstances in a hospital.

- Offer explanations and reassurances to the patient as you work even if he or she appears to be unconscious. Hearing may be present, and high levels of anxiety accompany accidents and assaults. Anxiety accompanies dyspnea and further distresses the patient.

- Explain to the patient with a simple rib fracture that time should heal the injury. Analgesics, rest, and the application of heat may reduce pain. Some institutions recommend taping the area or immobilizing the arm on the side of the injury in a sling, but these are basically comfort measures that do not affect the outcome of the injury. Multiple rib fractures indicate significant blunt trauma and are considered more serious.

- Do not allow the patient to eat or drink before he or she is examined by a physician. Immediate surgical intervention may be indicated, and oral intake will increase the risk of fatal aspiration during the perioperative period.

- Do not attempt to open a thoracic laceration to see how deep it is or if it penetrates the thoracic cavity; doing so could make the injury worse. Apply pressure over sites of direct bleeding to reduce blood loss, and transport the patient to a hospital for examination.

- Place your hands on each side of the patient's chest, and feel for chest excursions. Each side of the chest should move equally with the other.

On inspiration, dressing seals wound, preventing air entry.

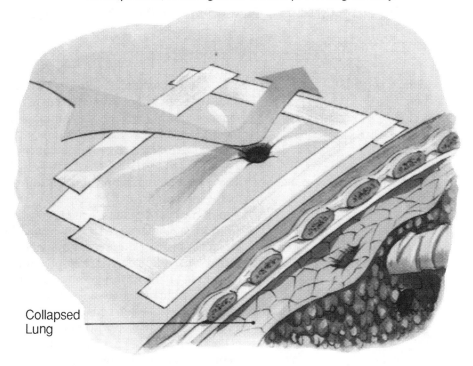

Collapsed
Lung

Expiration allows trapped air to escape through untaped section of dressing.

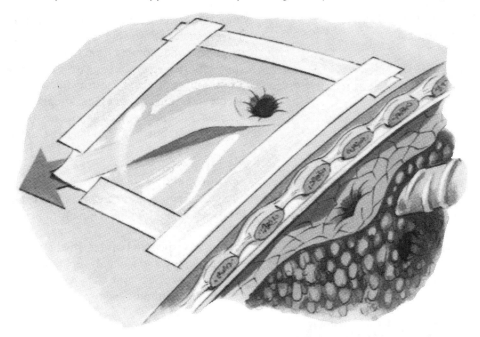

**Figure 7-5. Flutter-valve dressing for an open pneumothorax.** Reprinted by permission from Grant, H. D., Murray, R. H., Jr., & Bergeron, J. D. (Eds.). *Brady emergency care* (5th ed.). Englewood Cliffs, NJ: Prentice-Hall, 1990.

## Table 7-2
## Potential Nursing Diagnoses and Interventions for Patients with Thoracic Trauma

| Diagnosis | Interventions |
|---|---|
| Fluid volume deficit, potential, r/t thoracic trauma | Secure intravenous access with two large-bore intravenous lines and begin volume replacement as ordered, because rapid deterioration may occur. Monitor vital signs as indicated and report changes or trends. Administer blood products as ordered according to policy. |
| Suffocation, potential, r/t thoracic trauma | Check breath sounds for bilateral equality; check for bilateral and equal chest excursions; palpate for subcutaneous air. Report tracheal deviation, hemoptysis, distended neck veins, air leaks, and other signs to a physician. Have equipment for airway maintenance readily available in the event the patient's condition deteriorates; prepare for emergency intubation or cricothyroidotomy if airway obstruction develops. Administer oxygen as ordered. Monitor patient for signs of dyspnea and symptoms such as restlessness and anxiety that accompany respiratory distress. Reassure the patient, and notify a physician of changes in respiratory status. Prepare for emergency thoracotomy as necessary. Obtain or assist with collecting blood specimens for determination of arterial blood gases as indicated to monitor respiratory status. Obtain chest radiographs as ordered. |
| Breathing pattern, ineffective, r/t thoracic trauma | Monitor breath sounds, and note signs of respiratory distress such as a crowing sound on inspiration, bubbling or gurgling sounds coming from the thorax, and nasal flaring. Apply a flutter-valve dressing over an open chest wound to prevent more air from entering the wound; prepare for needle insertion to relieve tension pneumothorax; prepare for chest tube insertion or emergency surgery. Assist and support respirations as necessary. |
| Cardiac output, decreased, r/t structural problems | Start two large-bore intravenous lines and begin fluid resuscitation, monitor vital signs and report changes and trends to a physician Report any decrease in heart sounds or changes in electrocardiogram immediately to physician. |
| Gas exchange impairment | Monitor vital signs and cardiac rhythm as indicated; monitor oxygen therapy. Immediately report signs or symptoms of respiratory decompensation to a physician; monitor breath sounds and respiratory status. |

Note.—This is a sample of potential nursing diagnoses. It is not presented as or intended to be a complete care plan for the trauma patient. More complete information can be found in a medical-surgical nursing course and textbook. r/t = related to.

Adapted from Sparks, S. and Taylor, C. M. *Nursing diagnosis reference manual,* Springhouse, PA: Springhouse Corp., 1991, and Chitwood, L., *Ambulatory patient care,* San Diego: Western Schools, 1994.

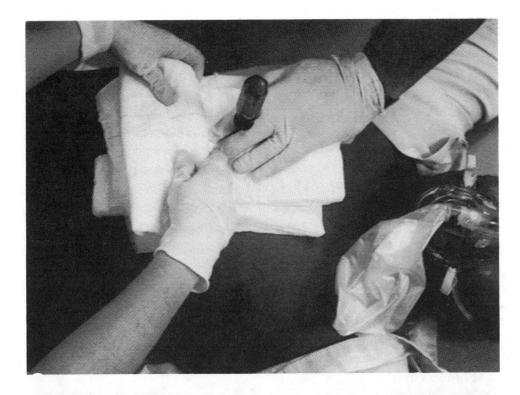

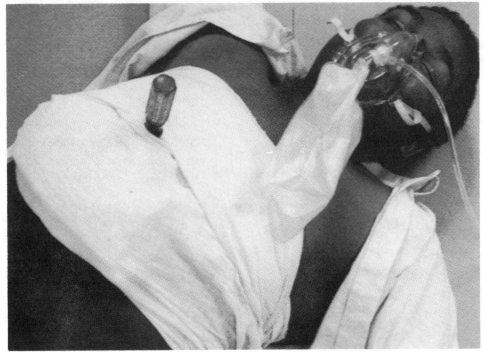

**Figure 7-6. Stabilizing and dressing an object impaled in the chest**. Reprinted by permission from Grant, H. D., Murray, R. H., Jr., & Bergeron, J. D. (Eds.). *Brady emergency care* (5th ed.). Englewood Cliffs, NJ: Prentice-Hall, 1990.

---

**Table 7-3**

**Indications for Emergency Thoracotomy**

Penetrating Stab Wounds to the Heart
- Entrance wound over cardiac region
- Cardiac tamponade

Massive or Progressive Hemothorax
- More than 1000 ml initially
- More than 800 ml in 4 hr

Esophageal Injury
- Odynophagia
- Mediastinal or cervical emphysema

Major Tracheal or Bronchial Injury
- Refractory pneumothorax
- Massive air leak

Source: Ordog, G. J. Wasserberger, J. Balasubramanium, S. and Shoemaker, W. . *The Journal of Trauma, 36,* 680–684, 1994.

---

- Palpate gently along the ribs for any structural deformities indicating fractures or crepitus, which might indicate air collecting under the skin because of a leak from the lung.

- Stabilize a flail segment of ribs with your hand or by using a bulky dressing. When spinal injury has been ruled out, allowing the patient to lie on the affected side limits movement of the segment and reduces pain. Be alert for the onset of shock and hypoxia.

- Note the turgor of the neck veins. Hypovolemia from bleeding into the chest cavity may collapse neck veins. Bulging distended neck veins can indicate obstruction of normal blood flow into the heart by increasing pressure in the thoracic cavity.

# SUMMARY

Because vital organs such as the heart are located in the chest, a swift response to thoracic trauma is one of the keys to reducing mortality. Management of thoracic injuries may mean simply transporting the patient with a single rib fracture to a physician or hospital. It also may mean performing critical interventions to open the airway, support breathing, and maintain the patient's circulation until arriving at a hospital. If the patient does not die immediately from major thoracic trauma, intervention can help save his or her life.

# CRITICAL CONCEPTS

- Assume that any penetrating thoracic trauma threatens the patient's life until it is proved otherwise.

- The probability of thoracic injury is high in any patient who has multiple trauma; 25% of all deaths caused by trauma are due to thoracic trauma.

- Monitor the electrocardiogram in any patient who has thoracic trauma. Cardiac changes may result from thoracic trauma; prompt recognition and treatment will enhance survival.

- Be prepared for life-threatening shock. Insert two large-bore intravenous catheters, begin fluid resuscitation, and administer supplemental oxygen as ordered.

- Hypoxia is often the cause of death in fatal thoracic trauma, so prompt recognition and swift intervention are the keys to the patient's survival. Getting the patient to the hospital quickly generally enhances survival rates.

# GLOSSARY

**Aortic rupture or dissection:** Rupture or tearing apart of the aorta. In aortic dissection, the layers of the vessel may tear apart and weaken the aorta, leading to leakage or rupture. This is generally rapidly fatal.

**Cardiac tamponade:** The collection of fluid in the pericardium, the sac surrounding the heart. Because the pericardium is not elastic, the heart is compressed, and its pumping is impaired by the constriction.

**Flail chest:** A condition in which a segment of thoracic ribs is fractured and moves independently of the rib cage, causing paradoxical movement.

**Myocardial contusion:** Bruising of the heart caused by blunt trauma; myocardial contusion causes damage and signs and symptoms similar to those associated with a heart attack or myocardial infarction.

**Pneumothorax:** A collection of air in the pleural cavity that impairs function of the lung.

**Traumatic asphyxia:** A condition associated with a crush injury of the chest that forces blood out of the heart and into the head and neck. The patient's head and neck swell, and the face and lips become cyanotic.

# EXAM QUESTIONS

## Chapter 7

### Questions 32 - 37

32. Which thoracic injury is characterized by the triad of hypotension, distended neck veins. and muffled heart sounds?

    a. Tension pneumothorax
    b. Aortic rupture
    c. Cardiac tamponade
    d. Esophageal tear

33. You are working in the emergency department when an ambulance radios that it is bringing in a patient who has two visible stab wounds over the heart. The patient is unstable, in shock, and near cardiac arrest. You anticipate the physician will do which of the following?

    a Perform an emergency thoracotomy.
    b. Pronounce the patient dead on arrival.
    c. Send the patient to the radiology department for computed tomography.
    d. Perform diagnostic peritoneal lavage.

34. A common potential nursing diagnosis for a patient with thoracic trauma is:

    a. Body image disturbance
    b. Fluid volume excess
    c. Grieving, anticipatory
    d. Gas exchange impairment

35. You are driving behind a car that strikes a man on a bicycle. The bicyclist lands on the hood of the car but is conscious and cooperative when you reach him. You expose the upper part of his body and note an obvious flail chest. Suddenly he becomes anxious, dyspneic, restless, and cyanotic. You suspect which of the following injuries?

    a. Myocardial contusion
    b. Tension pneumothorax
    c. Cardiac tamponade
    d. Pulmonary contusion

36. Bulging, distended neck veins ia a patient with thoracic trauma may indicate which of the following?

    a. Hypovolemia
    b. Pneumothorax
    c. Tacheobronchial disruption
    d. Aortic rupture

37. A flutter-valve dressing is used to treat which of the following thoracic injuries?

    a. Open pneumothorax
    b. Cardiac tamponade
    c. Flail chest
    d. Massive hemothorax

# CHAPTER 8

# ABDOMINAL TRAUMA

## CHAPTER OBJECTIVE

After completing this chapter, the reader should be able to differentiate between the basic structures and functions of the abdominal organs, recognize common causes of abdominal trauma, and suggest nursing interventions for patients with abdominal injuries.

## LEARNING OBJECTIVES

After studying this chapter, the reader should be able to

1. Recognize signs and symptoms of abdominal trauma.

2. Select methods commonly used to stabilize patients who have abdominal trauma.

3. List common types of abdominal trauma.

4. Specify common potential nursing diagnoses for patients with abdominal trauma.

## INTRODUCTION

Abdominal trauma is often not evident on physical examination, but death can occur in minutes because of internal bleeding. This chapter reviews basic anatomy and physiology of the abdominal organs and common mechanisms of injury that produce blunt and penetrating abdominal trauma. It also describes assessment of patients who have abdominal trauma, discusses common abdominal trauma and management of these injuries, and presents potential nursing diagnoses and strategies for the care of patients with abdominal trauma.

## BASIC ABDOMINAL ANATOMY AND PHYSIOLOGY

The abdominal cavity extends from the diaphragm down to the pelvis and is divided into three areas: the thoracic abdomen, the retroperitoneal abdomen, and the true abdomen. The organs in these specific areas are additionally classified as hollow or solid. Knowledge of the location and an understanding of the structure and function of the abdominal organs provide the foundation for assessment and management of patients who have abdominal trauma.

## Thoracic Abdomen

Some of the abdominal organs reside high in the abdomen under the ribs surrounding the chest or thorax. This part of the abdomen is referred to as the thoracic abdomen. Even though the ribs offer some protection, the thoracic abdominal organs can still be damaged by penetrating or blunt trauma. The intrathoracic abdominal organs include the following:

**Liver.** The largest of the abdominal organs (3–4 lb [1.4–1.8 kg]), the liver is solid, highly vascular, and one of the most vital organs in the body. It functions in metabolism, digestion, storage, and detoxification. In its position on the right side of the body (Figure 8-1), the liver can be shattered, fractured, lacerated, or contused during abdominal trauma. The liver is particularly vulnerable to rapid deceleration injuries caused by seat belts in motor vehicle accidents, to falls that tear major vessels, and to penetrating injuries caused by gunshots or stabbings. Both penetrating and blunt abdominal trauma can cause massive hemorrhage, resulting in death within minutes. The liver is the second most commonly damaged organ in blunt abdominal trauma.

**Spleen.** The highly vascular spleen is located on the left side of the body. It is the most commonly injured organ in blunt abdominal trauma (Sheehy & Jimmerson, 1994). Its function remains poorly defined, but it is known to be involved in blood production, blood destruction, and defense against disease. This solid organ stores several hundred milliliters of blood. Although useful to body function, the spleen is not a vital organ.

**Diaphragm.** The diaphragm is the muscle separating the chest from the abdomen. Attached to the ribs, sternum, and spine, it contracts to allow inspiration of air into the lungs. Both blunt and penetrating trauma can disrupt the integrity of the diaphragm and allow abdominal organs to slip through the tear and into the thoracic cavity. Signs and symptoms of diaphragmatic injury may be subtle or severe; immediate and life-threatening respiratory distress is possible.

**Stomach.** The stomach is a hollow organ located to the left of midline, under the liver and the diaphragm. Because it is hollow when empty, the stomach is compressible and can absorb some energy during trauma.

## Retroperitoneal Space

The peritoneum is the membrane lining the abdominal cavity. The kidneys, ureters, pancreas, and the part of the small bowel known as the duodenum are located in an area behind the peritoneum known as the retroperitoneal abdomen.

**Kidneys.** The kidneys are solid organs located at about the level of the waist. Although well protected in the retroperitoneal space, they may still sustain serious trauma that leads to massive blood loss.

**Ureters.** Muscular tubular structures, the ureters withstand blunt trauma well but may be injured in penetrating trauma.

**Pancreas.** The pancreas is located behind and beneath the stomach and the liver. Although generally well protected, it can be injured in either blunt or penetrating trauma; blunt injuries are more common.

**Duodenum.** The duodenum is the initial segment of the small bowel that begins at the stomach. It is hollow when empty and may be compressed against the spine in blunt abdominal trauma.

## True Abdomen

The remainder of the abdominal organs, including the small and large intestines and bladder, fill the true abdomen (Figure 8-2). In females, the uterus, fallopian tubes, and ovaries are also part of the true abdomen.

**Small and large intestines.** Because of their contents, rupture of the hollow small and large intestines leads to contamination of the abdominal cavity with fecal

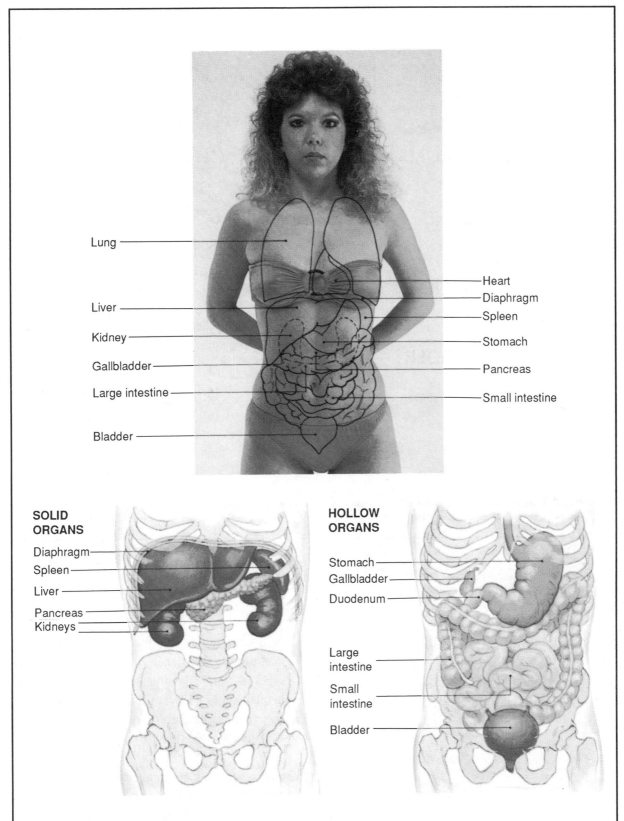

**Figure 8-1. Abdominal organs.** Reprinted by permission from Grant, H. D., Murray, R. H., Jr., & Bergeron, J. D. (Eds.). *Brady emergency care* (5th ed.). Englewood Cliffs, NJ: Prentice-Hall, 1990.

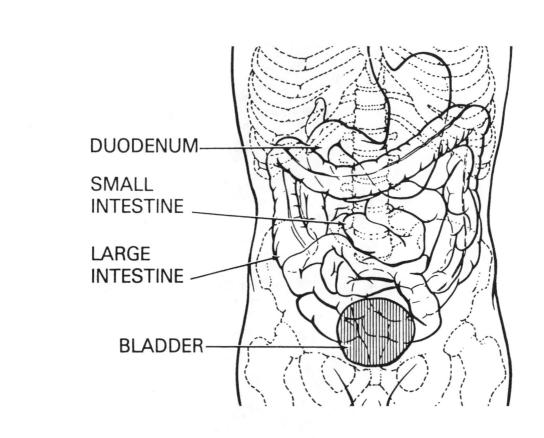

**Figure 8-2. True abdomen.** Reprinted by permission from Campbell, J. *Basic trauma life support: Advanced prehospital care* (2nd ed.). Englewood Cliffs, NJ: Prentice-Hall, 1988.

material and other toxins; serious peritonitis may occur. Blunt trauma to the abdomen compresses the abdominal organs against the spine, and rupture may occur.

**Bladder.** A muscular sac, the bladder lies in a protected site behind the symphysis pubis. However, it can still be injured by blunt or penetrating trauma, spilling urine into the abdominal cavity.

# MECHANISM OF INJURY

### Penetrating Trauma

Projectiles are responsible for most penetrating abdominal trauma, and penetrating abdominal trauma is usually intentionally inflicted. Because violence is frequently associated with use of alcohol and other drugs, treatment of these patients may be complicated by the effects of these drugs.

Penetrating abdominal trauma is usually caused by a knife or firearm and may lead to impalement, laceration, or rupture and puncture of the abdominal organs. The mortality rate associated with single stab wounds is low, and these wounds are usually not life threatening unless a major vessel is lacerated. The length and size of the weapon obviously affect how deep the wound is and how much damage is inflicted. However, gunshot wounds are generally more serious, as bullets shatter organs and spill intestinal contents into the abdominal cavity. Gunshot wounds frequently leave an entry and exit wound that allow the health care provider to assess probable structural damage and plan interventions accordingly. The damage left by a stab wound cannot be so easily estimated, and immediate treatment is usually based on the patient's signs and symptoms.

## Blunt Trauma

Blunt abdominal trauma may occur from rapid deceleration in a motor vehicle accident, during a fall, or when an object such as a bat or a fist strikes the abdomen. Falls, assaults, motor vehicle accidents, and sporting accidents account for much of blunt abdominal trauma. Rapid forward deceleration against a taut seat belt can rupture the intestines and bladder. Although seat belts themselves can cause blunt trauma in a crash, consider the alternative: Unrestrained passengers frequently sustain severe or fatal head and neck injuries, whereas patients generally recover from injuries caused by seat belts. Blunt trauma also damages internal organs by compressing the organs against the rigid spine, sometimes causing rupture. Unfortunately, blunt trauma often leaves little visible evidence of the injury, and bleeding is most often hidden. Blunt trauma with force sufficient to fracture the pelvis is often associated with damage to the bladder or urethra. Blunt trauma to the back and flanks may be associated with damage to the kidneys, although this often consists of a renal contusion that heals itself. Severe blunt trauma, however, can fracture the kidney.

# ASSESSMENT OF PATIENTS WITH ABDOMINAL TRAUMA

For any patient with abdominal trauma, follow the standard ABC assessment described in chapter 2. Abdominal trauma is seldom the sole injury; presume that unconscious trauma patients have a spinal injury until it is proved otherwise. Observe the accident scene and elicit a history of the injury while examining the patient. The mechanism of injury provides important information about potential injuries. Try to determine the object that caused the injury, the speed or force of the object, and the area of the abdomen hit by the object (Kitt & Kaiser, 1990). When examining the patient, note also any scars from previous abdominal surgery that may indicate preexisting health conditions. Be aware that abdominal injuries can go undetected because the injuries and bleeding are often internal rather than external.

## Signs and Symptoms of Possible Abdominal Trauma

Common signs and symptoms of abdominal trauma include the following:

- Abdominal pain.

- Guarding by the patient to protect tender abdominal areas.

- Bruising, crepitus.

- Abdominal distension.

- Bruising and swelling diagonally across the chest and across the pelvis caused by a seat belt and shoulder harness as a result of sudden deceleration.

## Signs Indicating Possible Internal Hemorrhage

Signs indicating possible internal hemorrhage in a patient with abdominal trauma include the following:

- Hypotension, tachycardia, and pallor.

- Rigid or distended abdomen.

- Obvious deformity of the abdomen, evisceration of the abdominal contents, or impalement of the abdomen.

- Hematemesis.

- Bruising and discoloration around the umbilicus (Cullen's sign), which may indicate hemoperitoneum, or blood in the peritoneal cavity.

- Bruising over the flank (Grey Turner's sign), which may indicate blood in the retroperitoneal space.

- Hematuria, blood, or semen (from disruption of the prostate) at the meatus.

- Inability to void.

## Diagnostic Tests for Abdominal Trauma

When the condition of a critically injured patient with abdominal trauma is unstable and rapidly deteriorating, some physicians may elect to go straight to surgery when the patient arrives at the hospital. However, ideally, the patient's condition is stabilized and evaluated under controlled circumstances. Some of the following diagnostic tests may be used to evaluate the injuries and determine the need for surgery.

**Diagnostic peritoneal lavage.** Diagnostic peritoneal lavage helps determine the presence of blood or intestinal contents in the peritoneal cavity. It is frequently done in the trauma suite or emergency department.

**Computed tomography.** Computed tomography (CT) is useful in examining the abdomen for defects and collections of fluid or air, although the patient must be transported to the CT scanner. Patients whose condition is critical and unstable may not tolerate the transfer. Those who are sent for CT require constant monitoring by skilled personnel who are ready to intervene immediately if the patient's condition deteriorates.

**Sonography.** Many trauma centers now obtain sonograms as a routine part of the diagnostic assessment of patients with abdominal trauma. This procedure can be performed with portable equipment in the trauma suite or emergency department.

**Radiography.** Radiographs can help detect free air or foreign objects in the abdomen.

**Local wound exploration.** After infiltration with local anesthesia, the wound may be explored in the emergency department or trauma suite. This allows the physician to assess the nature of the injury and determine if the patient should have surgery.

# COMMON ABDOMINAL TRAUMA

Common injuries due to abdominal trauma include the following:

**Lacerations and contusions of the abdomen.** Blunt and penetrating trauma to the abdomen cause pain, discoloration, and obvious or occult bleeding. Contusions may appear superficial, but marked damage to abdominal organs is possible. This is why knowing the mechanism of injury is so critical in assessing patients with abdominal trauma.

**Hepatic injuries.** The liver may be shattered or lacerated by either blunt or penetrating trauma. Suspect liver injury in patients who have rib fractures down the right side of the chest or who complain of abdominal pain and tenderness, especially in the right upper quadrant. If conscious, the patient may guard the abdomen against touch and complain of nausea. Injury to the liver can be fatal within minutes.

**Splenic injuries.** The spleen is the most commonly injured organ in blunt abdominal trauma (Kitt & Kaiser, 1990). Fractures of the lower left ribs, pain in the upper left quadrant, and pain referred to the left shoulder may indicate trauma to the spleen. Life-threatening hemorrhage can follow rupture of the spleen. Although tamponade may reduce the flow of blood, hemorrhaging may recur hours or even a few days after injury.

**Aortic injury.** The aorta can be injured by either blunt or penetrating trauma. Sudden decelerative forces may tear the aorta; compression against the spine on impact with the steering wheel may rupture the aorta. Exsanguination occurs within minutes after aortic rupture. Aortic trauma is frequently fatal: 80–90% of traumatic ruptures of the great vessels are fatal at the accident scene; 10–15% of traffic fatalities are due to aortic rupture (Strange, 1987).

**Diaphragmatic rupture.** Blunt or penetrating trauma may disrupt the diaphragm, allowing abdominal contents to enter the chest cavity. This generally causes impaired breathing. Sometimes, however, the injury is not even noticed until the abdomen is explored surgically. Signs of diaphragmatic injury include breath sounds that are decreased on one side of the chest and a shift in heart sounds. The patient may complain of dyspnea, and cyanosis may be evident, because the lungs can no longer function efficiently. More often, though, diaphragmatic injury is diag-

nosed at the hospital on the basis of radiographic findings.

**Gastrointestinal trauma.** Because it is compressible, an empty stomach is not as likely as a full stomach to be injured. However, patients with gastrointestinal trauma often complain of abdominal pain, tenderness, and perhaps nausea when the stomach or intestines are injured. Hematemesis may occur. Rupture of the intestines can cause a fulminant peritonitis, because intestinal contents are spilled into the abdominal cavity.

**Impalement.** Objects impaled in the abdomen often compress and tamponade affected vessels and organs and therefore reduce or stop bleeding. Traumatic injury from impalement depends on the type of instrument lodged in the body and the structures affected.

**Evisceration.** Severe penetrating trauma of the abdomen may leave the abdominal contents exposed outside the abdominal cavity. This is obviously a serious emergency.

**Ruptured bladder.** An empty bladder is less likely than a full bladder to be injured by trauma. For example, blunt trauma to the anterior part of the body, such as a blow from the steering wheel of a car or compression by a seat belt, may rupture a full bladder. Suspect a ruptured bladder if a patient has evidence of penetrating trauma in the suprapubic region (above the pubic bone) or indications of a fractured pelvis. See chapter 11 for more on the management of genitourinary trauma.

**Pelvic fracture.** The pelvis in humans is quite strong, and intense force is required to break it. Therefore, presume that any patient who has a pelvic fracture has associated abdominal injuries until it is proved otherwise. Pelvic fracture is a serious injury that may result in hypovolemia and death.

**Urethral disruption.** Pelvic fractures will sometimes interrupt or tear the urethra from the bladder, especially when blunt trauma forces the pubic bone backward into the urethra. See chapter 11 for more on the management of genitourinary trauma.

**Major renal trauma.** Fractured or lacerated kidneys and injuries to the renal pelvis can produce life-threatening internal hemorrhage, although the injury may not be obvious. However, suspect major renal trauma whenever a patient has serious blunt or penetrating abdominal trauma; anticipate hypovolemic shock from hemorrhage.

**Ureteral injury.** The ureters are seldom injured in blunt trauma. Ureteral injury most often is caused by a missile or foreign object that penetrates the abdominal cavity. Surgical repair is completed after more serious injuries are dealt with. Sheehy and Jimmerson (1994) state that trauma patients should void within 1 hr of admission; otherwise further evaluation is indicated. See chapter 11 for more on the management of renal trauma.

# NURSING STRATEGIES FOR PATIENTS WITH ABDOMINAL TRAUMA

For any patient with abdominal trauma, the goals are to establish the airway, breathing, and circulation and then get the patient to the hospital without delay. Trauma nurses usually insert two large-bore intravenous catheters, begin administration of fluids, and support the circulation while preparing and transporting the patient to the hospital. A pneumatic antishock garment to enhance venous return and support the blood pressure is often used also. Because a major cause of mortality in abdominal injury is delayed diagnosis and treatment (Campbell, 1988), rapid transport to the appropriate facility dramatically improves survival rates.

Table 8-1 gives potential nursing diagnoses and interventions for patients with abdominal trauma. The following general nursing strategies may also be useful. Your interventions should be within the scope of your professional license; commensurate with your skills and training; consistent with your state's nurse practice act; and when performed in a health care institution, adherent to that facility's standards of practice.

- Abdominal trauma usually does not exist alone; other injuries may be present. Assume that any patient who has multiple trauma has a spinal injury until it is proved otherwise.

- Look and feel for obvious deformities, tenderness, or tension in the abdomen. Pain from abdominal injuries may be referred to the shoulders.

- Expose the patient completely in order to conduct an accurate assessment. Cut the patient's clothes off; do not pull them off. Pulling them off can aggravate injuries. Ask a second rescuer to protect the patient's privacy; cover the patient promptly when the assessment is finished.

- Watch for indications of internal hemorrhaging. Signs and symptoms include hypovolemic shock, abdominal pain, abdominal distension, and increasing girth.

- Make stabilization of a pelvic fracture and any other life- or limb-threatening injury the first priority in a patient who has urethral disruption.

- Type and cross-match abdominal trauma patients for at least four units of blood, according to facility policy. Many major abdominal trauma patients will require at least this much blood for transfusion.

- Avoid administering pain medications until the patient has been examined by a physician, be-

**Table 8-1**

**Potential Nursing Diagnoses and Interventions for Patients with Abdominal Trauma**

| Diagnosis | Interventions |
| --- | --- |
| Fluid volume deficit | Secure intravenous access with two large-bore intravenous lines, and begin volume replacement as ordered even if the patient seems stable, because rapid deterioration may occur. Monitor the abdomen for tautness or distension, and report changes; also report onset of abdominal pain or changes in degree of pain. Assist with diagnostic tests and procedures to help determine the nature of the abdominal trauma. Monitor vital signs as indicated, and report changes or trends promptly. Collect specimens of body fluids for analysis as ordered and report results to a physician. |
| Infection, potential, r/t trauma | Use strict aseptic technique when caring for the patient, especially when suctioning the trachea, catheterizing the bladder, or administering parenteral medications. Administer antibiotics as ordered. Cover eviscerated organs with a wet sterile occlusive dressing until the injury can be evaluated by a physician; notify the surgical team of impending case. Monitor temperature and white blood cell count; report alterations or trends to a physician. Determine the date of the patient's last tetanus prophylaxis and report it to the physician for consideration of tetanus booster injection. |
| Tissue perfusion alteration r/t hypovolemia | Monitor vital signs as indicated, and report changes or trends to a physician; monitor skin color and temperature. Measure and record urine output; report decreases to a physician (in general, urine output should be a minimum of 1 mm/kg per hour). Send a urine specimen to the laboratory if ordered for analysis of hematuria and measurement of specific gravity. Administer fluids, colloids, and blood as ordered and according to institutional policy. Observe the patient for changes in mental status that might indicate brain perfusion or oxygenation is inadequate (hypoxia will cause restlessness, confusion, incoordination, and loss of consciousness). Administer oxygen to enhance oxygen delivery to tissues and organs. |
| Pain | Administer analgesics as ordered; offer quiet and simple explanations to the patient, because trauma increases anxiety and anxiety increases pain. Offer frequent reassurances and reinforce information given previously. |

Note.—This is a sample of potential nursing diagnoses. It is not presented as or intended to be a complete care plan for the trauma patient. More complete information can be found in a medical-surgical nursing course and textbook. r/t = related to.

Adapted from Sparks, S. and Taylor, C. M. *Nursing diagnosis reference manual,* Springhouse, PA: Springhouse Corporation, 1991, and Chitwood, L. *Ambulatory patient care,* San Diego: Western Schools, 1994.

cause the medications can mask symptoms. Use nonpharmacologic methods of pain relief such as reassurance, distraction, caring touch, stress reduction, and relaxation techniques when feasible.

- Assess and reassess the patient regularly. Deterioration may be rapid, and shock can develop quickly.

- Insert a Foley catheter cautiously if ordered, but only after other injuries are ruled out. Insertion of a Foley catheter could make a urethral injury worse.

- Do not spend time during the initial assessment listening for bowel sounds. This is generally a waste of the patient's precious golden hour, because the presence or absence of bowel sounds has little impact on initial management. Make better use of this time by securing venous access, replenishing lost fluids, and transporting the patient to the hospital.

- Patients with aortic trauma will generally be in obvious hemorrhagic shock. Prompt surgical intervention and fluid resuscitation may offer some hope for survival.

- Do not remove any object that has pierced and lodged in the abdomen, because it may reduce or block internal bleeding. Stabilize the object in place and transport the patient to a hospital immediately.

- Do not attempt to return eviscerated abdominal organs to the abdominal cavity. Cover the exposed organs with a sterile dressing moistened with sterile saline, and then place a dry dressing over that (Figure 8-3). Transport the patient to the hospital immediately.

- Do not allow the patient to eat or drink until he or she is examined by a physician. Immediate surgical intervention may be indicated for some abdominal trauma, and oral intake increases the risk of fatal aspiration or complications during the perioperative period.

- Reassure the patient that everything possible is being done. Pain is often intense, and other injuries are often present.

- Teach patients and their families about the importance of using seat belts, shoulder harnesses, and child restraint seats in motor vehicles. Although a seat belt can cause some trauma, the injuries are generally nonfatal; fatal or serious injuries are much more likely when no restraints are used.

- Keep the patient warm. Hypothermia causes defects in coagulation, increases oxygen requirements, reduces tissue perfusion, and hampers the success of resuscitation. Warming fluids and humidifying oxygen are methods of reducing heat loss; head wraps, blankets, and plastic or foil coverings also help maintain warmth.

# SUMMARY

Abdominal trauma may not be evident on visual inspection, but death can occur in minutes because of internal bleeding. Management of abdominal trauma generally is directed at preventing or intervening in shock and getting the patient to the hospital immediately. Knowledge of how the accident or assault took place provides important clues about the type of injury and helps guide the assessment. Abdominal trauma may range from a single uncomplicated stab wound to exsanguination and death from a fractured liver. Rapid assessment and prompt intervention are the keys to the patient's survival.

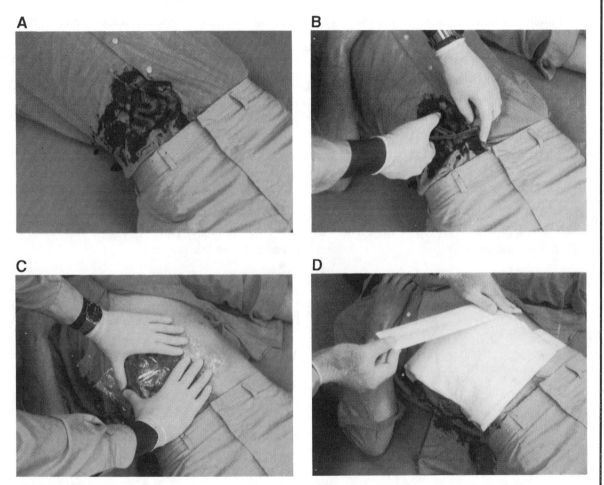

**A.** Open abdominal wound with evisceration. **B.** Cut away clothing from wound. **C.** Apply an occlusive dressing. **D.** Cover occlusive dressing to maintain warmth. *Note:* A saline-soaked dressing can be applied before the occlusive dressing.

**Figure 8-3. Management of eviscerated abdominal organs.** Reprinted by permission from Grant, H. D., Murray, R. H., Jr., & Bergeron, J. D. (Eds.). *Brady emergency care* (5th ed.). Englewood Cliffs, NJ: Prentice-Hall, 1990.

# CRITICAL CONCEPTS

- Assume that any trauma patient who is hypotensive, tachycardic, and pallid is bleeding into the chest or abdomen until it is proved otherwise.

- Maintain a high index of suspicion that an abdominal injury exists in any patient who has multiple trauma. Rapid recognition of internal hemorrhage may help save the patient's life.

- Transport any patient with serious or suspected abdominal trauma to a hospital immediately, as this increases the chances of survival.

- Be prepared for life-threatening shock in any patient who has serious abdominal trauma. Establish two large-bore intravenous lines, and begin fluid resuscitation.

# GLOSSARY

**Cullen's sign:** Bruising and discoloration surrounding the umbilicus.

**Diaphragmatic rupture:** Disruption of the diaphragm; includes tears, perforations, and lacerations. Diaphragmatic disruptions may allow abdominal contents to slip up into the chest cavity, which generally impairs breathing.

**Grey Turner's sign:** Bruising over the flank that may indicate hemoperitoneum.

**Internal hemorrhage:** Any hemorrhage into the abdominal cavity; generally hidden in blunt trauma. Signs and symptoms of internal hemorrhage include shock, abdominal pain, increasing abdominal girth, and a taut abdomen.

**Tamponade:** Pressure or compression on injured vessels that reduces hemorrhage.

# EXAM QUESTIONS

## Chapter 8

## Questions 38 - 41

38. The most commonly injured organ in blunt abdominal trauma is the:

    a. Bladder
    b. Liver
    c. Stomach
    d. Spleen

39. Bruising and discoloration around the umbilicus are called:

    a. Grey Turner's sign
    b. Cullen's sign
    c. Allen's indication
    d. Hoffman's sign

40. Which of the following is a common initial potential nursing diagnosis for a patient with abdominal trauma?

    a. Fluid volume deficit
    b. Fluid volume excess
    c. Hyperthermia
    d. Skin integrity impairment, potential

41. Your teenage son is playing touch football in the backyard when he falls face down on a sharp hand tool used for breaking up soil in the garden. The tool remains impaled in his abdomen. He is lying on the ground in pain and begging you to pull it out. What do you do after you tell the others to go call for help?

    a. Gently loosen and remove the tool from your son's abdomen, and then apply pressure.
    b. Stabilize the tool in place with towels and reassure your son while you wait for an ambulance.
    c. Turn your son on his side, quickly remove the tool, and apply pressure to the wound.
    d. Ask another person to locate your son's immunization records in the kitchen drawer in the house.

# CHAPTER 9

# ORTHOPEDIC TRAUMA

## CHAPTER OBJECTIVE

After completing this chapter, the reader should be able to differentiate between the basic structures and functions of the musculoskeletal system, recognize common causes of orthopedic trauma, and suggest nursing interventions for patients with orthopedic trauma.

## LEARNING OBJECTIVES

After studying this chapter, the reader should be able to

1. Recognize signs and symptoms of orthopedic trauma.

2. Select interventions for patients with orthopedic trauma.

3. List common types of orthopedic trauma.

4. Recognize special concerns in meeting the challenge of limb preservation in patients with orthopedic trauma.

5. Specify common potential nursing diagnoses for patients with orthopedic trauma.

## INTRODUCTION

Although a simple fracture is generally not life threatening, some orthopedic injuries, such as a fractured pelvis or femur, can cause death. Other injuries, such as dislocation of a hip or knee, can result in loss of the limb from arterial occlusion or in permanent disability. Nursing interventions in the care of patients with orthopedic trauma have substantial impact on outcome and recovery.

This chapter reviews basic anatomy and physiology of the musculoskeletal system, common mechanisms of injury that produce orthopedic trauma, and common orthopedic trauma. It also describes assessment of patients with orthopedic trauma and presents nursing strategies and interventions for the care of patients with orthopedic trauma.

## BASIC ANATOMY AND PHYSIOLOGY OF THE MUSCULOSKELETAL SYSTEM

The skeleton is composed of 206 bones (Figure 9-1). Tendons attach muscles to the bones and aid in movement. Bones are attached to other bones by tough ligaments that help keep joints stable. Some bones, such as the ribs, protect the soft tissues lying

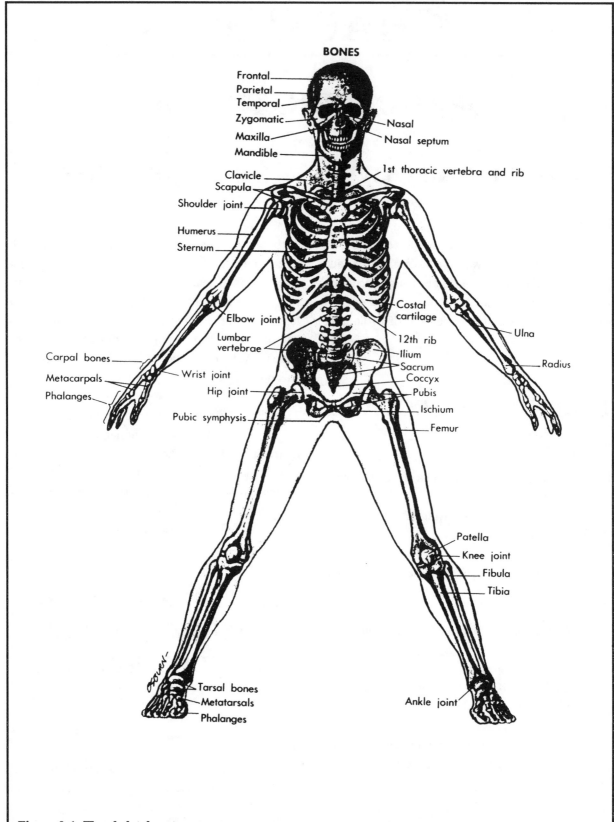

**Figure 9-1. The skeletal system**. Reprinted by permission from Miller, B.F., and Keane, C. B. *Encyclopedia and dictionary of medicine and nursing.*, Philadelphia: Saunders, 1972.

underneath them. Bones are ordinarily quite strong. In infants, the skull and thoracic cage are relatively elastic, so trauma must be significant to cause a fracture. However, as the body grows older, the bones become less dense and may fracture quite easily.

## Axial Skeleton

The axial skeleton composes the long axis of the body. It is formed from the sternum, ribs, spine, and skull.

## Appendicular Skeleton

The remaining bones in the body form the appendicular skeleton. Some of those categories of bones include the following:

- **Long bones:** The long bones are those that form the arms and legs: the femur, tibia, fibula, humerus, radius, and ulna. Fractures of the femur and humerus can result in life-threatening hemorrhage.

- **Short bones:** The short bones compose the hands and feet. Laceration of tendons and fractures of the short bones can result in limitations and disability.

- **Flat bones:** The ribs and shoulder blades are examples of flat bones.

# MECHANISM OF INJURY

Both penetrating and blunt trauma can cause orthopedic injury. The force of blunt trauma can fracture or dislocate bones. Whatever force causes trauma to the musculoskeletal system can also cause trauma to the surrounding tissues, usually the nerves and vessels near the bone. In some instances, the bones are sheared or torn from surrounding structures, result-ing in amputation. In other instances, the bone does not break, but the tendons, ligaments, and muscles are strained, sprained, or torn by the force of the trauma. According to Sheehy and Jimmerson (1994), with the same mechanism of injury, an older person's joint generally will fracture, whereas a younger person's will dislocate. Bones also can be fractured and tendons and ligaments ruptured by the twisting or rotational forces associated with participation in sports.

Penetrating trauma is caused by projectiles such as bullets or knives that shatter bones and lacerate muscles, tendons, and ligaments. A projectile that penetrates the body and passes through bone may drive bone fragments into the wound along with the foreign object, causing an additional injury. The ends of a fractured bone may also protrude through the skin and may become an open pathway for bacteria.

# ASSESSMENT OF PATIENTS WITH ORTHOPEDIC TRAUMA

As with any trauma patient, first evaluate the airway, breathing, and circulation. Orthopedic trauma may not be the only injury, but distorted limbs can be shocking. Do not be distracted by orthopedic injuries and neglect other life-threatening conditions. The goal is to intervene in life-threatening injuries first, limb-threatening injuries second, and then less serious injuries. Limb-threatening injuries must be carefully managed, however. Surrounding nerves and vessels also may be injured during musculoskeletal trauma, and these additional injuries could cause permanent disability. Orthopedic injuries in children especially can result in permanent disability and deformity.

Assessment continues as with any patient. Observe the accident scene and elicit a history of the injury while examining the patient. Include the following steps:

- Cut clothing away from the extremities, and then look carefully at them. Do not pull off the patient's clothing; doing so could aggravate the injury. Compare the injured extremity with the opposite limb; note skin temperature and color. Look for obvious injuries, deformities, and bleeding that may require intervention.

- Feel gently down each extremity, noting uneven surfaces, swelling, changes in skin temperature, grinding sensations, and complaints of pain from the patient. Palpate the distal pulses in each extremity to determine if circulation is impaired.

- Ask about previous musculoskeletal system disease, injuries, and surgical operations. The answers may provide clues about suspected orthopedic trauma.

Suspect bone fracture if any of the following occurs:

- The extremity is deformed.

- The patient states that he or she felt a bone break.

- The patient complains of moderate to severe pain.

- The area of injury is bruised or swollen.

Assessment of patients who have orthopedic trauma also requires an evaluation of the nerves and vessels in the injured area. Palpate the distal pulses in both extremities (Figure 9-2); they should be equal. Mark the point (e.g., with an X) where the maximal impulse is felt so that you can locate it later. Ask the patient if he or she can feel you touching the extremity, and if there is any numbness or tingling. If no

obvious deformity is present, ask the patient to wiggle the fingers or toes of the affected extremity; this provides information about damage to the nerves in the area.

# COMMON ORTHOPEDIC TRAUMA

## Fractures

When the continuity of a bone is disrupted, a fracture results. Many different types of fractures occur, but the specific type is not as important as the interventions used in selected injuries. Fractures may be open (the skin is broken over the fracture site) or closed (the skin remains intact). Obviously, open fractures provide a direct route for the entry of infectious organisms and foreign bodies and thus generally are considered more serious. Fractures that may be seen in trauma patients include the following:

**Pelvic fracture.** If gentle pressure applied to each side of the pelvis elicits pain, suspect a pelvic fracture. Other indications of a pelvic fracture include abdominal distension from internal bleeding, evidence of hypovolemic shock, and bloody urine. Pelvic fracture is second only to skull fracture in terms of complications and death (Grant et al., 1990).

**Femur fracture.** The femur is one of the strongest bones in the body. Substantial force is required to fracture it, so other musculoskeletal and soft-tissue injuries are often present. Fracture of a femur is a serious orthopedic injury. The fractured leg may appear to be shorter than the other leg and usually is rotated externally; that is, the foot and injured leg point away from the midline of the body. Trauma teams sometimes apply a pneumatic antishock garment to patients who have a fractured femur because blood loss may be heavy and because the compres-

A. Palpation of radial pulse.

B. Location of posterior tib-
ial and dorsalis pedis pulses.

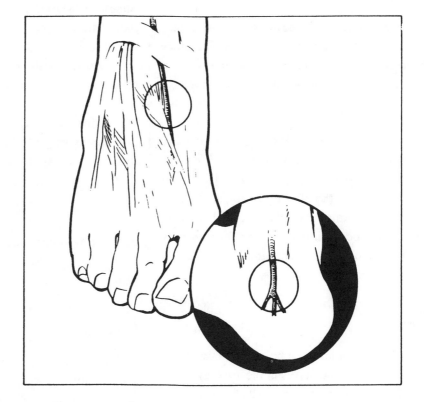

**Figure 9-2. Palpation of distal pulses.** Reprinted by permission from Campbell, J. *Basic trauma life support: Advanced prehospital care* (2nd ed.). Englewood Cliffs, NJ: Prentice-Hall, 1988.

sion applied by the garment helps splint the fracture. A Thomas half-ring splint is also often used to re-align the bone and promote circulation when a femur is fractured. Concurrent fracture of both femurs can cause life-threatening hemorrhage and death.

**Hip fracture.** Hip fractures are most common in eld-erly women and usually are caused by simple falls. Hip fractures also occur in motor vehicle accidents and other sudden deceleration incidents. Blood loss can be moderate to severe. The affected extremity may appear to be shorter than the other extremity. Discoloration and swelling may be present over the fracture site. A hip fracture is a serious injury that must be evaluated by an orthopedist.

**Humerus fracture.** The humerus is the longest and strongest bone in the upper extremity, and substan-tial force is required to fracture it; blood loss can be heavy. Neurovascular compromise may develop. This is a serious injury that requires evaluation by an or-thopedist.

**Wrist fracture.** Wrist fractures often occur when per-sons fall on their outstretched hands or when they throw up their hands to protect themselves against hitting the interior of the vehicle in a motor vehicle accident.

**Ankle fracture.** The bones of the lower legs often are fractured in sports accidents, motor vehicle acci-dents, and falls. If the injury was caused by rapid vertical deceleration (a fall), suspect spinal and heel injuries as well, because the energy would have been directed up the body on impact. Obvious deformity may be present, or the only indication of trauma may be swelling and pain.

## Dislocations

Any dislocation of a joint can be serious. Disruption of the blood supply and nerves in the area can result in loss of the limb or permanent disability. Even if the dislocated joint slips back into place, the patient still must be evaluated by an orthopedist.

**Hip dislocation.** A hip dislocation is a serious ortho-pedic emergency. The blood supply to the head or top of the hip may be impaired, causing necrosis and necessitating replacement with an artificial joint in the future. Pressure on the sciatic nerve can result in permanent disability. Hip dislocation often occurs in motor vehicle accidents when a person's knees strike the dashboard, and the energy then is directed back to the hips. Pain is often severe, and the leg may rest in an abnormal position.

**Knee dislocation.** When the bones forming the knee are dislocated or fractured, serious injury to the pop-liteal artery may occur. Therefore, arteriograms are obtained in the hospital whenever a patient has a dislocated knee. Serious knee injuries may necessi-tate amputation of the leg; consequently, knee dislo-cation is an orthopedic emergency (Campbell, 1988).

**Shoulder dislocation.** The shoulder is the most com-monly dislocated joint (Kitt & Kaiser, 1990). Shoul-der dislocations are most often sustained in athletic activities. Dislocations of the shoulder may become chronic and require surgical intervention.

**Elbow dislocation.** Like shoulder dislocations, elbow dislocations are generally associated with athletic activ-ity. Serious damage to nerves and vessels may occur.

## Impalement

Penetrating trauma may result in foreign bodies or objects impaling bones, muscles, or tendons. Disabil-ity or loss of the extremity may occur.

## Lacerations

Although simple lacerations often heal with only simple suturing, lacerations that penetrate the ten-dons and ligaments in the hands and feet can result in permanent disability if not thoroughly irrigated and repaired.

## Traumatic Amputations

Often sustained in industrial and recreation accidents, traumatic amputations are serious emergencies. Depending on the circumstances, the amputated parts can sometimes be replanted, so the parts should always accompany the patient to the hospital. Blood loss may be significant, and some disability and disfigurement are to be expected.

## Sprain

Tearing of a ligament that connects one bone to the other commonly is due to twisting forces and results in a sprain. Although sprains are not usually serious, the patient should be evaluated by a physician.

## Strain

Overstretching or overexerting a muscle, as in sports activities, can cause a strain of that muscle, which is associated with pain. The strain is generally in the area of the tendon, where the muscle attaches to the bone.

## Compartment Syndrome

Compartment syndrome develops most often with blunt trauma or crush injuries. It is due to an increase in pressure within a fascial compartment. The signs and symptoms include pain, parethesias, weakness, and an increase in intracompartmental pressure. These may develop a few hours to a few days after the injury. Surgical fasciotomy is usually necessary to relieve increased intracompartmental pressure. Otherwise, loss of the extremity may occur because vascular compression causes tissue necrosis.

# NURSING STRATEGIES FOR PATIENTS WITH ORTHOPEDIC TRAUMA

The goals with any patient with orthopedic trauma are to limit further damage, preserve the structure and function of the injured extremity to the extent possible, ensure perfusion and oxygenation, and transport the patient to a hospital for examination by an orthopedic specialist. Although many orthopedic injuries are not serious, some are associated with significant morbidity and mortality and may affect the patient's quality of life.

Table 9-1 gives potential nursing diagnoses and interventions. The following nursing strategies may also be useful. It is presumed with each that the patient's airway, breathing, and circulation have been established and that the patient is being transported to the hospital without delay. Your interventions should be within the scope of your professional license; commensurate with your skills and training; consistent with your state's nurse practice act; and when performed in a health care institution, adherent to that facility's standards of practice.

- Do not attempt to push exposed bones back into the wound; doing so could make the injury worse, contaminate the wound, and cause the patient pain.

- Establish venous access, administer fluids, and supply oxygen as ordered to any patient who has a fractured long bone or a suspected pelvic fracture, because shock may follow. Amounts of blood loss associated with certain fractures are listed in Table 9-2.

- Do not remove an object stuck in bone or muscle unless the object is interfering with the airway; doing so could make the injury worse.

**Table 9-1**

**Potential Nursing Diagnoses and Interventions for Patients with Orthopedic Trauma**

| Diagnosis | Interventions |
|---|---|
| Fluid volume deficit | Secure intravenous access with two large-bore intravenous lines and begin volume replacement as ordered when fracture of the pelvis or a long bone is suspected, because blood loss may be substantial. Monitor vital signs as indicated, and report changes or trends promptly. Collect blood specimens for analysis as ordered and report results to a physician. |
| Infection, potential, r/t trauma | Use strict aseptic technique when caring for the patient; administer antibiotics as ordered. Cover exposed bone with a dry sterile dressing; notify surgical team of probable impending case. Monitor temperature and white blood cell count; report alterations or trends to physician. Determine the date of the patient's last tetanus prophylaxis and report it to a physician for consideration of a tetanus booster injection. |
| Tissue perfusion alteration r/t orthopedic trauma | Assess and record neurovascular status and promptly report changes or trends to a physician, because orthopedic trauma can result in neurovascular compromise and can cause subsequent loss of the extremity or of normal function of the extremity. Palpate distal pulses and note skin temperature and report changes to a physician immediately. Prepare for surgery or vascular studies as indicted. Assist with the measurement of intracompartmental pressure as indicated. |
| Injury, potential, r/t sensory or motor deficit | Check and record neurovascular status at regular intervals; notify a physician of any changes indicating compromise or possible development of compartment syndrome. |
| Tissue integrity impairment r/t orthopedic trauma | Immobilize and splint any injured extremity as you found it. Move the patient carefully to avoid making the injury worse. Reassess the injured extremity after each move and at intervals. If cool packs are applied, check them and the extremity at regular intervals; do not apply ice to wounds. Keep the wound clean according to institution protocols; administer wound care as ordered; use aseptic technique. Notify the surgical team of a patient for possible replantation; follow protocols for preserving amputated parts for possible replantation. Check casts and splints for tightness that can precipitate compartment syndrome; record abnormal findings and report them to a physician. |

Note.—This is a sample of potential nursing diagnoses. It is not presented as or intended to be a complete care plan for the trauma patient. More complete information can be found in a medical-surgical nursing course and textbook. r/t = related to.

Adapted from Sparks, S. and Taylor, C. M. *Nursing diagnosis reference manual,* Springhouse, PA: Springhouse Corp., 1991, and Chitwood, L., *Ambulatory patient care,* San Diego: Western Schools, 1994.

| Table 9-2 | |
| :--: | :--: |
| **Estimated Blood Loss in Fractures** | |
| **Fracture of** | **Blood Loss (L)** |
| Humerus | 1.0–.2.0 |
| Elbow | 0.5–1.5 |
| Forearm | 0.5–1.0 |
| Pelvis | 1.5–4.5 |
| Hip | 1.5–2.5 |
| Femur | 1.0–2.0 |
| Knee | 1.0–1.5 |
| Tibia | 0.5–1.5 |
| Ankle | 0.5–1.5 |

Stabilize the object, and transport the patient to a hospital immediately.

• Retrieve amputated parts and transport them to the hospital with the patient. Replantation may be possible in some instances, and the parts may be used for grafts in others. Do not suggest to the patient that replantation may restore the severed parts, as this may not be possible (Campbell, 1988).

• In traumatic finger amputations, replantation of the thumb is generally a priority because of the function of this digit. Other amputated fingers are generally replanted on the stump that offers the best hope for maintaining structure and function.

• Apply pressure with a sterile dressing to the stump where amputation occurred, and elevate the stump if the potential for spinal trauma has been ruled out. This will help reduce blood loss and swelling.

• Place amputated parts in a dry container, lay the container on top of plain ice in a clean container, and transport the parts with the patient to the hospital. On the container, mark the time

the parts were amputated and the time they were placed on ice, because these times will help the transplantation team plan care.

• Do not soak amputated parts in any liquid; do not attempt to clean or rinse the parts; do not use dry ice for cooling; do not freeze the parts. Any of these actions could reduce the chance of successful replantation.

• Apply gentle pressure to any orthopedic injury that is bleeding, and await the arrival of an emergency team who can properly splint the fracture and transport the patient. If the patient must be moved, splint the fracture as you found it.

• Be aware that many accidents and assaults involve alcohol and other drugs, so the patient should be assessed for possible chemical addiction, use, or abuse. Refer the patient to the appropriate social agency, support system, counselor, social worker, or chaplain as indicated.

• Do not attempt to straighten a dislocated or fractured knee, hip, shoulder, or elbow. Splint the extremity as you found it, and transport the patient to a hospital for emergency care. See Figures 9-3 to 9-5.

• Pillows make excellent splints for suspected ankle fractures (Figure 9-6). If the ankle fracture is an isolated injury, and no other pathologic changes or indication of spinal trauma is present, elevate the ankle slightly and apply a cool pack to reduce swelling.

• Lay a fractured wrist on a firm surface such as a board to splint and immobilize the fracture, and then elevate the extremity (if the wrist fracture is an isolated injury), apply a cool pack, and transport the patient to the hospital.

• Splint a fractured extremity in the position you found it, as a general rule. Specially trained

**Figure 9-3. Splinting a hip fracture.** Reprinted by permission from Campbell, J. *Basic trauma life support: Advanced prehospital care* (2nd ed.). Englewood Cliffs, NJ: Prentice-Hall, 1988.

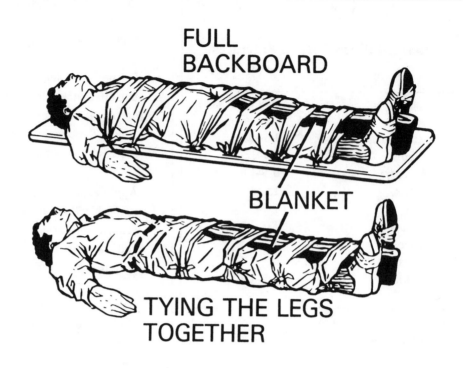

FULL BACKBOARD

BLANKET

TYING THE LEGS TOGETHER

**Figure 9-4. The dislocated shoulder loses its full lateral contour and appears indented under the point of the shoulder.** Reprinted by permission from Kitt, S., & Kaiser, J. *Emergency nursing: A physiologic and clinical perspective.* Philadelphia: Saunders, 1990.

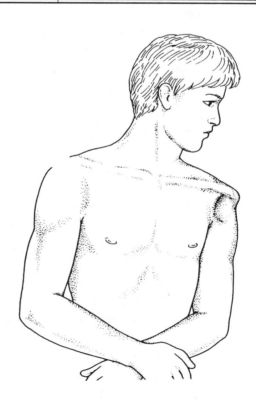

**Figure 9-5. Splinting fractures or dislocations of the elbow.** Reprinted by permission from Campbell, J. *Basic trauma life support: Advanced prehospital care* (2nd ed.). Englewood Cliffs, NJ: Prentice-Hall, 1988.

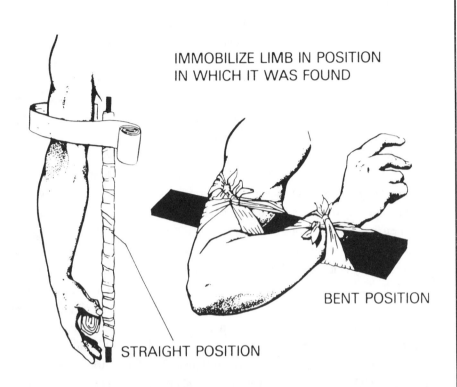

IMMOBILIZE LIMB IN POSITION
IN WHICH IT WAS FOUND

BENT POSITION

STRAIGHT POSITION

**Figure 9-6. Pillow splinting an injured ankle.** Reprinted by permission from Grant, H. D., Murray, R. H., Jr., & Bergeron, J. D. (Eds.). Brady emergency care (5th ed.). Englewood Cliffs, NJ: Prentice-Hall, 1990.

NOTE: Take care not to change the position of the ankle if there is a distal pulse.

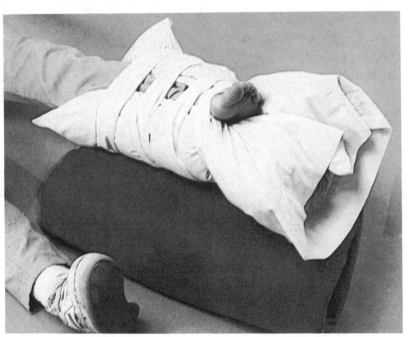

trauma professionals sometimes realign fractured extremities at the trauma scene, but unless you have these skills and special training, do not attempt this. Pillows, broomsticks, newspapers, and cardboard are a few of the items that can be used as splints when the patient must be moved before the arrival of a qualified emergency team. Splint to immobilize the joints above and below the suspected injury. For example, in a suspected elbow dislocation, splint the extremity from the shoulder to the hand.

- Check casts and splints at regular intervals to ensure that swelling has not occurred. Reassess the neurovascular status of the extremity frequently. Compartment syndrome and necrosis of the extremity can develop in a constricting cast or splint.

- Elevate a sprained or strained extremity if spinal injury has been ruled out; apply a cool pack. Both of these measures help reduce swelling and pain. Recheck under the cool pack at intervals to make certain the injured site has not changed and the pack is not too cool. Do not apply ice; this can impair tissue integrity.

- Do not spread open lacerations at the trauma scene to determine if underlying structures are damaged, because this can make the injury worse. Transport the patient to the hospital for evaluation by a physician.

- Immobilize a dislocated hip in the position you found it, and transport the patient immediately to the hospital for further evaluation.

- Administer oxygen to any patient who has multiple fractures or a fracture of a long bone. Increasing the amount of oxygen the patient inspires increases the amount of oxygen available to the body's tissues.

- Splint an extremity to prevent possible injury if you are uncertain whether orthopedic trauma exists.

- Reassess the injured extremity and palpate the distal pulse frequently and each time the patient is moved to make certain that the injury has not been aggravated by the movement.

- Do not apply a tourniquet to a bleeding extremity unless you have special training in this seldom-used technique. Direct pressure is usually more effective.

- Splint one leg with the other (Figure 9-3) and transport the patient to the hospital if you suspect a hip fracture. An elderly woman with a hip fracture may not complain of pain; do not allow this to lull you into the impression that the injury does not exist. Pain from a hip fracture may also be referred to the knee or pelvis, making it difficult to differentiate between a pelvic fracture and a hip fracture.

- Do not allow the patient to eat or drink until he or she is examined by an orthopedic surgeon. Immediate surgical intervention may be indicated, and oral intake increases the risk of fatal aspiration during the perioperative period.

- Offer explanations and reassurances to the patient as you work even if he or she appears unconscious. Hearing may be present, and high levels of anxiety accompany accidents and assaults.

- Reassure the patient that everything possible is being done. Orthopedic injuries with obvious deformities of an extremity distress patients.

# SUMMARY

Although simple fractures are seldom life threatening, some orthopedic injuries, such as a fractured pelvis or femur, can cause rapid blood loss and death. Other injuries, such as hip or knee dislocations, can result in loss of the limb or its function. The nurse's actions at the trauma scene play an integral role in the outcome of and recovery from orthopedic trauma.

# CRITICAL CONCEPTS

- Assess and stabilize the airway, breathing, and circulation before evaluating orthopedic trauma. Most orthopedic trauma does not threaten the patient's life.

- Palpate distal pulses, evaluate skin temperature, and check sensation frequently in an injured extremity and each time the patient is moved or the extremity is repositioned.

- Be aware that bilateral femoral fractures or a pelvic fracture can cause life-threatening hemorrhage and death.

- A dislocated hip or knee is a serious orthopedic emergency. The blood and nerve supply to the extremity may be impaired; permanent disability can result, or amputation of the extremity may be necessary.

- Retrieve amputated body parts and transport the parts to the hospital with the patient.

# GLOSSARY

**Compartment syndrome:** An increase in pressure within a fascial compartment; can result in tissue necrosis or loss of the extremity.

**Ligament:** Tough fibrous tissue that connects one bone to another.

**Replantation:** The surgical reattachment of amputated body parts, usually fingers or toes. Success rates vary.

**Sprain:** Partial tearing of a ligament, commonly due to a twisting motion.

**Tendon:** Fibrous tissue that connects a muscle to a bone.

# EXAM QUESTIONS

## Chapter 9

### Questions 42 - 46

42. An arteriogram is usually indicated in which of the following type of orthopedic trauma?

    a. Fracture of the radius
    b. Impalement of the tibia
    c. Shoulder separation
    d. Knee dislocation

43. Which of the following is a common potential nursing diagnosis for a patient with orthopedic trauma?

    a. Thermal regulation, ineffective
    b. Injury, potential
    c. Grieving, dysfunction
    d. Cardiac output, decreased

44. You are hiking in a park when you find another hiker who has fallen. Her left lower extremity has an obvious deformity. You must move her because a severe storm is coming, and you have no means of communication. Which of the following should you do before transporting her?

    a. Return the affected leg to proper alignment.
    b. Splint the extremity the way you found it.
    c. Apply an ice pack to her left hip.
    d. Straighten the leg and secure it with parallel sticks.

45. Compression from casts or splints can lead to which of the following?

    a. Adult respiratory distress syndrome
    b. Shock
    c. Fat embolism
    d. Compartment syndrome

46. Life-threatening hemorrhage may develop after fracture of which of the following?

    a. Femur
    b. Fibula
    c. Radius
    d. Elbow

# CHAPTER 10

# BURNS

## CHAPTER OBJECTIVE

After completing this chapter, the reader should be able to assess a burn patient, plan initial intervention, and transport the patient to the appropriate facility.

## LEARNING OBJECTIVES

After studying this chapter, the reader should be able to

1. Recognize signs and symptoms of burns.

2. Select methods to stabilize a burn patient.

3. Estimate the percentage of body surface area damaged by a burn.

4. Recognize special concerns in managing patients with burns.

5. Select common nursing diagnoses and interventions for burn patients.

## INTRODUCTION

Two million Americans are burned each year; 12,000 of these will die from their injuries (Campbell, 1988). Fires are the cause of most burn-related deaths, and scald injuries are the most common type of burn. The most common cause of death in the first 48 hr after a burn is respiratory complications; after that, the most common cause is sepsis (Sheehy & Jimmerson, 1994).

Burns often accompany other injuries. Disfigurement is common after serious burns, and long-term treatment and rehabilitation are often necessary. Because nursing care at the scene of the burn injury can shape the patient's future, knowledge of burn care is an essential basic trauma nursing skill. The first tasks are to remove the patient from the source of the injury and stop the burn process. Once the patient is removed from the source of the burn and is in a safe area, assessment, interventions, and transport can take place. The goal is to stabilize and safely transport the patient to an appropriate facility for treatment. Even patients who have major burns do not usually die within the first minutes or hours after injury, so burns that compromise the airway are often the most time-limited burn emergency you will encounter. One exception is electrical burns that can disrupt or halt cardiac activity and cause cardiopulmonary arrest.

This chapter reviews normal anatomy and physiology of the skin and the pathologic changes associated with common burns. It also discusses assessment and

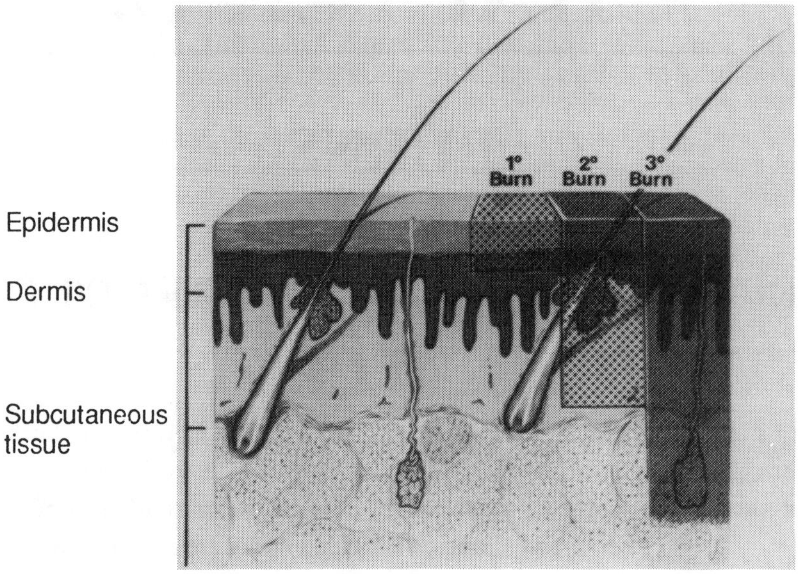

**Figure 10-1. Cross-sectional view of the skin.** Reprinted by permission from Campbell, J. *Basic trauma life support: Advanced prehospital care* (2nd ed.). Englewood Cliffs, NJ: Prentice-Hall, 1988, p. 211.

common types of burns and presents potential nursing diagnoses and interventions for burn patients.

# BASIC ANATOMY AND PHYSIOLOGY OF THE SKIN

As the body's covering, the skin is the largest organ in the body and is essential to life. The skin does the following:

- Protects the body against invasive organisms.

- Holds in body fluids.

- Retains and releases heat.

- Functions in maintenance of fluid and electrolyte balance.

- Serves as a sensory agent.

Knowledge of the basic structure and function of the skin is essential to assessment and management of burn patients. The skin that covers the subcutaneous tissue has two layers (Figure 10-1).

## Epidermis

The outer thin layer of skin that you can see and touch is called the epidermis. It is thickest in the skin covering the back and thinnest in the eyelids. Burns that injure the epidermis are referred to as first-degree burns.

## Dermis

Under the epidermis is the dermis, a mass of connective tissue composed of blood vessels, nerve endings, and hair follicles. Burns that injure both the epidermis and the dermis are referred to as second-degree or partial-thickness burns.

## Subcutaneous Tissue

Covered by the two layers of the skin, the subcutaneous tissue contains fatty tissues and blood vessels. Burns that damage tissue down to this level are called third-degree or full-thickness burns.

# MECHANISM OF INJURY

The mechanism of injury in burns is the application of heat, light, or electricity to the skin that subsequently disrupts the continuity and integrity of the skin. The destruction of skin and tissue that occurs may be minor or life threatening. Motor vehicle accidents and industrial or residential accidents may result in burns. Some sources of burns discussed in this chapter include sources of thermal injuries (flame, steam, hot liquids, and hot objects), chemicals, and electricity. In general, the longer the patient is in contact with the injuring agent, the worse the burn will be. Also affecting the extent and degree of resulting trauma are the type and temperature of the injuring agent. Patients also may have sustained other trauma in the accident that caused the burn; these other injuries may complicate a patient's status.

Burns can cause massive shifts of fluid within the body. Capillary permeability is altered, so fluid leaks from the vasculature into extravascular space, resulting in edema. This causes a functional hypovolemic state; shock may develop rapidly. Hypotension and shock can occur even when no blood loss is visible. Thermal injuries also can cause massive edema and occlusion of the airway.

## Thermal Burns

Although the skin protects the body from some changes in the temperature of the environment, high temperatures applied to the skin can sear through the skin and injure tissue even below the skin. Common causes of thermal burns include the following:

- **Flame exposure:** Burn injuries from flames occur when the patient's clothing or immediate environment ignites. Clothing and jewelry can melt and adhere to the hot skin. Injuries due to heat and smoke inhalation may be associated with a flame burn.

- **Contact exposure:** Boiling water gives off vapor as steam; serious burns can result from contact with the steam. Other contact burns can occur when a hot object meets or adheres to the skin. An example is spilling hot tar on the skin or picking up a hot pan.

- **Heat and smoke inhalation injury:** Injuries due to heat and smoke inhalation are often associated with flame injury. Inhaled hot air, smoke, and carbon can damage air passages, especially if a person is confined in an enclosed area during the accident.

## Chemical Burns

When caustic chemicals contact the skin or eyes, chemical injuries that destroy skin and tissue can occur. The chemical disrupts the body tissues until it is either expended or removed (Campbell, 1988).

## Electrical Burns

When power in the form of electricity races through the body, the major damage is often to the heart and muscles. Frequently, the patient has a burn on the body at the site where the electricity entered and another burn at the site where the electricity exited. These entry and exit wounds may appear minor, but the passage of electrical current through the body can cause cardiac or respiratory arrest, seizures, and violent muscle contractions that fracture bones.

# ASSESSMENT OF BURN PATIENTS

The assessment of any patient with a burn should follow the standard ABC plan from chapter 2. Evaluate the airway, breathing, and circulation. Be aware that other injuries are often associated with burns, such as chest trauma from a blast or explosion.

A hazard in assessing and managing burn patients is removing the patient from the source of the burn. Therefore, assessment begins with observation of the accident scene to determine if it is safe to approach the patient. Do not go to the patient until you are sure that your own safety is not compromised. When both you and the patient are in a safe place, take steps to stop the burn process. Then evaluate the airway, breathing, and circulation and assess the patient.

Burns are generally categorized as first-degree, second-degree, and third-degree; you may also see burns classified as partial-thickness and full-thickness. The extent of the body surface area burned is determined by the rule of nines. Figure 10-2 provides a guide to the predicted outcome for a burn patient, a chart depicting the rule of nines, and a summary of the characteristics of burns.

## Classification of Burns

Mortality and morbidity from burns are influenced by the patient's age, sex, and health before the accident in addition to the extent and depth of the burns and other associated injuries. The depth or degree of the burn is evaluated as follows:

- **First-degree burns:** When the epidermis or outermost layer of skin is injured, a first-degree burn results. The inflammatory response of the body is indicated by the reddened skin in the injured area. Injured nerve endings cause intense pain. Healing takes place in a few days in most cases. Simple sunburns are an example of first-degree burns.

- **Second-degree burns:** When both the epidermis and the dermis are injured, a second-degree burn exists. Pain is intense because of damage to nerves and tissue; the area is red and sometimes swollen. Blisters form in reaction to the injury, and weeping wounds may be present. Healing can take several weeks, depending on the depth of the burn. A burn from a hot liquid can cause a second-degree burn.

- **Third-degree or full-thickness burns:** Third-degree or full-thickness burns are dramatic and disfiguring, but paradoxically they cause no pain, because the nerve endings in the skin have been obliterated; both the epidermis and dermis are destroyed. The remaining tissue may appear charred or look white and dry. Because the skin is destroyed, skin grafts will be required.

## Rule of Nines

The rule of nines determines the extent of a burn. A standardized uniform method for the assessment of burn patients, the rule of nines allows the examiner to determine quickly and accurately the amount of body surface damaged by the burn. This is a general guideline, and burn professionals may modify the rule of nines for children, patients who are pregnant, and certain other patients. In general, the following percentages are used:

- Each upper extremity is counted as 9%; each lower extremity is counted as 18%.

- The torso is counted as 18% for the front and 18% for the back.

- The genitals and perineum count as 1%.

## Abbreviated Burn Severity Index*

The Abbreviated Burn Severity Index (ABSI) is a five-variable scale that may be used as a quick reference for evaluation of burn injury severity. The five variables are patient sex, age, presence of inhalation injury, presence of full-thickness burn, and percentage total body surface area burned. The score, which may be calculated in less than one minute, is derived by summation of the coded values for each of the five variables. The total score may then be related to severity of burn injury and to probability of survival. An ABSI score of six or greater, high-voltage electrical burns, burns associated with other major injuries, or full-thickness burns to the face, axillae, joints, hands, feet, or genitalia should be considered for treatment in a hospital with special expertise in burn care. Aids for evaluation of depth of burn and percentage of total body surface area burned are located on the back of this card.

| Sex | Female | 1 |
|---|---|---|
| | Male | 0 |
| Age | 0-20 Years | 1 |
| | 21-40 Years | 2 |
| | 41-60 Years | 3 |
| | 61-80 Years | 4 |
| | ≥81 Years | 5 |
| **Inhalation Injury Present** | | 1 |
| **Full-Thickness Burn** | | 1 |
| Total Body Surface Area Burned | 1%- 10% | 1 |
| | 11%- 20% | 2 |
| | 21%- 30% | 3 |
| | 31%- 40% | 4 |
| | 41%- 50% | 5 |
| | 51%- 60% | 6 |
| | 61%- 70% | 7 |
| | 71%- 80% | 8 |
| | 81%- 90% | 9 |
| | 91%-100% | 10 |

### Total Burn Score

| Score | Probability of Survival | Score | Probability of Survival |
|---|---|---|---|
| **2-3** | ≥99% | **8-9** | 50-70% |
| **4-5** | 98% | **10-11** | 20-40% |
| **6-7** | 80-90% | **≥12** | ≤10% |

*Adapted from Edlich RF, Rodeheaver GT, Halfacre SE, Tobiasen JA, Boyd DR. Systems conceptualization of burn care on a regional basis. *Topics in Emergency Medicine 3(3):7-15. 1961*

## Clinical Diagnosis of Depth of Burn Injury*

| | Full thickness | Deep partial thickness | Superficial partial thickness |
|---|---|---|---|
| **Appearance** | Brown with thrombosed veins | White | Pink with blisters |
| **Hair** | Absent | Absent | Present |
| **Biomechanical properties** | Depressed and leathery | Elevated soft and pliable | Elevated, soft, and pliable |
| **Sensation** | None | Pressure | Light touch, pinprick, and pressure |
| **Pain** | Painless | Painful | Exquisitely painful |

*Adapted from Tobiasen JM, Hiebert JM, Sacco WJ, Edlich RF. Burn injury severity scoring systems. *Current Concepts in Trauma Care 4(1)* 5-8. 1981

## Percentage of Total Body Surface Area Burned

**Rule of Nines†**

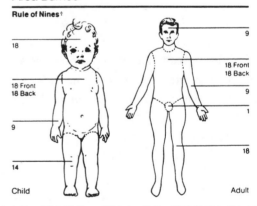

† Adapted from Edlich RF, Haynes BW, Larkam N, Allen MS, Ruffin W Jr., Hiebert JM, Edgerton MT: Emergency department treatment, triage and transfer protocols for the burn patient. *Journal of American College of Emergency Physicians 7(4):* 152-158. 1978

**Figure 10-2. Characterization of burns and their prognosis.** Reprinted by permission from Edlich, R. F., Glassberg, H. H., and Tobiasen, J. A. *Current Concepts in Trauma Care,* 7(1), 20, 1984.

- For small burns, many examiners use the size of the patient's hand as an estimate of 1% of the patient's body surface area.

## Burns in Children

When assessing a child who has burns or scald injuries, view both the injury and the trauma scene with suspicion unless it is obvious that the burns were indeed incurred in a fire or automobile or other accident. Burns in children may be associated with child abuse. If you suspect that a child's injuries may have been inflicted intentionally, have a second rescuer notify the police and ask them to investigate. See chapter 16 for more on trauma in children and issues of child abuse.

# COMMON BURN TRAUMA

### Flame Injuries

Flame injuries are common in house fires and may cause minor to mortal wounds. Burn injuries to the head and neck may compromise the airway because of massive tissue edema.

### Electrical Burns

Electrical burns can occur when an object held by a person contacts live wires, when lightning strikes the person, or even when a car topples a utility pole and power lines drape the vehicle. The primary concern is the patient's heart, which may be stopped or converted into life-threatening dysrhythmias by the electrical current. In addition, powerful muscle contractions can occur when the current strikes the body, and bones may be fractured. The electrical current also may initiate seizures.

### Chemical Burns

Chemical burns damage by contact with the skin. Management involves removing the chemical from contact with the patient, removing the patient from the scene, and flushing the chemical from the skin.

### Inhalation Injury

Air passages also can be injured by heat, smoke, or toxic fumes whenever a person's skin is burned by heat or chemicals. Assume that any patient who has a burn has sustained an inhalation injury until it is proved otherwise. Common inhalation injuries include the following:

- **Carbon monoxide poisoning:** Carbon monoxide is emitted in automobile exhaust and from some space heaters and is found in smoke from fires and even cigarettes; it can poison both patient and rescuer. The body's red blood cells have a greater affinity for carbon monoxide than for oxygen, so the oxygen content of the patient's blood drops, causing hypoxia as the oxygen in the blood is replaced with carbon monoxide. Death occurs eventually if the patient is not removed from the source of the carbon monoxide. Patients will not appear cyanotic despite the hypoxia; in fact, they may appear quite pink, and the blood will appear red. If conscious, the patient often will complain of a headache and may be confused. Because carbon monoxide is odorless, you will not even be aware of its presence.

- **Smoke inhalation:** When toxic fumes or vapors are inhaled, damage to the cells of the air passages occurs. Air exchange may be impaired. Suspect smoke inhalation injury in any burn patient who has burnt nares or soot in the mouth.

- **Heat inhalation:** A person who is trapped in a fire may sustain damage to the upper part of the airway from high temperatures; swelling of the airway and obstruction of air flow may occur.

This swelling may develop slowly. Suspect heat inhalation injury in any burn patient who has swollen lips, hoarseness, or respiratory distress. The airway, irritated by the heat injury, is prone to sudden closure from laryngospasm.

# NURSING STRATEGIES FOR BURN PATIENTS

Serious burns are a major injury and a devastating tragedy in a patient's life, and the initial intervention can have a critical impact on the patient's future. The challenges are to remove the patient from the source of the burn injury, stop the burn process, protect the patient from further injury, and stabilize and maintain his or her vital functions until arrival at an appropriate medical facility.

Table 10-1 gives potential nursing diagnoses and interventions for the care of burn patients. The following strategies may also be helpful. It is presumed with each that airway, breathing, and circulation are already established. Your interventions should be within the scope of your professional license; commensurate with your skills and training; consistent with your state's nurse practice act; and when performed in a health care institution, adherent to that facility's standards of practice. Before attempting to intervene for a burn patient, review the guidelines presented in Table 10-2.

- Approach with caution any patient who may have a chemical burn, because the presence of a chemical on the patient may not be obvious. Use protective clothing and gloves if at all possible when touching the patient.

- Do not apply butter or ointment to burns.

- Cool the patient immediately with cool water. This can reduce or halt the progression of thermal burns, because damage to the skin continues for a brief period even after the patient is removed from the source of the heat. Do not cool the patient for more than a few minutes; hypothermia and changes in the vital signs can result.

- Protect wounds and prevent loss of body warmth after cooling by covering the patient with a clean, preferably sterile, sheet and keeping the patient warm.

- Be aware that shock due to a burn usually develops slowly. The patient's golden hour is best spent getting him or her to the hospital instead of remaining at the trauma scene and attempting to secure intravenous access in burned extremities. The exceptions are patients who have other traumatic injuries or who have received an electrical burn. In these cases, cardiac dysrhythmias are common, and intravenous access facilitates the administration of resuscitative medications. Administer intravenous fluids for hypovolemic shock from other injuries if necessary.

- Flood the areas of a chemical burn with copious volumes of water immediately, and continue doing so for as long as possible before transporting the patient. Do not attempt to neutralize the first chemical by applying another chemical unless you have special training and skills in this, because it may only make the injury worse. Give the patient oxygen (preferably humidified) by mask during transport, because toxic fumes may have injured the patient's air passages. See chapter 12 for management of chemical burns to the eyes. Most states have poison control centers that may be a resource for specific antidotes.

- Move any patient who may have carbon monoxide poisoning to a place of safety, administer high concentrations of oxygen, and transport the patient to the hospital.

**Table 10-1**
**Potential Nursing Diagnoses and Interventions for Burn Patients**

| Diagnosis | Interventions |
|---|---|
| Injury, potential, r/t burn process | Stop the burn process to prevent further injury. Remove the source of injury or remove the patient from the scene of injury when possible. Remove the patient's clothes and jewelry, then cool and protect the patient by covering him or her with wet, cool (clean or preferably sterile) sheets. Do not apply ice, because that could make the injury worse. Do not overcool the patient, because that could result in hypothermia. |
| Airway clearance, ineffective, r/t edema | Maintain a patent airway; edema can rapidly occlude the airway in a burn patient. Monitor respiratory status vigilantly. Be prepared for rapid deterioration and potential need for intubation or surgical airway. Administer humidified oxygen until a physician orders its discontinuance. |
| Tissue perfusion impairment r/t fluid shifts due to thermal injury | Monitor vital signs, intake, and output carefully, and report changes or trends. Administer fluids as ordered. Monitor arterial blood gases and carbon monoxide levels as ordered. Administer high concentration of humidified oxygen to increase oxygen delivery to cells. Weigh patient as ordered. |
| Body image disturbance r/t burn | Be aware that a burn patient's appearance and functional status may be altered forever by the burn. Burn patients are generally alert and may receive unintended feedback about their appearance (e.g., from rescuers and health care providers) before they get a chance to see themselves, so limit bedside conversations and facial expressions (Strange, 1987) that could distress the patient or distort his or her self-image. |
| Fluid volume deficit, potential, r/t fluid shifts due to burn | Assess the patient for signs of hypovolemia, such as hypotension and tachycardia; note that burn patients may appear edematous and may show no evidence of blood loss. Secure intravenous access and administer fluids as ordered. Monitor vital signs frequently and report changes or trends immediately. Keep accurate records of amounts and types of infusions. Monitor urine output. |
| Hypothermia r/t stopping the burn process and injury to skin | Do not overcool the patient when stopping the burn process. Never apply ice to significant burns because it will cause vasoconstriction and further reduce blood supply to the injured area. Hypothermia can cause vital organ dysfunction and fluid shifts and make resuscitation more difficult. |
| Infection, potential, r/t burn injury to skin | Use sterile equipment and aseptic technique to avoid introducing bacteria to the patient's areas of injury. Practice strict asepsis. Isolate the patient protectively when indicated. Anticipate administration of a tetanus booster injection. Notify physician of changes in white blood count or vital signs; monitor results of cultures and notify physician promptly. |

Note.—This is a sample of potential nursing diagnoses. It is not presented as or intended to be a complete care plan for the trauma patient. More complete information can be found in a medical-surgical nursing course and textbook. r/t = related to.
Adapted from Sparks, S. and Taylor, C. M. *Nursing diagnosis reference manual,* Springhouse, PA: Springhouse Corp., 1991, and Chitwood, L., *Ambulatory patient care,* San Diego: Western Schools, 1994.

## Table 10-2
## Guidelines for Intervention in Burn Trauma

- Do not compromise your own safety when it comes to rescuing a burn patient. As noted by Grant et al. (1990), "'Heroic' efforts can place you and fellow rescuers in danger and may even delay proper care for the patient."

- If you determine that you can get to the patient safely, but you perceive that a threat may still exist, move the patient from harm as quickly as possible. Do not stop to assess or treat the patient until you are both in a secure location.

- When a building is on fire, there is a point at which everything in the room will spontaneously burst into flame as the temperature suddenly soars over 3,000°F; this "flashover" occurs without warning (Campbell, 1988). Do not get caught in the flashover: Extract your patient from a burning building immediately. Also be alert at motor vehicle accidents and industrial accidents; sudden eruptions of fuel tanks and combustion of vapors can occur.

- Do not attempt to move downed power wires or reach the victim of an electrical shock until the power source has been turned off and removed. Even seemingly harmless tools commonly proposed for use to push away power lines (such as a broom handle) may contain moisture or metal that will transmit the current to you.

- Poisonous substances and vapors may be present in the immediate environment or on the victim's clothing or skin. Proceed with caution even when you cannot see or smell these chemicals.

- Administer humidified oxygen to any patient who may have heat inhalation injury until a physician orders its discontinuance.

- Take the patient's rings off the fingers as soon as possible. Swelling after the burn can be significant; rings can obstruct circulation and may have to be cut off later.

- For any patient with an electrical burn, start electrocardiographic monitoring, secure intravenous access for injection of drugs as necessary, administer oxygen, and transport the patient to a hospital as soon as possible.

- Do not attempt to remove substances already melted onto the skin, such as hot tar. Removal may make the injury worse.

- Monitor burn patients frequently. Their condition may change, especially in burns of the airway that result in swelling and edema.

- Transport the patient to a hospital. All but the most minor burns should be evaluated by a physician.

- Do not allow the patient to eat or drink until he or she is seen by a physician. Immediate surgical intervention may be necessary, and oral intake increases the risk of a fatal aspiration during the perioperative period.

- Offer explanations and reassurances to the patient as you work even if he or she appears to be unconscious. Hearing may be present, and high levels of anxiety accompany accidents and assaults.

- Reassure the patient that everything possible is being done. Burns distress patients and their families, who fear death and disfigurement. The effects of burns can be quite dramatic and frightening.

# SUMMARY

Nursing care at the scene of a burn injury can shape the patient's future. The first tasks are to remove the patient from the source of the injury and stop the burn process. Once the patient is in a safe area, assessment, interventions, and transport can take place. The goal is to stabilize and safely transport the patient to an appropriate facility for treatment.

# CRITICAL CONCEPTS

- Never compromise your own safety to reach a burn victim. Doing so may endanger your life and delay rescue of the original victim.

- Airway compromise or closure may occur rapidly as edema develops in a burn patient.

- Electrical burns may disrupt or halt cardiac activity and cause respiratory arrest.

- The first priority with a burn patient is to stop the burn process.

- Remove clothing and jewelry from burned areas, because they can retain heat and aggravate the burn, but do not attempt to remove anything (e.g., clothing or hot tar) that has already adhered to the skin.

# GLOSSARY

**Burn:** The application of heat, light, or electricity to the skin that subsequently disrupts the continuity and integrity of the skin.

**Dermis:** The layer of connective tissue that lies under the epidermis.

**First-degree burn:** A burn that damages the epidermis or outermost layer of the skin.

**Full-thickness burn:** A burn that extends down through the epidermis and dermis into the subcutaneous tissue.

**Inhalation injury:** Damage to the air passages caused by inhalation of toxic fumes, hot air, or carbon monoxide.

**Second-degree burn:** A burn that damages the epidermis and extends into the dermis.

# EXAM QUESTIONS

## Chapter 10

## Questions 47 - 51

47. Which of the following may develop rapidly in a burn patient who initially appeared stable?

    a. Infection
    b. Airway edema
    c. Hypothermia
    d. Impaired mobility

48. A teenage girl is sniffing gasoline fumes and accidently drops her cigarette into the container. She is burned entirely on the front and back of both legs aid the genitals. Using the rule of nines, you estimate that the percentage of her body surface area that has been burned is:

    a. 49%
    b. 37%
    c. 27%
    d. 18%

49. Hypotension that develops along with edema in a burn patient is most likely caused by:

    a. Inadequate volume replacement
    b. Fluid shifts
    c. Burn eschar constricting the chest
    d. Cardiac failure

50. A common potential nursing diagnosis for a patient with a full-thickness thermal burn is:

    a. Pain
    b. Infection, potential
    c. Self-esteem, chronic low
    d. Noncompliance

51. Treatment of a heat inhalation injury would likely include administration of which of the following?

    a. Cardiotonic agents
    b. Humidified oxygen
    c. Antibiotics
    d. Oxygen-free radicals

# CHAPTER 11

# GENITOURINARY TRAUMA

## CHAPTER OBJECTIVE

After completing this chapter, the reader should be able to differentiate between basic structures and functions of the genitourinary system, recognize common causes of genitourinary trauma, and plan appropriate nursing care for patients with genitourinary trauma.

## LEARNING OBJECTIVES

After studying this chapter, the reader should be able to

1.  List common types of genitourinary trauma.

2.  Indicate special concerns in managing patients who have genitourinary trauma.

3.  Select common potential nursing diagnoses and interventions for patients with genitourinary trauma.

## INTRODUCTION

Because the genitourinary organs are protected by their location in the body, genitourinary trauma, with a few exceptions, is seldom life threatening and often exists as one of many injuries. This chapter reviews normal anatomy and physiology of the genitourinary system and common mechanisms of injury in genitourinary trauma. It also describes common genitourinary trauma, reviews assessment of patients with genitourinary trauma, and presents common potential nursing diagnoses and interventions.

## BASIC ANATOMY AND PHYSIOLOGY OF THE NORMAL GENITOURINARY SYSTEM

The urinary system (Figure 11-1) consists of the two kidneys, the two ureters, the bladder, and the urethra. Urine is produced by the kidneys and flows down the ureters to the bladder, where it is held until it is eliminated from the body via the urethra.

### Kidneys

About 4 in. (10.2 cm) long and 1 in. (2.5 cm) thick, the kidneys are located just above the level of the waist and behind the peritoneum. Blood flows to the kidneys from the renal arteries that branch off the aorta. The renal veins return the blood to the inferior vena cava, where it circulates to the heart. The kidneys perform the vital, life-saving functions of filtering wastes from the blood, maintaining acid-base balance, and regulating sodium and water balance in the body. As vital organs, the kidneys receive preferential treatment by the body during shock: Blood is diverted from other organs to maintain perfusion of the kidneys, the heart, and the brain. The kidneys' position in the abdomen offers substantial protection against trauma. However, blunt or penetrating trauma may disrupt, fracture, or lacerate a kidney and cause irreversible damage and life-threatening blood loss. A single kidney easily can manage the body's waste removal needs if the other kidney is lost.

## Ureters

Urine produced by each kidney is propelled down to the bladder by the rhythmic contractions of the ureters. These 12-in. (30.5 cm) tubular muscular structures can withstand blunt trauma well but may be injured in penetrating trauma.

## Bladder

A muscular hollow sac, the bladder lies in a protected site behind the symphysis pubis. Two openings in the bladder receive urine from the ureters; a third empties urine into the urethra. Collection, storage, and expulsion of urine are the bladder's functions. Bladder capacity is 250–500 ml in adults.

## Urethra

The urethra is the final structure in the urinary system. In adult males, the urethra is about 8 in. (20.3 cm) long, runs through the penis, and serves as a passage for both urine and reproductive fluids. In females, the urethra is shorter (about 1.5 in. [3.8 cm]) and exits near the opening to the vagina.

# MECHANISM OF INJURY

Projectiles are responsible for most penetrating genitourinary trauma. The projectile may be a knife or a missile, such as a bullet. Penetrating trauma may result in impalement, laceration, rupture, or puncture of the genitourinary organs, all of which may cause loss of both structure and function. The ureters are

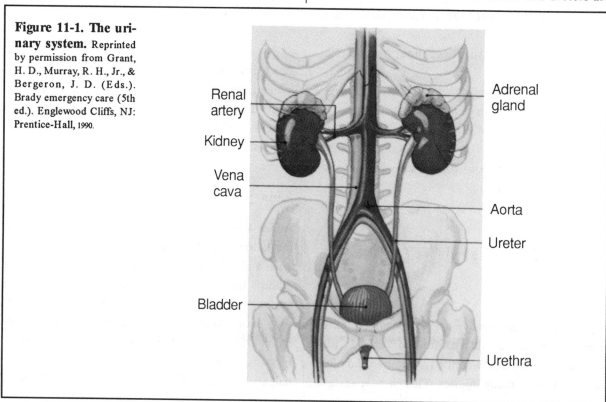

**Figure 11-1. The urinary system.** Reprinted by permission from Grant, H. D., Murray, R. H., Jr., & Bergeron, J. D. (Eds.). Brady emergency care (5th ed.). Englewood Cliffs, NJ: Prentice-Hall, 1990.

Renal artery

Kidney

Vena cava

Bladder

Adrenal gland

Aorta

Ureter

Urethra

damaged more often by penetrating trauma than by blunt trauma. Penetrating injury to the urinary system is extremely common in gunshot wounds of the upper part of the abdomen and stab wounds of the flank (Guerriero, 1984). Injuries to the genitalia may occur in an industrial setting as a result of clothing being caught in fast-moving machinery, and burns may result in severe disfigurement and loss of function of this portion of the body.

Blunt trauma also may damage any of the genitourinary structures, although the external genitalia and urinary system are well protected from trauma: the bladder by the solid symphysis pubis and the kidneys and ureters by padding in the torso from fat, muscles, ribs, and the spine. Nevertheless, genitourinary trauma may occur from rapid deceleration in a motor vehicle accident, during a fall, or when an object such as a bat or a fist strikes the abdomen or flank or external genitalia. Blunt trauma of force sufficient to fracture the pelvis often is associated with damage to the bladder and urethra. Blunt trauma to the back and flank may be associated with kidney damage, although this often consists of a simple renal contusion that heals itself. Severe blunt trauma, however, may fracture the kidney.

# ASSESSMENT OF PATIENTS WITH GENITOURINARY TRAUMA

For any patient with an injury to the genitourinary system, follow the standard ABC assessment plan from chapter 2. Evaluate the airway, breathing, and circulation, because genitourinary trauma seldom exists as the sole injury. Direct attention first to injuries that threaten life or limb; once the airway and circu-

lation are established, and bleeding is controlled, go back to evaluate the genitourinary trauma.

Assessment proceeds as with any patient. Observe the scene of the accident or injury and elicit a history of the injury while assessing the patient. In addition to obtaining an accurate history and posing the routine questions asked of every trauma patient, be especially careful to protect the patient's dignity and privacy. Shield the patient from bystanders' view when removing the patient's clothing to evaluate genitourinary trauma. Cover the patient again as soon as you have completed your assessment.

Genitourinary injuries may go undetected until radiologic studies are done. A rectal examination and palpation of the prostate in male patients are often the first steps to confirming genitourinary trauma. Do not let the absence of external signs of injury lull you into a false sense of security. Internal hemorrhage from a fractured kidney can be substantial, and a ruptured bladder is a serious injury. Although mortality associated with urologic trauma is low, morbidity is high (Guerriero, 1984), so early detection and intervention often are critical to the outcome.

Because the injuries are often internal, it is difficult to determine with a physical examination if trauma to the genitourinary system exists. Nevertheless, genitourinary trauma is likely if any of the following occurs:

- The patient complains of pain in the pelvic or suprapubic region.

- The external genital structures have an obvious deformity.

- The urine is bloody.

- The patient cannot void despite apparently adequate fluid replacement.

- Blood is present at the meatus. In male patients, also check for the presence of semen at the meatus. This can be due to prostatic damage from a pelvic fracture.

- Swelling or bruising of the scrotum or over the flank is present.

- The patient sustained blunt or penetrating abdominal trauma.

# COMMON GENITOURINARY INJURIES

## Ruptured Bladder

A full bladder can be ruptured by blunt or penetrating trauma. When empty, the bladder lies low in the pelvis and seldom ruptures. Blunt trauma to the anterior part of the body, such as a blow from the steering wheel of a car or compression by the seat belt, also may rupture the bladder. Evidence of penetrating trauma in the suprapubic region (above the pubic bone) or signs of a fractured pelvis suggest a ruptured bladder. Figures 11-2 and 11-3 depict examples of bladder trauma. A ruptured bladder requires surgical intervention.

## Urethral Disruption

Pelvic fractures (Figure 11-4) sometimes interrupt or tear the urethra from the bladder, especially when blunt trauma from the front of the patient forces the pubis backward into the urethra. Females seldom sustain urethral injuries; such injuries are more common in males because of the increased length of the urethra and its anatomic position in males. The first priority should be stabilization of the pelvic fracture and any other life- or limb-threatening injuries. In general, wait until urethral damage has been ruled

out before attempting to catheterize a trauma patient who has a pelvic fracture or genital injury. Catheterization may result in further damage to a traumatized urethra. Surgical intervention is necessary for urethral disruption, although it often is postponed until other injuries are treated.

## Major Renal Trauma

Fractured or lacerated kidneys and injuries to the renal pelvis can produce life-threatening internal hemorrhage, although the injury is not often obvious. However, suspect major renal trauma whenever a patient sustains major blunt or penetrating abdominal trauma, and anticipate hypovolemic shock from hemorrhage. Figure 11-5 is a schematic representation of the steps for managing blunt renal trauma. See chapter 8 for more on management of abdominal trauma.

## Ureteral Injury

The ureters seldom are injured by blunt trauma. Injury most often is caused by a missile or foreign object that penetrates the abdominal cavity. Signs of ureteral trauma usually are noted only on radiologic examinations in the hospital. Surgical repair is indicated after more serious injuries have been stabilized.

## Lacerations and Contusions of the External Genitalia

Blunt trauma to the external genitalia causes contusions and subsequent pain. The penis may be lacerated or severed. Figures 11-6 and 11-7 are guidelines for the care of other genital injuries.

**Figure 11-2. Bladder rupture caused by blunt trauma.** Reprinted by permission from Guerriero, W. G., and Devine, C. J., Jr. *Urologic injuries.* E. Norwalk, CT: Appleton-Century-Crofts, 1984.

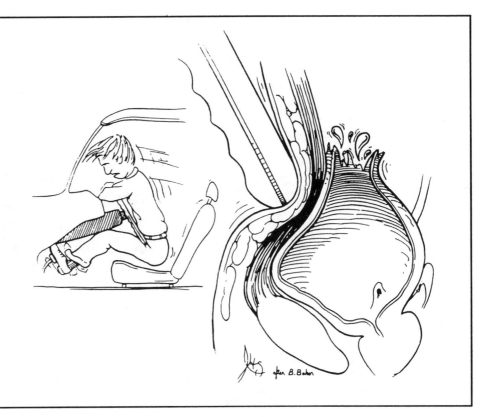

**Figure 11-3. Mechanisms of extraperitoneal bladder rupture. A. Penetration of bladder with spicule of bone with pelvic fracture. B. Stab wound. C. Gunshot wound to bladder.** Reprinted by permission from Guerriero, W. G., and Devine, C. J., Jr. *Urologic injuries.* E. Norwalk, CT: Appleton-Century-Crofts, 1984.

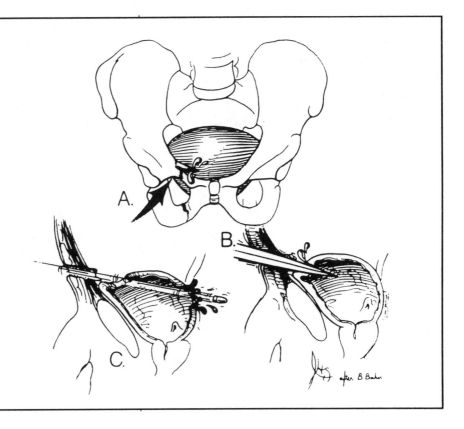

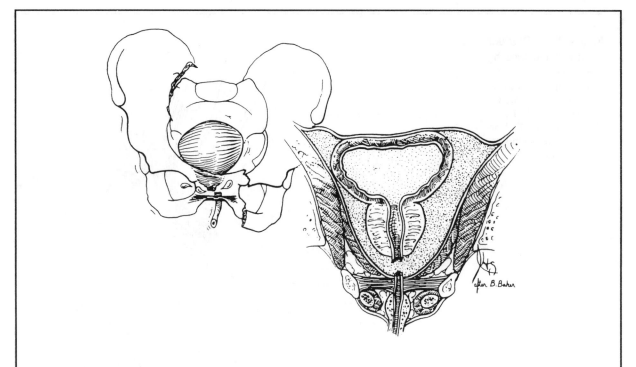

**Figure 11-4. Urethral disruption caused by pelvic fracture.** Reprinted by permission from Guerriero, W. G., and Devine, C. J. Jr. *Urologic injuries.* E. Norwalk, CT: Appleton-Century-Crofts, 1984.

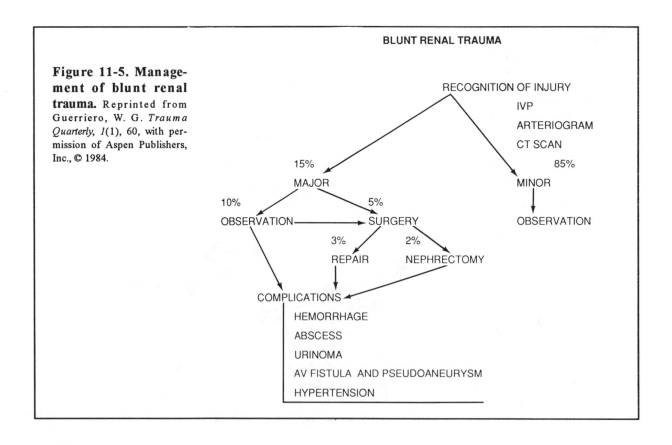

**Figure 11-5. Management of blunt renal trauma.** Reprinted from Guerriero, W. G. *Trauma Quarterly, 1*(1), 60, with permission of Aspen Publishers, Inc., © 1984.

BLUNT RENAL TRAUMA

RECOGNITION OF INJURY

IVP

ARTERIOGRAM

CT SCAN

15%                    85%

MAJOR                  MINOR

10%          5%

OBSERVATION ────→ SURGERY          OBSERVATION

        3%        2%

      REPAIR      NEPHRECTOMY

COMPLICATIONS

HEMORRHAGE

ABSCESS

URINOMA

AV FISTULA  AND PSEUDOANEURYSM

HYPERTENSION

**MALE REPRODUCTIVE SYSTEM**

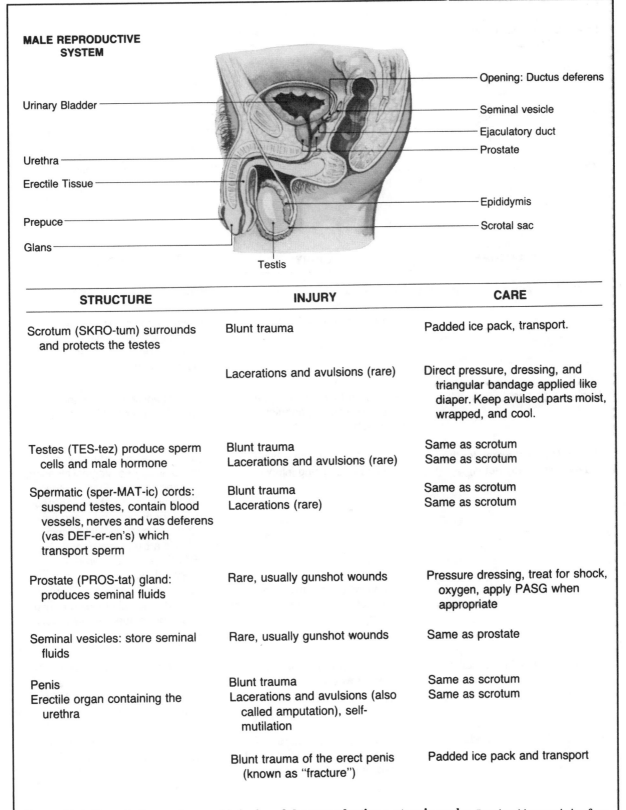

| STRUCTURE | INJURY | CARE |
|---|---|---|
| Scrotum (SKRO-tum) surrounds and protects the testes | Blunt trauma | Padded ice pack, transport. |
| | Lacerations and avulsions (rare) | Direct pressure, dressing, and triangular bandage applied like diaper. Keep avulsed parts moist, wrapped, and cool. |
| Testes (TES-tez) produce sperm cells and male hormone | Blunt trauma<br>Lacerations and avulsions (rare) | Same as scrotum<br>Same as scrotum |
| Spermatic (sper-MAT-ic) cords: suspend testes, contain blood vessels, nerves and vas deferens (vas DEF-er-en's) which transport sperm | Blunt trauma<br>Lacerations (rare) | Same as scrotum<br>Same as scrotum |
| Prostate (PROS-tat) gland: produces seminal fluids | Rare, usually gunshot wounds | Pressure dressing, treat for shock, oxygen, apply PASG when appropriate |
| Seminal vesicles: store seminal fluids | Rare, usually gunshot wounds | Same as prostate |
| Penis<br>Erectile organ containing the urethra | Blunt trauma<br>Lacerations and avulsions (also called amputation), self-mutilation | Same as scrotum<br>Same as scrotum |
| | Blunt trauma of the erect penis (known as "fracture") | Padded ice pack and transport |

**Figure 11-6. Description and care of injuries of the reproductive system in males.** Reprinted by permission from Grant, H. D., Murray, R. H., Jr., & Bergeron, J. D. (Eds.). *Brady emergency care* (5th ed.). Englewood Cliffs, NJ: Prentice-Hall, 1990, p. 364.

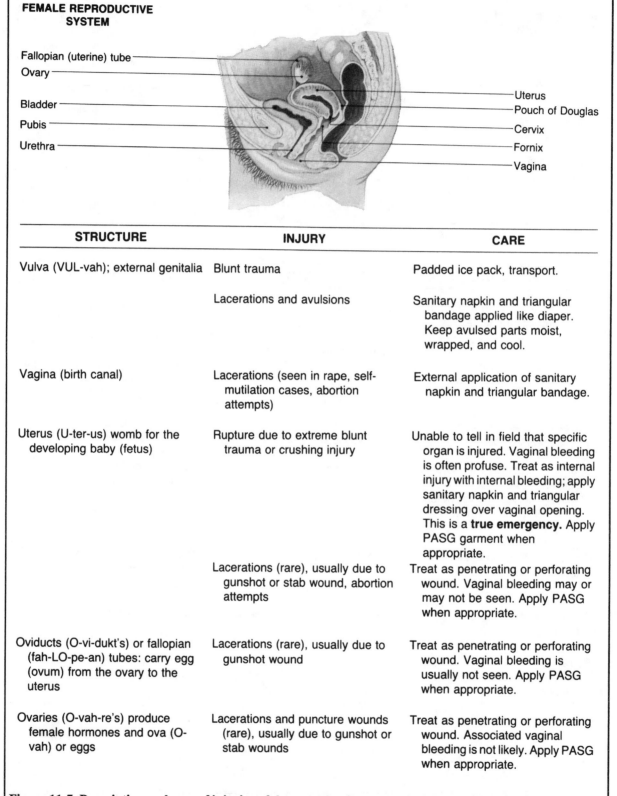

**FEMALE REPRODUCTIVE SYSTEM**

Fallopian (uterine) tube
Ovary

Bladder
Pubis
Urethra

Uterus
Pouch of Douglas
Cervix
Fornix
Vagina

| STRUCTURE | INJURY | CARE |
|---|---|---|
| Vulva (VUL-vah); external genitalia | Blunt trauma | Padded ice pack, transport. |
| | Lacerations and avulsions | Sanitary napkin and triangular bandage applied like diaper. Keep avulsed parts moist, wrapped, and cool. |
| Vagina (birth canal) | Lacerations (seen in rape, self-mutilation cases, abortion attempts) | External application of sanitary napkin and triangular bandage. |
| Uterus (U-ter-us) womb for the developing baby (fetus) | Rupture due to extreme blunt trauma or crushing injury | Unable to tell in field that specific organ is injured. Vaginal bleeding is often profuse. Treat as internal injury with internal bleeding; apply sanitary napkin and triangular dressing over vaginal opening. This is a **true emergency.** Apply PASG garment when appropriate. |
| | Lacerations (rare), usually due to gunshot or stab wound, abortion attempts | Treat as penetrating or perforating wound. Vaginal bleeding may or may not be seen. Apply PASG when appropriate. |
| Oviducts (O-vi-dukt's) or fallopian (fah-LO-pe-an) tubes: carry egg (ovum) from the ovary to the uterus | Lacerations (rare), usually due to gunshot wound | Treat as penetrating or perforating wound. Vaginal bleeding is usually not seen. Apply PASG when appropriate. |
| Ovaries (O-vah-re's) produce female hormones and ova (O-vah) or eggs | Lacerations and puncture wounds (rare), usually due to gunshot or stab wounds | Treat as penetrating or perforating wound. Associated vaginal bleeding is not likely. Apply PASG when appropriate. |

**Figure 11-7. Description and care of injuries of the reproductive system in females**. Reprinted by permission from Grant, H. D., Murray, R. H., Jr., & Bergeron, J. D. (Eds.). *Brady emergency care* (5th ed.). Englewood Cliffs, NJ: Prentice-Hall, 1990.

# NURSING STRATEGIES FOR PATIENTS WITH GENITOURINARY TRAUMA

The first goal in a patient with genitourinary trauma is to maintain the airway, breathing, and circulation. Although most genitourinary injuries are not life threatening, they are potentially serious, have significant morbidity, and may affect the patient's life-style and self-image. Because these injuries often do not exist as a single entity, assess and stabilize the patient for life- or limb-threatening injuries before proceeding with management of genitourinary trauma. The ultimate goals are to preserve both structure and function of the genitourinary system and have the patient examined by a urologist.

Table 11-1 gives potential nursing diagnoses and interventions for care of patients with genitourinary trauma. The following nursing strategies may also be useful. It is presumed with each that airway, breathing, and circulation are already established. Your interventions should be within the scope of your professional license; commensurate with your skills and training; consistent with your state's nurse practice act; and when performed in a health care institution, adherent to that facility's standards of practice.

- Apply a padded ice pack to injured external genitalia to reduce swelling; transport the patient to a hospital for examination. Check the temperature of the area periodically to make certain that the pack is not too cold and that the status of the injury has not changed. For lacerations of the penis or vagina, cover the injuries with a sterile dressing or sanitary napkin and apply a padded ice pack.

- Work quickly and professionally to reduce the embarrassment that patients with genitourinary trauma often feel during examination. Expose the area completely for your assessment while a second rescuer protects the patient's privacy. Cover the patient promptly the assessment is finished.

- Encourage the patient to void if possible, and collect a urine specimen for analysis. Abnormal findings, such as red blood cells in the urine, can help in the detection of unseen trauma. Do not attempt to catheterize the patient if you suspect genitourinary trauma may be present. Leave this procedure to the urologist.

- Do not allow the patient to eat or drink until seen by a urologist. Immediate surgical intervention may be indicated for some genitourinary trauma, and oral intake will increase the risk of fatal aspiration during the perioperative period.

- Reassure the patient that everything possible is being done. Injuries to the external genitalia distress many patients, who fear sexual dysfunction and perceive alterations in their self-image.

# SUMMARY

Because the genitourinary organs are protected by their location in the body, genitourinary trauma, with a few exceptions, is seldom life threatening and often exists as one of many injuries. With appropriate intervention by a urologist or nephrologist, morbidity can be minimized, and outcome may be good. However, some patients may require counseling if genitourinary trauma alters their self-image or results in sexual dysfunction.

**Table 11-1**

**Potential Nursing Diagnoses and Interventions for Patients with Genitourinary Trauma**

| Diagnosis | Interventions |
|---|---|
| Fluid volume deficit r/t trauma | Monitor the patient for signs of shock; anticipate the onset of shock in any patient who has a pelvic fracture. Secure venous access and start fluid replacement as ordered. Anticipate emergency surgery to halt blood loss in the event of kidney damage. |
| Infection, potential | Minimize risk of infection by observing asepsis and proper handwashing. Keep the patient's genitourinary area clean; use sterile technique when catheterizing. Encourage fluid intake as allowed. |
| Body image disturbance | Accept patient's perception of self; provide reassurance that he or she can overcome this challenge. Show the patient how body functions are stabilizing or improving. Give him or her an opportunity to voice feelings. Arrange for the patient to meet others who have had similar experiences. Refer the patient to support groups and counselors as necessary. |
| Urinary elimination pattern alteration | Monitor intake and output; assess voiding pattern; note color and characteristics of urine and report any changes. Provide supportive measures such as fluids and analgesics when ordered. Explain urologic condition to the patient and the patient's family. Encourage them to ask questions, and answer the questions according to their level of understanding. |
| Injury, potential | Do not catheterize the bladder of the patient until cleared to do so by a physician. Prepare the patient for radiologic studies as indicated. Administer supplemental oxygen as ordered to the patient in shock to increase oxygen delivery to vital organs. |
| Pain | Apply ice (monitor temperature carefully) to external genital injuries that result in contusions, bruising, or swelling. Administer analgesics as ordered. |

Note.—This is a sample of potential nursing diagnoses. It is not presented as or intended to be a complete care plan for the trauma patient. More complete information can be found in a medical-surgical nursing course and textbook. r/t = related to.

Adapted from Sparks, S. and Taylor, C. M. *Nursing diagnosis reference manual,* Springhouse, PA: Springhouse Corp., 1991, and Chitwood, L., *Ambulatory patient care,* San Diego: Western Schools, 1994.

# CRITICAL CONCEPTS

- Suspect genitourinary injury in any patient who has penetrating trauma to the abdomen, pelvic fractures, or blunt abdominal trauma.

- Assess and stabilize the patient's airway, breathing, and circulation before evaluating genitourinary trauma, because such trauma is seldom life-threatening.

- Although the mortality rate associated with genitourinary trauma is low, the morbidity rate is high.

- If a kidney was fractured or lacerated during abdominal trauma, be prepared for shock or hypovolemic hemorrhage. Note that most genitourinary trauma is internal and not visible.

- Do not attempt to catheterize a patient who has a pelvic fracture. The urethra may be damaged, and attempts to pass a catheter may make the injury worse.

# GLOSSARY

**Bladder rupture:** A breaking or tearing open of the bladder; may result from blunt or penetrating trauma. An empty bladder is seldom ruptured; this injury is associated with full bladders.

**Kidney fracture:** A breaking open or rupture of the kidney caused by trauma.

**Urethral disruption:** Tearing or rupture of the urethra; commonly associated with a pelvic fracture. This injury occurs more often in males than in females.

# EXAM QUESTIONS

## Chapter 11

## Questions 52 - 55

52. Which of the following is the most likely injury in a patient with a stab wound of the flank?

    a.  Thoracic spine injury
    b.  Ruptured bladder
    c.  Lacerated urethra
    d.  Kidney and ureteral damage

53. Blunt trauma that fractures the pelvis is often associated with damage to which organ or organs?

    a.  Liver
    b.  Bladder and urethra
    c.  Colon
    d.  Spleen and right lung

54. A potential nursing diagnosis for a patient with genitourinary trauma is:

    a.  Dysreflexia
    b.  Incontinence, total
    c.  Infection, potential
    d.  Self-esteem, chronic low

55. Patients with genitourinary trauma should not be catheterized until they have been evaluated by a physician because cathertization could aggravate which of the following?

    a.  Urethral trauma
    b.  Kidney failure
    c.  Ureteral fracture
    d.  Bladder spasms

# CHAPTER 12

# OCULAR TRAUMA

## CHAPTER OBJECTIVE

After completing this chapter, the reader should be able to differentiate between the basic structures and functions of the eye, recognize common causes of ocular trauma, and select nursing diagnoses and interventions for patients with ocular trauma.

## LEARNING OBJECTIVES

After studying this chapter, the reader should be able to

1. Recognize signs and symptoms of ocular trauma.

2. Select methods to stabilize patients who have ocular trauma.

3. Indicate special concerns in meeting the challenge of sight preservation in patients with ocular trauma.

4. Choose common nursing diagnoses or interventions for patients with ocular trauma.

## INTRODUCTION

Ocular trauma, although seldom life threatening, is distressing to the patient, because vision can be lost and personal appearance may be altered. This chapter reviews basic normal anatomy and physiology of the eye and the mechanism of injury in ocular trauma. It also describes common ocular injuries and provides common potential nursing diagnoses and interventions.

## BASIC NORMAL OCULAR ANATOMY AND PHYSIOLOGY

The eye itself is referred to as the globe; it rests in a bony structure called the orbit. Only a small portion of the globe is visible; most of it is housed in the protection of the bones that form the skull and face. Six extraocular muscles control the movement of the eye in all directions.

Vision is made possible by the rays of light that pass through the cornea to focus on the retina. The nerve tissue in the retina transmits information from the light to the optic nerve. The optic nerve relays the information to the occipital lobe of the brain, where the impulses are translated into images by the brain.

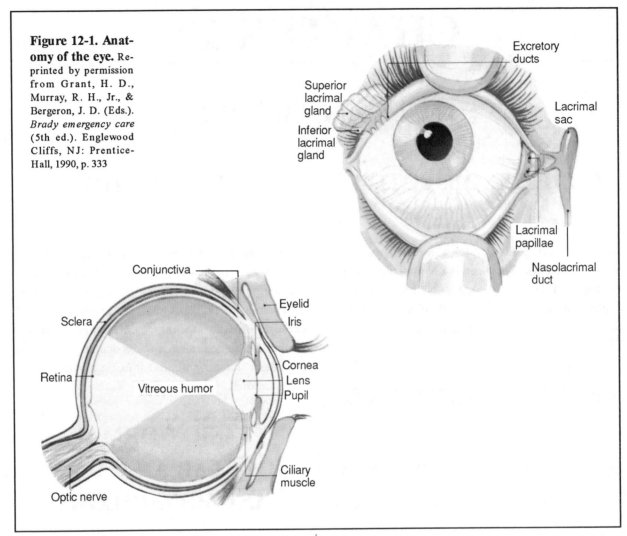

**Figure 12-1. Anatomy of the eye.** Reprinted by permission from Grant, H. D., Murray, R. H., Jr., & Bergeron, J. D. (Eds.). *Brady emergency care* (5th ed.). Englewood Cliffs, NJ: Prentice-Hall, 1990, p. 333

The major ocular structures (Figure 12-1) include the following:

## Globe

About 1 in. (2.5 cm) in diameter, the globe usually is thought of as two cavities: the large posterior chamber and the smaller anterior chamber, both of which are filled with fluid.

## Sclera

As the outermost tissue of the eye, the sclera helps form the shape of the globe and holds the fluids found in the eye. The sclera is the white part of the eye, but it is clear at the front of the eye.

## Cornea

The clear portion of the sclera at the front of the eye forms the cornea. The cornea is exquisitely sensitive; the lacrimal glands produce tears to moisten and protect it. It is through the cornea that the iris, or colored portion of the eye, can be seen. The iris dilates or constricts in response to light.

## Lens

Behind the cornea, iris, and pupil is the lens, which resides in a cavity filled with aqueous humor, a thin, clear fluid. The lens bends rays of light so they are focused on the retina for vision.

## Retina

The innermost lining of the eye is the retina, which is formed from nervous tissue. Trauma to the head can cause detachment of the retina and subsequent blindness, although skilled ophthalmologists can reattach the retina in some cases. When increased intracranial pressure compresses the tiny veins from the optic nerve, the retina's optic disk swells, a condition known as papilledema.

## Aqueous Humor

A clear fluid found in the anterior portion of the eye, aqueous humor can be replenished by the body if an injury causes it to leak out.

## Conjunctiva

The inside of the eyelids is formed from the conjunctiva, a thin pink membrane that can become swollen and inflamed in a condition known as conjunctivitis.

## Vitreous Humor

The vitreous humor is a gelatinous substance that fills the posterior chamber of the eye. This substance cannot be replenished by the body. It is instrumental in maintaining the shape of the globe.

# MECHANISM OF INJURY

Projectiles are responsible for most penetrating ocular trauma. The projectile may be a knife, a missile such as a bullet or a bottle rocket used in fireworks, or another foreign body. Penetrating ocular trauma may lead to impalement, laceration, or puncture of the globe, all of which may result in loss of the eye and vision. Blunt ocular trauma can produce simple corneal abrasions or contusions, retinal detachment, or even loss of the eye. Injuries from blunt trauma

result when the eyes and orbits rapidly decelerate and forcefully contact a hard surface. The blow may come from hitting the dashboard of the car in a crash, from falling, or from having the eyes or head struck with an object such as a bat or fist. In some cases, ocular trauma involves burns to the eyes by contact with a caustic substance.

# ASSESSMENT OF PATIENTS WITH OCULAR TRAUMA

For any patient with an injury to the eye, follow the standard ABC assessment plan from chapter 2. Evaluate the airway, breathing, and circulation. Because eye injuries are seldom life threatening, direct attention first to injuries that threaten life or limb. Once the airway and circulation are established, and bleeding is controlled, go back for the secondary survey. Any patient who has ocular trauma also may have an injury to the head or cervical spine or other trauma to the structures of the head and neck. These injuries should be evaluated and stabilized first.

Assessment proceeds as with any patient. Observe the scene of the accident or injury and elicit a history of the injury while assessing the patient. In addition to obtaining an accurate history and asking the routine questions you should ask of every trauma patient, for patients with ocular trauma it is important to know the following:

• What was the patient's visual acuity before the trauma? Has visual acuity changed since the injury?

• Does the patient have a history of glaucoma, diabetes, or other medical conditions?

- Does the patient wear contact lenses or glasses?

Signs and symptoms of ocular trauma vary with the type of trauma, but may include the following:

- Pain.

- Redness and swelling of the conjunctiva.

- Tearing.

- Possible decrease in visual acuity and light perception.

- Possible change in the shape and contour of the globe.

- Obvious disruption of the globe, orbit, eyelids, or cornea.

If any of the following signs are noted, suspect serious head trauma or brain damage (Grant et al., 1990):

- One or both eyes protrude.

- The pupils are not equal in size or do not react to light. (Some drugs can alter pupil size.)

- One or both of the orbits are fractured.

- The sclera is red from bleeding.

- The patient cannot move one or both eyes.

- The eyes cross or turn in different directions independent of each other.

# COMMON OCULAR TRAUMA

Although eye injuries are seldom life threatening, they are distressing to patients, who justifiably are concerned with potential loss of vision and alterations in personal appearance. All but the most minor ocular trauma should be evaluated by a specialist in eye care.

## Foreign Body in the Eye

When a foreign body is present in the eye, the patient generally complains of intense pain in the eye, and redness and tearing are often present. The foreign body may be superficial and visible on the surface of the cornea. However, it also can penetrate the globe and be intraocular. In some cases, a Wood's lamp and fluorescein stain are necessary to visualize the object.

## Corneal Abrasions

When the cornea is scraped, the abrasion may be minor or serious. Suspect a corneal abrasion if the cornea does not appear smooth and shiny. Even a minor abrasion can cause intense pain. Although painful, superficial corneal abrasions usually will heal themselves.

## Chemical Burns

When caustic substances contact the eyes, serious injury usually occurs. Signs and symptoms vary according to the degree of trauma; pain is intense in most cases, and the eye often is reddened. Some tissue destruction may be evident. The patient usually will relate a history of contact with a caustic substance, or you may receive clues from the scene or from bystanders. This is a serious emergency.

## Contusions and Lacerations

When the orbit, globe, or eyelids are injured, the tissues around the eye may swell and become discolored. Signs and symptoms vary according to the degree of trauma. Again, suspect head or neck injury in any patient who has contusions or lacerations around the eyes. Cuts of the eyelids can be minor. However, lacerations may affect the movement of the eyelids and disrupt the lacrimal system. Most lacerations of the eyelids require suturing, and any bruises or contusions of the orbit or globe should be evaluated by a physician.

## Hyphema

When the orbit or globe sustains blunt trauma, intraocular hemorrhage may occur. This is known as a hyphema. Clots may form inside the eye, blocking the flow of aqueous humor and increasing intraocular pressure, or the sclera may appear bloody. Patients with hyphema often complain of pain and a decrease in their visual acuity.

## Retinal Detachment

When blunt trauma to the head tears or separates the retina from its underlying layer, blindness often results. The patient may complain of a decrease in visual acuity or odd perceptions of flashing lights.

## Perforation of the Globe

When penetrating trauma perforates the eye or ruptures the globe, loss of the eye often results. Any patient with a perforated globe should be transported to the hospital immediately. Seepage of blood, vitreous humor, or intraocular contents from the eye may be noticeable.

# NURSING STRATEGIES FOR PATIENTS WITH OCULAR TRAUMA

The first goal for any patient with ocular trauma is to maintain the airway, breathing, and circulation. Although ocular injuries are seldom life threatening, they are distressing to patients, who justifiably are concerned with loss of vision and potential alterations in personal appearance. Table 12-1 gives potential nursing diagnoses and interventions for the care of patients with ocular trauma. The following nursing strategies may also be useful. It is presumed with each that airway, breathing, and circulation are already established. Your interventions should be within the scope of your professional license; commensurate with your skills and training; consistent with your state's nurse practice act; and when performed in a health care institution, adherent to that facility's standards of practice.

- Any patient who has ocular trauma also may have injuries of the head, cervical spine, or neck. Examine and stabilize life-threatening injuries before proceeding with the management of ocular trauma.

- Remember that the goal of care is to preserve both vision and the eyes.

- Do not, in general, attempt to remove an object on or in the cornea. This should be done by an ophthalmologist.

- Simple sterile patches over both eyes may help reduce discomfort until the patient can be seen by a physician. Patching both eyes may help limit movement of both eyes and reduce pain.

- Do not attempt to remove an object that impales the eye. Stabilize the object with bandages on

## Table 12-1
## Potential Nursing Diagnoses and Interventions for Patients with Ocular Trauma

| Diagnosis | Interventions |
|---|---|
| Poisoning, potential, r/t caustic substance contact with eyes | If the patient's eyes have had contact with a caustic substance, begin flushing the eyes immediately and continue until directed to stop by an ophthalmologist. Flush from the inner to the outer aspect of the eye; flush without ceasing until an ophthalmologist can take over. |
| Injury, potential, r/t ocular trauma | Transport the patient to a hospital for evaluation by an ophthalmologist. When an object is impaled in the eye, do not remove it; stabilize the object and transport the patient to a hospital. Do not attempt to replace a protruding eye into the socket. |
| Fear r/t unfamiliarity and concern for potential loss of vision | Offer simple, quiet explanations and act in a professional manner to build the patient's confidence. Present information at a level consistent with the patient's level of understanding. Remember that when a patient is under stress, explanations often must be repeated. Offer frequent reassurance and answer the patient's questions. Accept all questions as valid; do not minimize concerns. |
| Body image disturbance r/t ocular trauma | Explain that you are doing everything possible to help minimize or limit the trauma; reassure the patient often. Give the patient an opportunity to verbalize feelings; explain how his or her condition is being stabilized and what treatments can be expected. |
| Powerlessness r/t loss of vision | State your name and your role in the patient's care. Encourage the patient to express concerns, and then answer his or her questions. Accept the patient's feelings as valid, and do not minimize or negate them. |
| Pain | When not contraindicated by other trauma, the patient may benefit from lowered lights, elevation of the head of the bed, and administration of analgesics or ointments as ordered. Corneal abrasions are quite painful although the injury may appear insignificant. Because the eyes move together, it may reduce pain if both eyes are patched even if only one eye is injured. |
| Sensory or perceptual alteration: visual | Offer clear, simple explanations as you work; explain to the patient what is happening. Describe the environment; tell the patient the names and roles of other rescuers. |

Note.—This is a sample of potential nursing diagnoses. It is not presented as or intended to be a complete care plan for the trauma patient. More complete information can be found in a medical-surgical nursing course and textbook. r/t = related to.

Adapted from Sparks, S. and Taylor, C. M. *Nursing diagnosis reference manual,* Springhouse, PA: Springhouse Corp., 1991, and Chitwood, L., *Ambulatory patient care,* San Diego: Western Schools, 1994.

each side of it, and transport the patient immediately to the nearest hospital.

- Flush the eyes immediately with running water in any patient who has experienced a chemical burn to the eyes. Do not wait until the patient reaches a hospital. Begin flushing the eyes with sterile water or fluid from an intravenous solution of saline or lactated Ringer's solution; use tap water if these are not available. A bulb syringe can be used if necessary. During transport, continue to flush the eyes. Flush from the inner to the outer part. If contact lenses are present, remove them during the flushing, preferably with a small suction device designed for that purpose. Do not attempt to neutralize the offending solution; simply continue the flush until an ophthalmologist can assume treatment of the injury.

- Lay a sterile dressing over a laceration to reduce further contamination and aid absorption of blood, but do not apply pressure, because that could rupture a damaged globe or squeeze out vital vitreous humor.

- Do not attempt to replace a protruding eye into the orbit. Any pressure on the eye could cause additional loss of the vitreous humor, which cannot be replaced by the body. Protect the eye during transport by placing a sterile eye patch loosely over it. Any foreign body impaling the eye should be left in place and guarded from further movement that could cause additional damage to the eye.

- Provide a quiet environment to help calm the anxious patient. If the patient is experiencing photophobia, consider reducing light levels to reduce pain once the assessment is complete. Elevate the head of the bed to reduce the swelling and congestion in the eye if it is not contra-

indicated by other injuries. Do not elevate the head until spinal injury has been ruled out by a physician in a hospital.

- A simple sterile eye patch can help reduce discomfort until the patient can be seen by a physician.

- Be aware that you should in general leave the patient's contact lenses in place, but be certain to report the presence of the lenses to staff members who are receiving the patient.

- Gently close the eyes of any unconscious patient who does not have ocular trauma. An unconscious patient cannot protect the eyes by blinking or by withdrawing from painful contact. If the eyes will not stay closed, they can be taped shut. Be careful not to damage the eyes during transport or while caring for other injuries.

- For all but the most superficial ocular trauma, refer the patient to an ophthalmologist.

- Do not allow the patient to eat or drink until seen by an ophthalmologist. Immediate surgical intervention may be indicated for some ocular trauma, and oral intake will increase the risk of fatal aspiration during the perioperative period.

# SUMMARY

Ocular trauma, although seldom life threatening, is distressing to the patient, because vision can be lost and personal appearance may be altered. Unless the globe has been ruptured or penetrated, outcome and restoration or maintenance of sight are often good. Some alterations in appearance frequently persist after lacerations are sutured.

# CRITICAL CONCEPTS

- Suspect injuries to the head and cervical spine in any patient who has ocular trauma.

- Assess and stabilize the airway, breathing, and circulation first; ocular trauma is seldom life threatening.

- Reassure any patient who has ocular trauma. Eye injuries frighten patients, who are concerned about loss of vision and alterations in appearance and who may not be able to see because of injuries or eye patches.

# GLOSSARY

**Aqueous humor:** The clear watery fluid that fills the area of the eye between the cornea and the lens; it can be replenished by the body.

**Cornea:** The clear portion of the sclera at the front of the eye.

**Globe:** The eyeball.

**Hyphema:** Bleeding into the anterior chamber of the eye; usually caused by blunt trauma.

**Orbit:** The bony structures that form the protective casing for the eyeball or globe.

**Retina:** The innermost lining of the eye, formed from nervous tissue.

**Sclera:** The white fibrous covering of the eyeball.

**Vitreous humor:** The clear gelatinous substance that fills the area of the eyeball between the lens and the retina; it cannot be replenished by the body.

# EXAM QUESTIONS

## Chapter 12

## Questions 56 - 59

56. An important action that may preserve vision in a patient with a chemical burn of the eye is:

    a. Continuous flushing of the eyes
    b. Bandaging both eyes
    c. Getting the victim to an optometrist quickly
    d. Taping the eyes shut

57. Your children are playing in the yard on July 4th when a bottle rocket impales your daughter's eye. Only the stem of the rocket is visible. You call for an ambulance. While awaiting its arrival, which of the following should you do?

    a. Stabilize the object in place.
    b. Gently slide the object out of the eye.
    c. Flush the eye with tap water.
    d. Patch the unaffected eye.

58. You are leaving a restaurant when you see one man strike another in the face and then flee. The victim falls to the ground, but then gets back up saying he keeps seeing flashing lights. What ocular injury is most likely?

    a. Hyphema
    b. Retinal detachment
    c. Ruptured globe
    d. Corneal abrasion

59. A potential nursing diagnosis for a patient with ocular trauma is:

    a. Sleep pattern disturbance
    b. Aspiration, potential for
    c. Fear, related to unfamiliarity
    d. Thermoregulation, ineffective

# CHAPTER 13

# MAXILLOFACIAL AND NECK TRAUMA

## CHAPTER OBJECTIVE

After completing this chapter, the reader should be able to differentiate between structures of the face and neck, recognize common causes of maxillofacial trauma, and select nursing diagnoses and interventions for patients with maxillofacial and neck trauma.

## LEARNING OBJECTIVES

After studying this chapter, the reader should be able to

1. Recognize signs and symptoms of maxillofacial and neck trauma.

2. Select methods to stabilize and transport patients who have maxillofacial trauma.

3. Identify special concerns in meeting the challenge of airway management in patients who have maxillofacial and neck trauma.

4. Differentiate among head, ocular, neck, and maxillofacial trauma.

5. Select common nursing diagnoses and interventions for patients with maxillofacial and neck trauma.

## INTRODUCTION

Maxillofacial trauma is often just one of several injuries sustained by a trauma patient. Although the injury may appear severe, maxillofacial trauma is not usually life threatening unless the airway is compromised. However, patients with trauma to the neck are at high risk. The airway, the carotid arteries, the jugular vessels, the cervical spine, and the spinal cord are all contained in the neck; death or permanent paralysis can be the ultimate outcome of trauma. Spinal cord injuries are discussed in chapter 6; this section focuses on neck injuries other than injuries of the spine and spinal cord. Head injuries are discussed in chapter 5.

This chapter reviews basic normal anatomy and physiology of the face, jaw, and neck and the mechanism of injury. It also describes assessment of patients with maxillofacial and neck trauma, reviews common maxillofacial and neck injuries, and presents common potential nursing diagnoses and interventions for patients with neck and maxillofacial trauma.

# BASIC NORMAL MAXILLOFACIAL ANATOMY AND PHYSIOLOGY

A complex structure, the skull is composed of 11 paired sets of bones and 6 additional single bones. Divided into two regions, the skull consists of the cranial vault and the facial bones. The mandible is the only bone that moves. The bony orbits house the eyes. The nose protrudes from the face and is the facial structure injured most often. Facial structures are formed from 14 bones, all of which touch the maxillae. The nose and mouth open into the pharynx. The pharynx opens into the esophagus and the larynx, which opens into the trachea and then the lungs. The trachea is surrounded by soft tissues consisting of muscles and major vessels that provide the blood supply of the head.

The structures of the face, jaw, and neck house some of the upper part of the airway, which serves as a critical passageway to and from the lungs. The orbits protect the eyes. The mandible and teeth are essential for chewing. Major maxillofacial and neck structures include the following:

## Maxillae

The maxillae are actually two bones that meet in the midline of the face. They form the floor of the orbits and the roof of the mouth and therefore support the upper teeth.

## Mandible

The strongest bone in the face, the mandible anchors the lower teeth. Two projections called the rami point up toward the ears and join the body of the mandible at an angle. Upward pressure on the rami often helps relieve an obstructed airway.

## Zygomatic Bone

The zygomatic bone forms the cheekbone and parts of the orbits.

## Nasal Bones and Cartilage

The shape of the nose is formed by the thin nasal bones and cartilage.

## Teeth

Hard, bonelike structures emanating from the mandible and maxillae, the teeth are essential for chewing and speech. They also maintain shape in the lower face, which is why it can be more difficult to ventilate an edentulous patient by mask. In maxillofacial trauma, the teeth can become dislodged and obstruct the airway.

## Hyoid Bone

A U-shaped bone attached to the base of the tongue, the hyoid bone does not touch any other bone in the body. Because it is attached to the tongue, this bone often plays a role in airway obstruction.

## Pharynx

A muscular structure, the pharynx begins at the base of the skull. This airway may become obstructed if food, blood, or foreign bodies lodge in it. Opening into the esophagus and larynx, the pharynx also plays a role in speech.

## Larynx

The larynx is constructed from a series of cartilaginous structures and muscles that assist in speech. However, its most critical function is as an air passage.

## Epiglottis

A floppy mucosa-covered piece of cartilage, the epiglottis is attached to the thyroid cartilage, which commonly is referred to as the Adam's apple, and is part of the larynx. In unconscious or trauma patients, the epiglottis may flop over the opening to the trachea and obstruct the airway.

## Trachea

Serving as the passageway for air from the upper part of the airway to the main bronchi that branch out into the lungs, the trachea is composed of C-shaped rings of cartilage joined by tough membranes. If the upper part of the airway is obstructed, skilled professionals may incise between the rings of the trachea to open an air passage.

## Major Vessels

Laceration of any of the major vessels of the head may result in life-threatening hemorrhage. Also, air may be sucked in through venous vessels and result in a fatal air embolism.

**Carotid arteries.** The carotid arteries run bilaterally alongside the trachea. Chemoreceptors in the arteries respond to changes in blood chemistry such as hypoxia, causing reflex increases in pulse rate, blood pressure, and respiratory rate. Interruption of the carotid blood supply will result in brain damage. Palpation of the carotid arteries yields information about the patient's circulatory status: If a carotid pulse can be palpated, the patient's systolic blood pressure should be at least 60 mm Hg.

**Jugular veins.** The large jugular veins drain blood from the head and neck. The internal jugular vein can be cannulated in order to obtain information about the fluid status of the body; the external jugular vein can be cannulated for intravenous administration of fluid.

# MECHANISM OF INJURY

Projectiles are responsible for most penetrating maxillofacial trauma. The projectile may be a knife or a missile such as a bullet. Penetrating maxillofacial or neck trauma may lead to lacerations, impalement, or puncture of the cheek or eye. Disruption of the major blood vessels in the neck may occur, and brain damage or exsanguination can result.

In an accident, unrestrained occupants (especially front-seat passengers) in motor vehicles may crash through the windshield and then be pulled back through the shattered glass as the car decelerates. The result can be severe facial and scalp lacerations; soft-tissue trauma; and facial, neck, or skull fractures. Because the scalp and facial skin are highly vascular, bleeding is often profuse. Although the effect is quite dramatic, blood loss from scalp or facial lacerations is not usually life threatening.

Blunt maxillofacial or neck trauma can produce injury ranging from simple nasal fractures to major head injury or collapse of the airway. Injuries from blunt trauma occur when maxillofacial structures or the neck forcefully contacts a hard surface in rapid deceleration. Blunt maxillofacial and neck trauma often occur in motor vehicle accidents, sports accidents, or falls or when the face or jaw is struck in an assault with an object such as a bat or fist. Figure 13-1 shows potential complications of facial trauma.

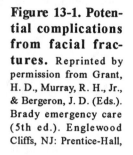

**Figure 13-1. Potential complications from facial fractures.** Reprinted by permission from Grant, H. D., Murray, R. H., Jr., & Bergeron, J. D. (Eds.). Brady emergency care (5th ed.). Englewood Cliffs, NJ: Prentice-Hall,

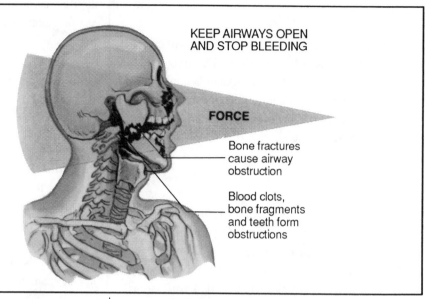

KEEP AIRWAYS OPEN
AND STOP BLEEDING

FORCE

Bone fractures cause airway obstruction

Blood clots, bone fragments and teeth form obstructions

# ASSESSMENT OF PATIENTS WITH MAXILLOFACIAL TRAUMA

For any patient with an injury to the maxillofacial or neck structures, follow the standard ABC assessment plan. Evaluate the airway, breathing, and circulation. Direct attention first to serious injuries that threaten life or limb. Once the airway and circulation are established, and bleeding is controlled, begin a secondary survey of the maxillofacial area and the neck. Maxillofacial injuries are seldom life threatening unless the airway is compromised. In fact, it is not uncommon to wait hours or even days to intervene with surgical repairs. See chapter 6 for a discussion of injuries to the cervical spine.

Maxillofacial trauma is often one of a number of injuries, so assume that any patient who has trauma to the face also has injury to the head or cervical spine; this chapter presumes that a patient with any of these injuries has been stabilized first. Next, turn your attention to assessment of the maxillofacial trauma. Proceed as with any patient. Observe the accident scene and elicit a history of the injury while assessing the patient.

Suspect maxillofacial and neck trauma in any patient who has any of the following:

• Obvious fractures, deformities, or distortion of the face or neck (Figure 13-2).

• Asymmetry of the face or neck.

• Pain.

• Swelling, which may be severe, and discoloration, especially under the eyes (Raccoon eyes) or of the sclera, or bruising or swelling behind the ears at the base of the skull (Battle's sign). Raccoon eyes and Battle's sign are indications of a fracture in the base of the skull (Figure 13-3).

• Misalignment of the upper and lower teeth (not always a reliable sign).

• Difficulty in speaking or in moving the jaw.

• Damage to the teeth, loose or missing teeth, bleeding from the mouth.

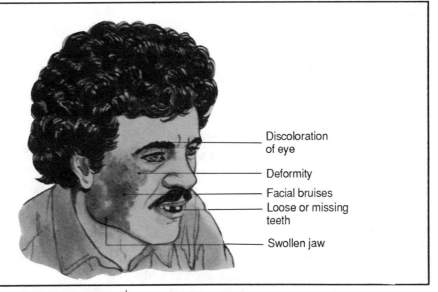

**Figure 13-2. Signs of facial fractures.** Reprinted by permission from Grant, H. D., Murray, R. H., Jr., & Bergeron, J. D. (Eds.). *Brady emergency care* (5th ed.). Englewood Cliffs, NJ: Prentice-Hall, 1990, p. 333.

Discoloration of eye

Deformity

Facial bruises

Loose or missing teeth

Swollen jaw

- Blood or fluid (possibly cerebrospinal fluid) draining from the nose; hemorrhage from the major vessels in the neck.

# COMMON MAXILLOFACIAL AND NECK TRAUMA

## Facial Trauma

Maxillofacial trauma causes distortion of the facial structures and copious bleeding. It is often caused by blunt trauma sustained in an assault or motor vehicle accident. Broken teeth and blood may obstruct the airway, and it may be difficult to ensure a patent airway because of fracture of the mandible. Bleeding or facial trauma may make endotracheal intubation impossible; the airway will have to be opened below the level of the epiglottis. This involves puncturing or incising the cricothyroid membrane in the neck, a technique that should be performed only by those who are skilled in its execution.

## Le Fort Fractures

Named after the surgeon who identified them, Le Fort fractures are three different types of mid-face fractures that are common after blunt facial trauma. They include a fracture of the maxillae above the teeth, a triangular fracture from the upper teeth to an area between the eyes, and a serious fracture involving separation of the facial bones from the cranium.

## Mandibular Fractures

Significant force from blunt trauma is necessary to fracture the mandible. However, mandibular fractures are a fairly common injury in motor vehicle accidents and assaults, although falls and sports injuries also may cause such fractures. Unless the mandible is shattered to the point that the airway is obstructed, no immediate intervention is indicated. See the section on dental injury for information on the care of damaged teeth.

## Zygomatic Arch Fractures

Although the cheekbones may be fractured by blunt trauma, this is not a critical injury unless the orbits or eyes are damaged by the blow.

## Nasal Fractures

As the most prominent feature of the face, the nose is easily fractured. Blunt trauma directed at the front of the face may cause posterior displacement of the bones; blunt trauma from the side may cause lateral displacement. Nasal fractures most commonly are caused by motor vehicle accidents, sports injuries, falls, and assaults. The nose may be bleeding, and some swelling often occurs.

## Avulsions

Avulsions result when structures are torn from the foundation that secures them to the body. The scalp most frequently is torn from the skull; profuse bleeding results. Suspect a skull fracture and neck injury when a patient's head sustains trauma that causes an avulsion.

## Facial Lacerations

Cuts to the eyelids can be minor; however, lacerations may affect the movement of the eyelids and disrupt the lacrimal system. Most lacerations of the eyelids will require suturing, and any bruises or contusions of the orbit or globe should be evaluated by an ophthalmologist.

## Contusions

The eyes may be swollen from blunt facial trauma or from tissue edema in response to the trauma. In general, all eye injuries should be evaluated by an ophthalmologist.

## Injury to Major Vessels

Penetrating trauma of the neck is a serious emergency. Severe, life-threatening hemorrhage or air embolism may occur, and bleeding is difficult to stop because of the pressure within the vessels.

## Carotid Artery Injury

As the major arteries in the neck, the carotid arteries supply the blood for perfusion and oxygenation of the brain. When bright red blood spurts in a pulsat-

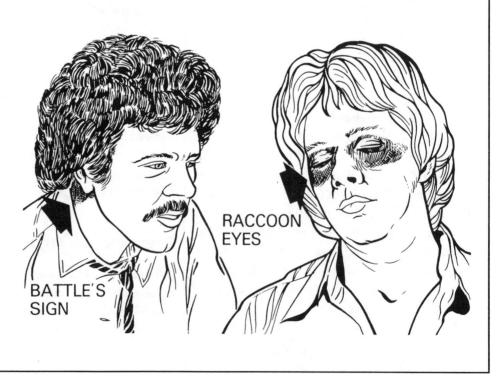

**Figure 13-3. Signs of basilar skull fracture: Battle's sign and raccoon eyes.** Reprinted by permission from Campbell, J. *Basic trauma life support: Advanced prehospital care* (2nd ed.). Englewood Cliffs, NJ: Prentice-Hall, 1988.

BATTLE'S SIGN

RACCOON EYES

ing flow from a neck wound, the carotid artery may be damaged, and a life-threatening situation exists.

## Jugular Vein Injury

Dark red blood streaming from an open neck vein is a serious emergency because of potential blood loss and potential air entrainment into the venous system.

## Dental Injury

Teeth often are damaged in facial trauma. Loose teeth can be inhaled into the throat or lungs and obstruct the airway. Dentures and other dental appliances may be knocked out or swallowed. Any patient with dental trauma should be evaluated by a dentist or an oral surgeon.

## Tracheal Injury

Blunt or penetrating trauma to the neck may produce tracheal injury and close the airway. Hypoxia and death follow within minutes.

# NURSING STRATEGIES FOR PATIENTS WITH MAXILLOFACIAL AND NECK TRAUMA

The first goal for any patient with maxillofacial trauma is to maintain the airway, breathing, and circulation. Although maxillofacial injuries that do not compromise the airway are seldom life threatening, these injuries are distressing to patients, who justifiably are concerned with potential alterations in personal appearance. Table 13-1 gives potential nursing diagnoses and interventions for the care of patients with maxillofacial and neck trauma. The following

nursing strategies may also be useful. It is presumed with each that airway, breathing, and circulation are already established. Your intervention should be within the scope of your professional license; commensurate with your skills and training; consistent with your state's nurse practice act; and when performed in a health care institution, adherent to that facility's standards of practice.

- Do not shave the eyebrows of a patient who has facial trauma. They provide a landmark for repair, and they may not grow back (Sheehy & Jimmerson, 1994).

- Apply direct pressure with a sterile dressing over bleeding sites except as follows: where obvious deformity indicates fractures, over ruptured or penetrated eyes, and where cerebrospinal fluid is flowing or brain tissue is exposed.

- Presume that injuries to the cervical spine exist in any patient with maxillofacial trauma who lost consciousness from the blow. Immobilize the head and neck as described in chapter 6.

- Apply pressure to bleeding from the neck to reduce blood loss but do not occlude the airway. Never apply a tourniquet to the neck; airway compromise and brain damage will result.

- When possible, lay a dressing moistened with saline over avulsed tissue to reduce contamination and drying of the tissues.

- Retrieve avulsed tissue, such as an ear, from the trauma scene, cover it with a sterile moist dressing, wrap it in plastic, label it, and transport it to the hospital with the patient. In some cases, surgeons may be able to reattach the part.

- Nasal fractures often result in blood running into the stomach and subsequent vomiting. Offer the patient gauze bandages to catch any drainage, and transport him or her to a hospital. Do

## Table 13-1
## Potential Nursing Diagnoses and Interventions
## for Patients with Maxillofacial or Neck Trauma

| Diagnosis | Interventions |
|---|---|
| Airway clearance, ineffective, r/t trauma | Maintain a patent airway; blood and loose teeth may make this more difficult. Wear protective eyewear and a mask in case the patient coughs and sprays blood. Injured tissue may swell and obstruct the airway gradually, so vigilance is essential. |
| Suffocation r/t internal factors (bleeding into the airway) | Have suction equipment available when possible; use a rigid tonsil suction device to clear vomitus and blood from the airway. When spinal injury has been ruled out at the hospital, raise the head of the bed of a conscious patient to decrease swelling and facilitate respiration. |
| Body image disturbance r/t maxillofacial trauma | Allow the patient and support persons to express concerns about facial trauma. Answer questions; accept the patient's perception of self. When possible, involve the patient and the patient's family in planning care. |
| Injury, potential for repeated trauma | Counsel victims of domestic violence, and refer them to social and legal services; suggest counseling and support groups. Suggest anger management and substance abuse counseling when appropriate. Teach use of seat belts, shoulder harnesses, and child restraint devices. |
| Verbal communication impairment r/t trauma | Use communication aids when possible for any patient who cannot speak. Provide hospitalized patients with an emergency call system and respond quickly and in person. |
| Breathing pattern, ineffective r/t maxillofacial trauma | Monitor respiratory status frequently, because blood or foreign material can quickly obstruct the airway. Keep wire cutters at the bedside if the patient has had his or her jaw wired shut after mandibular surgery (Bartkiw & Pynn, 1993). |

Note.—This is a sample of potential nursing diagnoses. It is not presented as or intended to be a complete care plan for the trauma patient. More complete information can be found in a medical-surgical nursing course and textbook. r/t = related to.

Adapted from Sparks, S. and Taylor, C. M. *Nursing diagnosis reference manual,* Springhouse, PA: Springhouse Corp., 1991, and Chitwood, L., *Ambulatory patient care,* San Diego: Western Schools, 1994.

not obstruct the flow of blood; that might result in airway obstruction or increased intracranial pressure in the event that a skull fracture exists.

- Be prepared to suction blood and vomitus. Blood filling the pharynx can compromise the airway, and vomiting often occurs as blood drains into the stomach.

- Save loose and dislodged teeth when time and priorities permit. Make a note of the time, wrap the loose teeth in moist dressings or place them in a container of saline or cool milk, label the container, and transport it with the patient. Dislodged teeth can sometimes be reimplanted successfully.

- Do not attempt to force injured eyelids open to check the pupils; doing so may aggravate ocular injury. Lay a cool moist compress over the contusion; follow-up treatment can be administered by a physician.

- Offer strong emotional support to patients who have maxillofacial trauma. They may experience alterations in their self-image because of the injury.

- Do not attempt to remove an object impaled in the patient's head, even if it is in the brain or eye, unless it is obstructing the airway. Stabilize the object with bandages on each side of it, and transport the patient immediately to the hospital. If an impaling object is obstructing the airway, it should be removed or death may result. Be prepared for increased bleeding, because the object most likely was placing pressure on vessels and therefore decreasing blood flow at the wound.

- Elevate the head of the bed of the conscious patient to reduce swelling, bleeding, and congestion, if it is not contraindicated by other injuries and a physician has ruled out spinal injury.

- Do not lift or move the patient's head to examine for further injury or to apply bandages until injury to the cervical spine has been ruled out by a physician.

- Do not remove the Philadelphia cervical collar until ordered to do so by a physician. Conscious patients may complain that the collar is uncomfortable, but it must remain in place until a cervical injury has been ruled out in the hospital.

- Do not allow the patient to eat or drink until seen by a physician. Immediate surgical intervention may be indicated for some maxillofacial trauma, and oral intake will increase the risk of a fatal aspiration during the perioperative period.

- Apply firm pressure over a bleeding site in the neck (do not occlude the airway), administer oxygen, prepare for the onset of shock if bleeding is brisk, and transport the patient immediately to the hospital. Keep the site covered when possible. Air can be sucked into an open jugular vein and circulated to the heart (air entrainment); the final result could be a fatal air embolism.

- Never insert a nasogastric tube or nasal airway in a patient with suspected mid-face or skull fractures. The tube or airway could penetrate the cranium and enter the brain.

# CRITICAL CONCEPTS

- Suspect injuries to the head and cervical spine in any patient who has maxillofacial or neck trauma.

- Maxillofacial trauma is generally not life threatening unless the airway is compromised.

- Blunt and penetrating trauma to the neck can cause death within minutes from hemorrhage and airway obstruction.

- Never insert anything into the nose of a patient with suspected mid-face, nasal, or skull fractures or leakage of cerebrospinal fluid. The device could penetrate the brain.

- Offer referrals to legal, social welfare, counseling, drug abuse, and anger management resources to patients who have been involved in assaults. Counsel victims of motor vehicle accidents about use of seat belts.

# GLOSSARY

**Air entrainment:** Pulling of ambient air into an open vein, such as an open jugular vein. This can lead to a fatal air embolus as the air is circulated to the heart, lungs, and brain.

**Avulsion:** Stripping or pulling away of tissue from body structures.

**Battle's sign:** Bruising behind and under the ear; may indicate a basilar skull fracture.

**Raccoon eyes:** Discoloration and bruising under the eyes; may indicate a basilar skull fracture.

# EXAM QUESTIONS

## Chapter 13

### Questions 60 - 65

60. One possible indication of a basilar skull fracture is:

    a. Battle's sign
    b. Avascular necrosis
    c. Carotid artery laceration
    d. obvious deformity of the crown

61. Your neighbor falls in his driveway, knocking out his four upper front incisors. You instruct another rescuer to gather up the dislodged teeth and do which of the following?

    a. Discard the teeth in a tightly covered trash can.
    b. Place the teeth in a container of cool milk for transport with the patient.
    c. Take the teeth on ahead to the patient's dentist's office.
    d. Put the teeth in a paper bag and store for later study by the patient's dentist.

62. Which of the following may cause rapid development of airway obstruction in a patient who has maxillofacial trauma?

    a. Bleeding and tissue swelling
    b. Bone fragments entering the trachea
    c. Loss of cerebrospinal fluid through a basilar skull fracture
    d. Delayed loss of consciousness

63. A common potential nursing diagnosis for a patient with maxillofacial trauma patient is:

    a. Pain, chronic
    b. Airway clearance, ineffective
    c. Nutrition, altered: more than body requirements
    d. Noncompliance

64. A rider is thrown from his horse, striking his head on a railing. Fluid is flowing from his nose, and swelling and discoloration develop under his eyes. Which of the following injuries is most likely?

    a. Basilar skull fracture
    b. Air embolus form a torn jugular vein
    c. Mandibular fracture
    d. Dental injury

65. While playing outside, your neighbor's daughter trips and falls face down on the sidewalk. She has blood flowing freely from her nose. Which of the following should you do?

    a. Pinch her nostrils tight together and hold this pressure until the bleeding stops.
    b. Have her remain flat on the sidewalk, elevate her legs to enhance circulation, and call an ambulance.
    c. Place a dressing moistened with saline over her eyes and send her to her home to lie down.
    d. Hold a towel under her nose to catch the flow without occluding the nasal air passage.

# CHAPTER 14

# TRAUMA IN THE ELDERLY

## CHAPTER OBJECTIVE

After completing this chapter, the reader should be able to describe changes in anatomy and physiology that occur with aging, recognize common causes of trauma in the elderly, and initiate appropriate nursing intervention for elderly trauma patients.

## LEARNING OBJECTIVES

After studying this chapter, the reader should be able to

1. Identify leading causes of death in the elderly.

2. Recognize special concerns associated with trauma in the elderly.

3. Recognize common types of trauma that occur in the elderly.

4. Indicate common characteristics of elderly patients who are victims of abuse.

5. Choose common nursing diagnoses and interventions for elderly trauma patients.

## INTRODUCTION

The estimated number of senior citizens in the United States is 56 million, or about 13% of our population. That is expected to increase to 17% by 2020 (Fleming, 1993). The elderly suffer fewer injuries, but their mortality rate from trauma is the highest of all age groups (Sheehy & Jimmerson, 1994) because medical complications are more common (Fleming, 1993). So, the changes that occur with aging influence the mortality and morbidity of trauma patients.

Elderly drivers are more likely to die from injuries per mile driven, and they have higher fatal crash rates than any other drivers except teenagers (Fleming, 1993). The prevalence of fractures, especially of the hip and to a lesser degree the extremities, increases dramatically after age 55 (*Introduction: Injury Prevention*, 1990). The goal is to prevent trauma and minimize the impact of trauma when it does occur.

This chapter reviews the alterations in normal anatomy and physiology that occur with aging and describes common types of trauma in the elderly. It also reviews assessment and management of these injuries; discusses issues of abuse of the elderly; and presents common nursing diagnoses, interventions, and strategies. For the purposes of this discussion, *elderly* is defined as any patient who is more than 65 years old.

# CHANGES IN ANATOMY AND PHYSIOLOGY WITH AGING

As the body ages, physiologic functioning is diminished (Figure 14-1). Most of these changes reduce the body's ability to respond to the challenges of trauma; some increase the propensity to injury. An older patient simply is not as resilient as a younger patient. Changes in anatomy may also occur, such as arthritis that leads to kyphosis or limited range of motion of the joints.

## Cardiovascular Changes

The cardiovascular system progressively deteriorates with age. The blood pressure gradually increases, the vessels show a tendency to hardening, and the system has less reserve. The heart rate is generally slower; tachycardia does not always accompany shock.

## Respiratory Changes

Changes in the respiratory system with aging can be significant:

- **Airway:** Teeth may be lost with aging; full sets of dentures are not uncommon. Artificial ventilation with a mask can be difficult in an edentulous patient because the cheeks have no shape and air leaks around the mask.

- **Ventilation and perfusion:** Reduced efficiency in gas exchange results in decreased arterial oxygen.

- **Thorax:** Whereas the chest wall in children is compliant and flexible, the rib cage and chest wall in the elderly are less elastic. The vital capacity of the lungs decreases.

## Metabolic and Hepatic Changes

The basal metabolic rate slows. The liver's ability to clear toxins is diminished, and the effects of hypoxia are more pronounced.

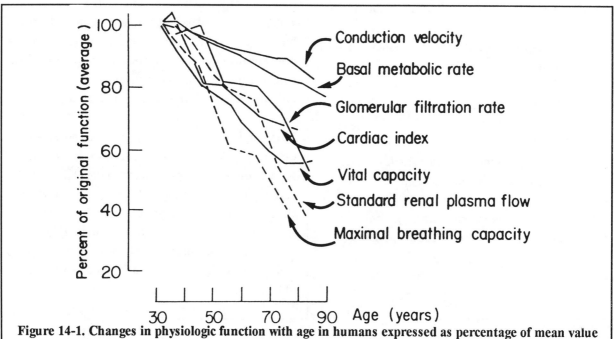

**Figure 14-1. Changes in physiologic function with age in humans expressed as percentage of mean value at age 30 years.** Reprinted by permission from Miller, R. (Ed.). *Anesthesia* (2nd ed., Vol. 2). New York: Churchill Livingstone, 1981.

## Renal Changes

The kidneys show a decline in function with aging. The elderly tend to lose salt and retain potassium.

## Changes in Thermoregulation

The elderly are prone to heat loss and chilling and become dehydrated sooner than the young.

## Skeletal Changes

Bone density decreases in the elderly, and osteoporosis is often present. Although more pronounced in women, osteoporosis means that the elderly are prone to fracture from trauma, especially fractures of the hips, wrists, and ribs. Recovery from fractures is slow and prolonged; pelvic fractures can be life threatening. The prevalence of arthritis also increases, making the elderly less mobile and complicating their recovery.

# MECHANISM OF INJURY AND COMMON CAUSES OF TRAUMA IN THE ELDERLY

Because they can not react as quickly as younger persons, the elderly are more likely to sustain trauma, both blunt and penetrating. With the limited reserves of an aging body, their recovery is often prolonged. Although cancer, heart disease, and stroke are the leading causes of death among the elderly, accidents rank fourth. Traumatic deaths in the elderly most often are caused by motor vehicle accidents, falls, and burns. The death rate associated with motor vehicle accidents increases with age (Table 14-1). Additionally, abuse of the elderly has become more widely known, revealing that trauma in the elderly is sometimes intentional rather than accidental.

### Table 14-1
### Passenger Car Driver Deaths per 100,000 Persons, 1992

| Age | Male | Female |
|---|---|---|
| 16–19 | 21 | 9 |
| 20–24 | 23 | 8 |
| 25–29 | 17 | 6 |
| 30–34 | 14 | 5 |
| 35–39 | 12 | 5 |
| 40–44 | 11 | 4 |
| 45–49 | 10 | 5 |
| 50–54 | 11 | 4 |
| 55–59 | 10 | 4 |
| 60–64 | 11 | 4 |
| 65–69 | 12 | 4 |
| 70–74 | 16 | 6 |
| 75–79 | 19 | 7 |
| 80–84 | 28 | 7 |
| 85+ | 26 | 4 |

Reprinted by permission from Fleming, A. (Ed.). *Facts, 1993*. Arlington, VA: Insurance Institute for Highway Safety, 1993.

Although motor vehicle accidents are the most common cause of trauma in the elderly, falls are also common and can be associated with a medical condition. For example, an elderly person who falls and fractures a hip may have had an episode of bradycardia resulting in syncope. Orthostatic hypotension, the drop in blood pressure that occurs when a person rises from a sitting or supine position, is another common factor with a fall. Alcohol also remains a causative factor in trauma of the elderly. The goal of assessment is to gather as much information as possible about the accident (or assault) and about the patient's medical history. Assessment may be hampered by the patient's limited hearing and mobility.

# NURSING STRATEGIES FOR THE CARE OF ELDERLY TRAUMA PATIENTS

The first goal with an elderly trauma patient is to preserve the patient's life and prevent further injury. Table 14-2 gives potential nursing diagnoses and interventions for the care of elderly trauma patients. The following nursing strategies may also be useful. It is presumed with each that airway, breathing, and circulation are already established. Your intervention should be within the scope of your professional license; commensurate with your skills and training; consistent with your state's nurse practice act; and when performed in a health care institution, adherent to that facility's standards of practice.

- Follow the standard ABC plan of assessment. Elderly patients initially are treated no differently from any other trauma patient in this regard. Be aware of the decreased reserve and limited function of the elderly patient's body,

and stay vigilant for clues to changes in the patient's condition.

- Observe the accident scene and elicit a history of the injury while assessing the patient. Try to obtain information from relatives or bystanders, because any information about the mechanism of injury or preexisting medical conditions may be valuable.

- Administer oxygen. An elderly patient's oxygen reserve is usually limited.

- Watch for loose teeth and dental appliances. Artificial airways can dislodge them, and the teeth or appliances can be inhaled. Dentures can obstruct airflow if they slip out of place. Sweep dislodged teeth from the mouth; monitor the status of loose teeth at intervals.

- Generally, leave the patient's dentures in place when you use a bag-valve-mask device for artificial ventilation; the dentures help create a seal around the mask. Make a note of the dentures and be certain to check their security at intervals; always inform the emergency team accepting the patient of the presence of the dentures. Remove and save a patient's dentures if endotracheal intubation is necessary.

- Keep the patient warm. The elderly lose heat quickly, and heat loss can have deleterious effects on resuscitation efforts.

- Ask family members to gather up all bottles of medication the patient may have been taking, if possible. Transport the drugs to the hospital with the patient; they can provide essential clues in the detection and management of the patient's condition.

- Elicit as much of the patient's medical history as possible. The patient's health before the trauma

**Table 14-2**
**Potential Nursing Diagnoses and Interventions for Elderly Trauma Patients**

| Diagnosis | Interventions |
|---|---|
| Airway clearance, ineffective, r/t trauma | Maintain a patent airway. It may be more difficult to secure a good seal with a mask in patients who are edentulous. Be aware that the elderly often have dental appliances such as partial plates or may have loose or decayed teeth that can obstruct the airway or be swallowed. |
| Tissue perfusion, altered, r/t aging cardiovascular system | Administer intravenous fluids as ordered, but note that elderly patients are vulnerable to fluid overload and that compensatory mechanisms may be compromised by age. Anticipate invasive circulatory monitoring in any elderly patient who is critically injured. |
| Thermoregulation ineffective r/t aging | Keep the patient warm by covering him or her with blankets, because the elderly lose heat easily, but do not obscure observation of injuries. Use head wraps and warming blankets as indicated; consider warming fluids where possible. Hypothermia reduces the chance of successful resuscitation. |
| Verbal communication impairment r/t aging | Allow the patient ample time for response; intelligence does not decrease with age, but the speed of thought processing does (Sheehy & Jimmerson, 1994). Face the patient; speak slowly and clearly; use short, simple phrases; and ask yes or no questions. Do not shout. |
| Cardiac output, decreased, r/t reduced stroke volume due to aging or trauma | Monitor electrocardiogram, and administer treatment as ordered for life-threatening arrhythmias. Administer oxygen. Note that the elderly often take cardiotonic agents such as beta-blockers that may diminish the body's sympathetic response to trauma. |

Note.—This is a sample of potential nursing diagnoses. It is not presented as or intended to be a complete care plan for the trauma patient. More complete information can be found in a medical-surgical nursing course and textbook. r/t = related to.

Adapted from Sparks, S. and Taylor, C. M. *Nursing diagnosis reference manual,* Springhouse, PA: Springhouse Corp., 1991, and Chitwood, L. *Ambulatory patient care,* San Diego: Western Schools, 1994.

will have considerable impact on the management of and recovery from the trauma.

• Be aware that hip fractures sometimes cause so little pain that elderly patients may even deny that the injury exists.

• Identify yourself to the patient, and stay at the patient's eye level when possible. Use gestures and facial expressions to enhance what you are saying. Speak in low tones, and use short sentences (Jubeck, 1994).

• Reassure the patient often, and offer frequent explanations. Disorientation and confusion are more common in the elderly than in younger persons.

- When possible, transport the patient to a high-risk facility that has complete geriatric and social services.

- Do not allow the patient to eat or drink until he or she is seen by a physician. Immediate surgical intervention may be indicated, and oral intake increases the risk of fatal aspiration during intubation or anesthesia.

- Be aware that an elderly patient may turn violent; this violence is often unexpected because of the patient's age. Trauma, hypoxia, and pain can cause elderly patients to become combative and agitated. Recommendations include not turning your back on a potentially violent patient and not taking on more than you can handle (Williams & Powers, 1994).

# ABUSE OF THE ELDERLY

Although child abuse has spawned volumes of research, abuse of the elderly has only recently been exposed. Sadly, abuse of the elderly likely will increase as our population ages. For the purpose of this discussion, abuse of the elderly is defined as deprivation of the necessities of life such as food or medical care; physical injury; and sexual, emotional, or physical maltreatment.

Abuse of the elderly can be difficult to discern and document because older persons are naturally more prone to falls and accidents. Triggering factors for abuse include the following (*Injury Prevention*, 1989):

- Impairment and physical dependence.

- Psychopathologic aspects of the abuser.

- Poor internal family dynamics.

- External stress such as poverty or unemployment.

- Demographic or social changes.

The typical abused elderly person is a white widow with limited income who lives with relatives and is perceived as a source of stress to them. Abused elderly live with their abuser in 75% of cases (*Injury Prevention*, 1989).

To date, no comprehensive programs have been developed to detect conclusively and prevent abuse of the elderly. Recommendations include public education programs to increase awareness and reporting of abuse, school education programs to dispel myths about aging, and community projects to help families meet the needs of their elderly members.

If you suspect that an elderly patient was abused, do the following:

- Notify the authorities and let them sort out the facts. Many metropolitan areas have teams with special training and skills to manage this situation.

- Transport the patient to the hospital for further evaluation of the injuries, even if under other circumstances the injuries would not seem to warrant further care.

- Do not divulge your suspicions to anyone other than the appropriate authorities. This is privileged medical information, and the family has a right to privacy.

- Keep accurate records, and document your findings and actions.

- Report your suspicions if you are in doubt, so a professional counselor and investigator can make the final determination.

# SUMMARY

Because mortality from accidental injury is higher in older persons, understanding the special needs of elderly trauma patients enhances the probability of a good outcome. Most of the changes that occur with aging mean limited reserves and a reduced margin of error.

# CRITICAL CONCEPTS

- Many of the changes that occur with aging diminish the body's ability to respond to the challenge of trauma.

- The death rate associated with motor vehicle accidents is higher for the elderly than for other age groups, partly because of the medical complications that often follow trauma.

- Treating the elderly means greater attention to detail because the margin of error is less than with younger patients.

- Fractures are common in elderly trauma patients, and these fractures are often serious, with prolonged healing phases.

- The elderly may survive the initial traumatic injury but then succumb to medical complications from the trauma.

- Ask the authorities to investigate trauma in the elderly that may have been inflicted intentionally.

# GLOSSARY

**Elderly abuse:** Deprivation of the necessities of life such as food or medical care; physical injury; and sexual, emotional, or physical maltreatment.

# EXAM QUESTIONS

## Chapter 14

## Questions 66 - 71

66. The leading causes of death in the elderly are:

    a   Heart disease, pulmonary failure, stroke, and accidents
    b.  Heart disease, cancer, stroke, and accidents
    c.  Cancer, heart failure, kidney failure, and stroke
    d.  Smoking, blood diseases, accidents, and hip fractures

67. The prevalence of which of the following increases dramatically after age 55?

    a.  Coma
    b.  Sepsis
    c.  Fractures
    d.  Stroke

68. Which of the following is more common in elderly trauma patients than in younger trauma patients?

    a.  Complete recovery
    b.  Spinal fracture
    c.  Cardiac arrest
    d.  Medical complications

69. The most common fracture in the elderly is of the:

    a.  Humerus
    b.  Hip
    c.  Tibia
    d.  Lumbar vertebrae

70. A common potential nursing diagnosis for an elderly trauma patient is:

    a.  Defensive coping
    b.  Thermoregulation, ineffective
    c.  Parental role conflict
    d.  Fluid volume excess

71. Which of the following is characteristic of most abused elderly patients?

    a.  They are assaulted by strangers.
    b.  They live with their abuser.
    c.  They are injured when attempting to fight back.
    d.  They are killed by their abuser.

# CHAPTER 15

# OBSTETRIC AND GYNECOLOGIC TRAUMA

## CHAPTER OBJECTIVE

After completing this chapter, the reader should be able to specify the normal alterations in anatomy and physiology that occur during pregnancy, recognize common causes of obstetric and gynecologic trauma, and select nursing diagnoses and initiate nursing care for trauma patients who are pregnant. The reader should also be able to recognize trauma caused by sexual assault and plan intervention for female victims of sexual assault.

## LEARNING OBJECTIVES

After studying this chapter, the reader should be able to

1. Recognize common obstetric trauma.

2. Specify the rationale for using cricoid pressure when artificial ventilation is required in a pregnant trauma patient.

3. Recognize changes in anatomy and physiology that occur with pregnancy.

4. Indicate common nursing diagnoses for persons who have been sexually assaulted.

5. Indicate common nursing diagnoses for patients with obstetric trauma.

## INTRODUCTION

Injury in a pregnant patient is "trauma for two" (Coursin, 1993). The goal of trauma care for pregnant patients is to reduce mortality and morbidity for both mother and infant by maintaining the mother's oxygenation and perfusion. This chapter presents two different types of trauma unique to women: obstetric trauma and gynecologic trauma. Gynecologic trauma often is caused by violent sexual assault, and other types of injuries may be present also. The sensitivity displayed by the nurse and others involved in providing care will have a dramatic effect on the pregnant patient's psychologic and emotional recovery. Although males also are assaulted sexually, this chapter covers trauma unique to females, because females are the most frequent victims. It discusses sexual assault as the primary form of gynecologic trauma, but gynecologic trauma also can be caused by falls, straddle injuries, and motor vehicle accidents. The chapter also describes alterations in normal anatomy and physiology that occur during pregnancy and presents potential nursing diagnoses and interventions for patients with gynecologic and obstetric trauma.

# NORMAL ALTERATIONS IN ANATOMY AND PHYSIOLOGY DURING PREGNANCY

Both the anatomy and physiology of the female change during pregnancy. Most of these changes are the body's adaptations to preserve and nurture the developing fetus. An awareness of these changes is essential when care is provided to the pregnant trauma patient. Figure 15-1 shows the fetus in utero. Table 15-1 summarizes the physiologic alterations that occur during pregnancy.

## Cardiovascular and Hematologic Changes

Cardiovascular changes can be quite dramatic during pregnancy. Most are designed to meet the needs of the developing fetus and to sustain the mother through a normal blood loss of about 500 ml during routine vaginal delivery and 1 L during cesarean delivery.

**Cardiac output.** Cardiac output increases by about 40% as a result of the increased stroke volume and increased heart rate (Bonica, 1980). The sacral veins are engorged, making the pregnant patient more prone to life-threatening hemorrhage from a pelvic fracture.

**Blood pressure.** The systolic blood pressure dips, usually to 5-15 mm Hg below nonpregnant levels. Some pathologic conditions of pregnancy, such as preeclampsia, cause an increase in blood pressure.

**Heart rate.** The heart rate increases 15-20 beats per minute.

**Hematocrit.** The number of red cells increases, but the hematocrit actually decreases because of the dilutional effect of the increased plasma volume.

**Clotting.** The blood has an increased tendency to clot, which helps protect against blood loss but also increases the risk of clots in the bloodstream.

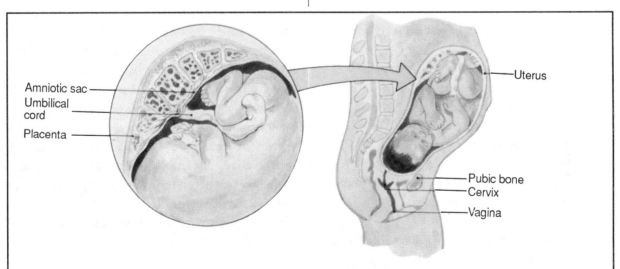

Amniotic sac
Umbilical cord
Placenta
Uterus
Pubic bone
Cervix
Vagina

**Figure 15-1. The structures of pregnancy.** Reprinted by permission from Grant, H. D., Murray, R. H., Jr., & Bergeron, J. D. (Eds.). Brady emergency care (5th ed.). Englewood Cliffs, NJ: Prentice-Hall, 1990, p. 437.

## Table 15-1

### Physiologic Alterations in Pregnancy

**Cardiovascular**
Cardiac output increases by 1–2 L/min
Pulse increases 15–20 beats/per minute
Systolic blood pressure decreases 5–15 mm Hg

**Respiratory**
Hypocarbia ($pCO_2 = 30$ mm Hg)
secondary to increased tidal volume and
minute ventilation

**Hematologic**
Hematocrit increases 30–35%
Plasma volume increases by up to 50%

**Gastrointestinal**
Delayed gastric emptying

## Respiratory Changes

Pregnancy causes dramatic changes in the anatomy and physiology of the respiratory system (Bonica, 1980).

**Diaphragm.** As the fetus grows, the uterus rises out of the pelvis and displaces the diaphragm upward by about 4 cm. Total lung volume is slightly decreased.

**Air passages.** The air passages become engorged from the increased blood flow. The mucosa may be swollen and edematous, making intubation of the trachea difficult. Intense bleeding may occur from placement of a nasal airway.

**Respiratory rate.** The respiratory rate increases.

**Oxygen consumption.** Oxygen consumption and basal metabolism increase to meet the needs of the fetus. Hypoxia develops rapidly in a pregnant patient.

**Carbon dioxide concentration.** The $pCO_2$ is decreased because of the increased ventilation rate.

## Gastrointestinal Changes

As the uterus expands, it displaces the stomach and intestines. Gastric emptying is delayed, putting the patient at increased risk for aspiration pneumonia.

## Renal Changes

Renal blood flow and the glomerular filtration rate increase.

## Uterine Changes

The uterus, normally the size and shape of a pear, expands as the fetus grows. The nonpregnant uterus receives about 2% of the cardiac output and has a capacity of about 2 ml; the gravid uterus consumes about 20% of the cardiac output (Campbell, 1988) and contains about 1 L of amniotic fluid.

Because conception and gestation necessarily have specific terminology, commonly used terms are reviewed here.

**Amniotic sac.** The amniotic sac is the membrane that holds the fluid in which the fetus floats. The sac and fluid are commonly called the "bag of water."

**Amniotic fluid.** The fluid contained within the amniotic sac is called the amniotic fluid.

**Fetus.** The fetus is the developing human offspring that begins as an embryo. An embryo becomes a fetus after about 8 weeks' gestation.

**Gestation.** Gestation is the time from conception to birth, or the duration of pregnancy. It normally lasts 38-40 weeks. Fetuses have survived intact when born as early as 24-26 weeks of gestation.

**Gravid.** Pregnant.

**Placenta.** Commonly referred to as the afterbirth, the placenta is a structure that embeds in the wall of the uterus and provides metabolic exchange (e.g., oxygen, carbon dioxide, and nutrients) between the mother and the fetus.

**Parturient.** A woman in childbirth.

**Umbilical cord.** The umbilical cord is composed of three vessels that exchange blood between the fetus and the mother. It is covered by a gelatinous substance.

# MECHANISM OF INJURY

The most common cause of trauma in pregnant women is motor vehicle accidents. Other common causes are falls, penetrating injuries, domestic violence, and burns or smoke inhalation (Sheehy & Jimmerson, 1994). Trauma in a pregnant patient can result in injury to both the patient and the fetus, although the risks vary according to the stage of gestation. Pregnant women experience trauma more frequently than nonpregnant women do; estimates are that trauma complicates 6-7% of all pregnancies (Campbell, 1988). Relatively minor mishaps and trauma that occur during the early stages of pregnancy include injuries caused by fainting or fatigue. Injuries associated with full-term pregnancy include falls from imbalance caused by the gravid uterus.

During the first trimester, the fetus is not often injured directly because the uterus is still relatively small and shielded by the bony pelvis. However, the fetus is vulnerable to hypoxia and hypotension caused by injuries sustained by the mother. During the third trimester, the uterus and fetus, which have risen up out of the pelvis, more often are injured directly.

Blunt trauma from rapid forward deceleration as in a head-on motor vehicle accident directs energy through the abdomen of the pregnant patient and compresses the abdominal contents against her spinal column. During the third trimester, this deadly force can rupture the uterus or separate the placenta from the wall of the uterus. Either injury can result in massive hemorrhage and the death of both the mother and the fetus. Any trauma strong enough to fracture the maternal pelvis often fractures the fetal skull also. In pregnant patients, blunt trauma most often is incurred in a motor vehicle accident or caused by a blow to the abdomen; some women do not wear seat belts because of a misguided concern for the fetus. However, the most common cause of death in pregnant women injured in motor vehicle accidents is head trauma (Campbell, 1988), a complication usually prevented by use of seat belts with shoulder harnesses. The prevalence of head, neck, and chest trauma is even lower in vehicles equipped with air bags.

Penetrating trauma in pregnant patients most often is caused by gunshots or knives. Whether the fetus is harmed depends on the point of contact and the stage of pregnancy. As the uterus grows, the stomach and small intestines are displaced upward and backward, so the uterus provides the mother some protection against penetrating abdominal trauma. According to Fabian and Patterson (1985), multiple organ injuries from gunshots occur less frequently in pregnant women than in nonpregnant women. However, the fetus often is wounded because the mother's internal organs are displaced behind the uterus. The fetal mortality rate in penetrating trauma to the uterus is 70%.

# ASSESSMENT OF PATIENTS WITH OBSTETRIC OR GYNECOLOGIC TRAUMA

The assessment of any pregnant trauma patient should follow the standard ABC plan. Evaluate the airway, breathing, and circulation as in any trauma patient. Special concerns in assessing patients who have gynecologic trauma are mentioned later.

Observe the scene of the accident and elicit a history of the injury while assessing the patient. Information from those at the trauma scene can provide clues about the injury and help guide the assessment.

Because the most common cause of fetal death during trauma is maternal death (Campbell, 1988), the first goal is to decrease the mortality and morbidity of both mother and child by maintaining the mother's oxygenation and perfusion. Plan to support the mother's respiration and circulation, prevent aspiration, and transport her to a hospital with obstetric facilities. When possible, assess the condition of the fetus and the placental circulation by feeling for fetal movement and listening for fetal heart tones.

Also, it is helpful to know the following:

- The duration of the pregnancy or the due date.

- Whether this is the first, second, or other pregnancy.

- Any known complications of the pregnancy.

- Any abnormal medical conditions such as hypertension, diabetes, or heart disease.

- The patient's normal blood pressure and resting pulse rate.

Signs of serious obstetric trauma include the following:

- **Hypovolemic shock:** A pregnant patient generally has a lower blood pressure and a faster pulse rate than a nonpregnant woman. Pregnant patients are also well prepared to withstand blood loss, so hemorrhage may be significant before signs and symptoms are evident. However, by term, a pregnant patient is experiencing nearly maximal cardiac output and has little ability to compensate further in the event of hypovolemia (Sheehy & Jimmerson, 1994).

- **Taut, firm fundus:** The fundus of the uterus generally cannot be palpated until the second trimester, but it should feel relatively soft. If the uterus is filled with blood, it will feel firm, or even literally "hard as a board." The fundus also feels firm during labor contractions.

- **Vaginal bleeding:** Flow of blood from the vagina may indicate separation of the placenta from the wall of the uterus or penetration or rupture of the uterus. All are ominous conditions for the fetus.

- **Decreased fetal heart rate and movement:** Although it is difficult to detect fetal heart tones by auscultation without a special fetal stethoscope, it is sometimes possible to place a standard stethoscope over the mother's abdomen and hear the fetal heartbeat. Place your hands on the mother's abdomen to feel for fetal movement. Assess fetal heart rate and movement at regular intervals in order to establish a baseline against which any changes can be compared.

Signs of gynecologic trauma include the following:

- **Vaginal bleeding:** Vaginal bleeding can be caused by blunt trauma between the legs or uterine or abdominal trauma. The rectum, urethra, and bladder also can be injured by blunt or penetrating trauma inflicted during an assault or accident.

- **Swelling of the vulva and perineum:** Blunt trauma to the external genital tract can cause pain, swelling, bleeding, and hematomas.

- **Lacerations:** Lacerations of the external genital tract, vulva, perineum, cervix, uterus, bladder, urethra, and internal organs can be caused by gynecologic trauma. Bleeding can be profuse and can be life threatening, depending on the extent of the injury.

# COMMON OBSTETRIC TRAUMA

As discussed before, the fetus is well protected and usually does not suffer direct trauma until the third trimester of pregnancy, when the uterus is enlarged and vulnerable. Most obstetric trauma is relatively minor, but serious trauma calls for swift detection of problems and quick interventions. Also, women are more frequently abused when pregnant, so health care providers should be wary of suspicious injuries. Serious obstetric trauma includes the following:

## Uterine Rupture

Blunt trauma from a motor vehicle accident or a blow or kick to the abdomen may cause compression and subsequent rupture of the uterus. Bleeding will be severe, and both maternal and fetal mortality are high.

## Placental Separation

Blunt trauma can cause separation of the placenta from the uterus. This is known as abruptio placentae and is heralded by bleeding and abdominal pain. Mortality and morbidity are related to the degree of separation and the time between separation and delivery of the infant. Blood can also collect between the placenta and the wall of the uterus (Figure 15-2), so minimal vaginal bleeding may be noted although serious blood loss occurs.

## Gunshot or Stab Wounds

Penetration of the gravid uterus by a projectile exposes the fetus to direct injury by contact with the object or indirect injury as a result of maternal injury. Surgery for both mother and child is often necessary to repair damage.

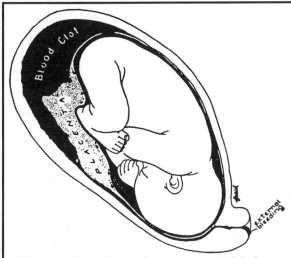

**Figure 15-2. Abruptio placentae with large blood clot between placenta and uterine wall**. Reprinted by permission from Reeder, S., Mastroianni, L., Jr., Martin, L. L., and Fitzpatrick, E. *Maternity nursing* (13th ed.). Philadelphia: Lippincott, 1976.

### Pelvic Fracture

Blunt trauma can fracture the pelvis of the mother and the skull or other bones of the fetus. Trauma of sufficient force to fracture the maternal pelvis often damages the fetus, too. Blood loss in pelvic fracture is generally significant and may affect oxygen delivery to the fetus.

### Impalement

The gravid uterus and protruding abdomen may be more prone to impalement injuries. Both mother and fetus may sustain internal injuries.

# NURSING STRATEGIES FOR PATIENTS WITH OBSTETRIC TRAUMA

The first goal for any patient with obstetric trauma is to maintain the airway, breathing, and circulation. Table 15-2 gives potential nursing diagnoses and interventions for the care of patients with obstetric trauma. The following nursing strategies may also be useful. It is presumed with each that airway, breathing, and circulation are already established. Your interventions should be within the scope of your professional license; commensurate with your skills and training; consistent with your state's nurse practice act; and when performed in a health care institution, adherent to that facility's standards of practice.

- Administer a high concentration of oxygen to the mother to increase the amount of oxygen delivered to the fetus.

- Evaluate uterine muscle tone by palpating the fundus at regular intervals to determine the onset of labor or uterine rigidity that could indicate bleeding. Monitor fetal heart rate when possible.

- Monitor the patient for vaginal bleeding, which may be sudden, severe, and initially hidden by blankets or clothing. Protect the patient's privacy and dignity during this assessment.

- Do not put anything into the vagina of a pregnant trauma patient. Do not perform a vaginal or pelvic examination unless you have special training and skills in obstetric nursing and the presence of excessive vaginal bleeding or other unusual signs indicate a pressing need. Pelvic examinations can introduce harmful microorganisms into the genital tract or aggravate existing injuries. Simply place a clean pad against the perineum and change it as necessary. Do not discard soiled pads; save them for the obstetrician who may want to examine any expelled tissue and use the pads to estimate blood or amniotic fluid loss.

- Ask another rescuer to apply cricoid pressure (Figure 15-4) if artificial ventilation becomes necessary; this is an effort to combat the potential for aspiration of gastric contents. A serious or fatal aspiration pneumonia that occurs in

**Table 15-2**

**Potential Nursing Diagnoses and Interventions for Patients with Obstetric Trauma**

| Diagnosis | Interventions |
|---|---|
| Gas exchange impairment r/t altered oxygen supply | Administer high concentrations of oxygen to the patient until directed otherwise by a physician. Displace the uterus to the patient's left to reduce aortocaval compression. Remember that intubation of pregnant patients may be difficult and be prepared to use alternative methods of airway management. |
| Fluid volume deficit r/t active loss | Administer intravenous fluids and medications as ordered to combat shock; estimate blood loss frequently. Remember that blood pressure is slightly lower and heart rate slightly higher in pregnancy. Displace the uterus to the patient's left to reduce aortocaval syndrome. Save perineal pads for the obstetrician. |
| Fear r/t concern for potential loss of pregnancy | Offer frequent reassurance and answer the patient's questions. Accept all questions as valid; do not minimize concerns. Reassure the patient that everything possible is being done for both her and her baby; do not offer false reassurances. Explain what you are doing, and accept the patient's feelings without judgment. |
| Suffocation, potential, r/t possible aspiration | Consider all obstetric patients to have a full stomach, and ask another rescuer to apply cricoid pressure if artificial ventilation becomes necessary. Maintain pressure until an endotracheal tube cuff is inflated, and you have verification that the tube is in the trachea. To avoid possible rupture of the esophagus or stomach, release the cricoid pressure if the patient begins to vomit or retch. |
| Cardiac output, decreased, r/t mechanical obstruction | Guard against supine hypotensive syndrome (aortocaval compression) in which the gravid uterus compresses the aorta and vena cava (Figure 15-3), because this can reduce blood flow. Displace the uterus to the patient's left side. |
| Injury, potential, r/t radiographs or medications | Inform all caregivers of the patient's pregnancy. Avoid administration of teratogenic drugs such as benzodiazepines. Avoid radiographs when possible; shield pelvis and abdomen with lead apron when possible. |

Note.—This is a sample of potential nursing diagnoses. It is not presented as or intended to be a complete care plan for the trauma patient. More complete information can be found in a medical-surgical nursing course and textbook. r/t = related to.

Adapted from Sparks, S. and Taylor, C. M. *Nursing diagnosis reference manual,* Springhouse, PA: Springhouse Corp., 1991, and Chitwood, L., *Ambulatory patient care,* San Diego: Western Schools, 1994.

pregnant patients was first identified by Mendelson in 1946 and can occur from inhalation of as little as 25 ml of gastric secretions (Shnider and Levinson, 1979). Pressure on the cricoid cartilage will compress the esophagus and help prevent reflux of gastric contents into the lungs. However, anytime the patient begins to retch or vomit, the pressure should be released immediately, because rupture of the esophagus could occur. Cricoid pressure should be maintained until the trachea is effectively sealed from the esophagus by a cuffed tracheal tube.

- Begin fluid resuscitation as ordered, and transport the patient immediately to the hospital if uterine rupture, placental separation, or pelvic fracture is suspected. Be aware that pregnant patients generally require far more fluid in resuscitation than nonpregnant ones do (Coursin, 1993).

- If the patient has penetrating trauma, apply direct pressure to any sites of bleeding, begin fluid resuscitation, and transport her to the hospital immediately.

- Do not remove any object that has become lodged in the abdomen. Doing so could aggravate the injury and stimulate hemorrhage. Stabilize the object and transport the patient to a hospital immediately.

- Administer intravenous fluids as indicated to combat shock, but be aware that blood pressure is slightly lower during pregnancy and heart rate is normally higher, so detection of hypovolemic shock requires astute observation skills. In general, begin fluid therapy if you have any doubt about the patient's volume status; pregnant patients generally tolerate fluid load well.

- Guard against supine hypotension syndrome (aortocaval compression) that can occur in pregnant patients beginning about halfway through gestation. The syndrome occurs when the pregnant patient lies flat on her back and the gravid uterus compresses the aorta and vena cava (Figure 15-3). Fainting may occur in the mother, and fetal bradycardia may develop. For this reason, pregnant women are advised against lying supine after the 20th week of gestation. You can prevent this syndrome by displacing the uterus manually (push the uterus to the patient's left side to displace it from its position over the vena cava); propping up the right side of a spine board (to displace the uterus to the left) on which the patient has been secured; or, if she has no known spinal injury, instructing the patient to lie on her left side.

- Identify the fundus and mark the height with a pen on the patient's abdomen to assist in evaluating any changes that might be due to the uterus filling with blood.

- See Figure 15-5 for a diagram of emergency delivery.

- Be aware that sonograms and radiographs may be obtained of any pregnant trauma patient who arrives at a hospital or physician's office complaining of abdominal pain. Some forms of obstetric trauma may not have obvious external signs or symptoms, and ultrasound (sonography) can confirm the status of the placenta and fetus. X-rays are most harmful in the early stages of pregnancy. The risks must be weighed against the benefits when procedures that use x-rays are used to help diagnose trauma during pregnancy. When possible, shield the torso of the pregnant patient (or patient of childbearing age) with a lead apron.

- Transport pregnant patients who have moderate to severe injuries to a level 1 trauma facility or to a hospital with high-risk perinatal facilities whenever possible. All equipment and staff nec-

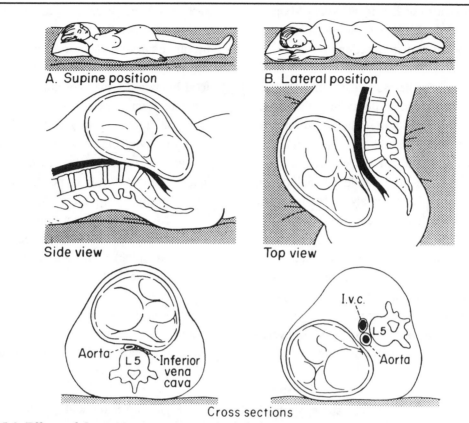

A. Supine position

B. Lateral position

Side view

Top view

Aorta — L 5 — Inferior vena cava

I.V.C. — L 5 — Aorta

Cross sections

**Figure 15-3. Effects of the pregnant uterus on the inferior vena cava (I.V.C.) and the aorta in the supine (A) and lateral (B) positions.** Reprinted by permission from Bonica, J. J. (Ed.). *Obstetric analgesia and anesthesia* (2nd ed. rev.). Amsterdam: World Federation of Societies of Anesthesiologists, 1980.

essary to care for the patient and a high-risk newborn should be in place at these facilities.

• Continue CPR even if the patient appears to be mortally wounded; it is slightly possible that the infant might survive after emergency cesarean delivery. In some cases, an immediate postmortem cesarean delivery may even be performed in the emergency department or trauma suite in an effort to save the fetus.

• Be aware that when trauma causes the death of the fetus, spontaneous vaginal delivery of the dead fetus usually occurs within hours. If trauma damages the uterus, surgeons usually make every effort to preserve the uterus and future fertility.

• Question all female trauma patients of childbearing age about the possibility of pregnancy,

because radiographs and medications given during treatment could have a teratogenic effect on a fetus.

• Intubation may be difficult because of engorgement and edema of the airway structures. Trauma professionals may find it necessary to access the trachea directly by incising the neck if the first few attempts at intubation are not successful.

• Do not allow the patient to eat or drink until she is seen by an obstetrician or gynecologist. Immediate surgical intervention may be indicated, and oral intake increases the risk of a fatal aspiration during the perioperative period.

• Offer explanations and reassurances to the patient as you work even if she appears to be un-

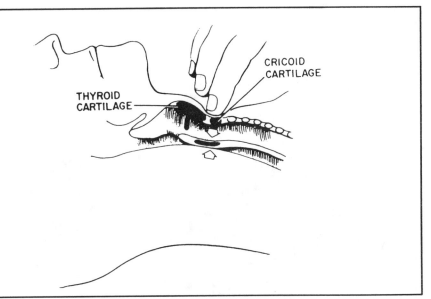

**Figure 15-4. Using posterior pressure on the cricoid cartilage to occlude the esophagus can be effective in blocking regurgitation but not active vomiting.** Reprinted by permission from Hamelberg, W., and Bosomworth, P. B. *Aspiration pneumonitis.* Springfield, IL: Charles C Thomas, 1968.

conscious. Hearing may be present, and high levels of anxiety accompany accidents and assaults.

- Reassure the patient that everything possible is being done for both her and her baby. Trauma in pregnant patients distresses patients and their families, who fear for the life of both the mother and the baby.

# NURSING STRATEGIES FOR PATIENTS WITH GYNECOLOGIC TRAUMA

Common gynecologic trauma is seen in straddle injuries, some types of falls, and sexual assault. Gynecologic trauma sustained during sexual assault requires special expertise and finesse on the part of the rescuer. According to Vachss (1993), police reports indicate that a woman is raped every six minutes in the United States. Consequently, the probability of providing care to a victim of a sexual assault is increasing. Juveniles are increasingly affected: A 1992 study of 11 states by the Justice Department (Thomas, 1994) found that 10,000 female rape victims were less than 18 years old; at least 3,800 of those were less than 12 years old. Most (46%) of these children were attacked by their relatives (Thomas, 1994). Experts also think that a substantial number of attacks go unreported.

Sexual assault is many women's most dreaded nightmare; as the rescuer, your actions and comments can have enormous influence on the patient's recovery. For any person who has been sexually assaulted, follow the ABCs and manage life- and limb-threatening injuries first. Once those injuries are controlled, or if serious injuries do not exist, begin intervention to reduce the patient's emotional distress and evaluate any minor gynecologic trauma. Many cities and hospitals have specially trained nurses or clinicians who examine the patient; gather evidence; administer treatment, including prophylaxis and specific therapy for sexually transmitted diseases; and refer the patient for follow-up support and counseling.

Table 15-3 gives potential nursing diagnoses and interventions for patients with gynecologic trauma. The following strategies may also be useful. Your interventions should be within the scope of your professional license; commensurate with your skills and training; consistent with your state's nurse practice act; and when performed in a health care institution, adherent to that facility's standards of practice.

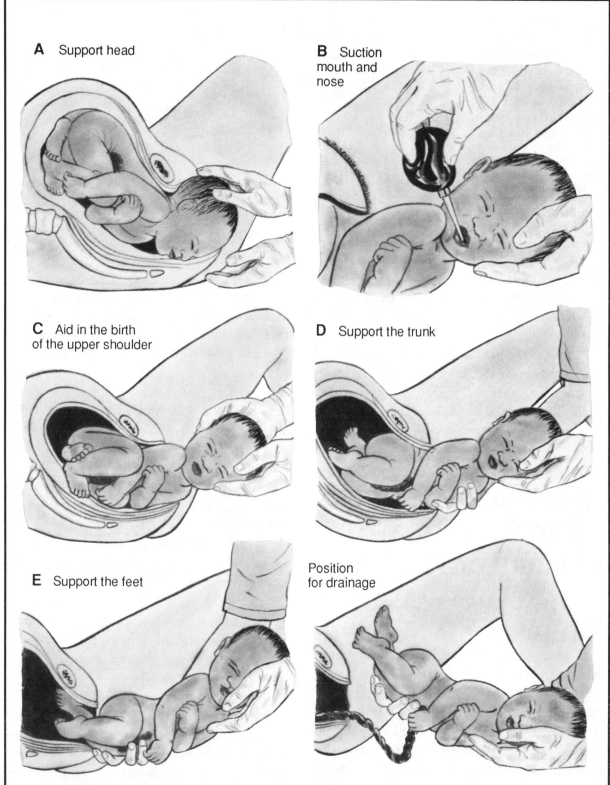

A   Support head

B   Suction mouth and nose

C   Aid in the birth of the upper shoulder

D   Support the trunk

E   Support the feet

Position for drainage

**NOTE:**   Assist the mother by supporting the baby throughout the entire birth process.

**Figure 15-5. Emergency delivery.** Reprinted by permission from Grant, H. D., Murray, R. H., Jr., & Bergeron, J. D. (Eds.). *Brady emergency care* (5th ed.). Englewood Cliffs, NJ: Prentice-Hall, 1990.

## Table 15-3

## Potential Nursing Diagnoses and Interventions for Patients with Gynecologic Trauma

| Diagnosis | Interventions |
|---|---|
| Posttrauma response r/t assault | Provide the patient with psychological support; do not leave her alone. Reorient her as necessary, speak softly, and reassure her frequently that she is safe now. Avoid care-related activities and stimuli that may intensify anxiety or stimulate fear. Offer to call support persons such as a minister, friends, family members, or a counselor. Allow the patient to express her feelings such as anger or fear; listen without offering judgments. Provide privacy. |
| Rape-trauma syndrome | Follow medical and institutional protocols to manage physical injuries and protect the patient's health and legal rights. Provide emotional support and be available to listen. Accept the patient's feelings as valid. Provide her with privacy during the examination and interview by police; protect confidentiality. Ensure the patient's safety by taking whatever measures are necessary to secure it. Refer her to appropriate support groups, such as sexual assault recovery groups. |
| Powerlessness | Accept as normal the feelings of powerlessness of anyone who has been sexually assaulted, because rape is about domination and power, not sex. Be present during this time and tell the patient you can be powerful for her until she feels stronger. Remind her that she is safe. Explain all impending events so she has no surprises. Modify the environment when possible to make the patient feel more in control or safer. Identify and accommodate her spiritual needs. |
| Family process alteration r/t incest | Report sexual assaults to the authorities as required by law. Explain to the person assaulted that incest is never his or her fault; it is a crime, not a punishment, and is therefore the responsibility of the perpetrator. Arrange for and participate in family conferences to facilitate effective family coping. Act as an advocate for the incest victim. |
| Self-esteem, situational low | A person who is raped often feels ashamed and humiliated. Explain to the patient that she was not at fault, that nothing about her has changed. Assess her mental status through communication and observation. Provide her with positive feedback for verbal reports and behaviors that indicate a return to a positive self-appraisal. Refer her to a counselor, minister, social service agency, and support groups. |

Note.—This is a sample of potential nursing diagnoses. It is not presented as or intended to be a complete care plan for the trauma patient. More complete information can be found in a medical-surgical nursing course and textbook. r/t = related to.

Adapted from Sparks, S. and Taylor, C. M. *Nursing diagnosis reference manual*, Springhouse, PA: Springhouse Corp., 1991, and Chitwood, L., *Ambulatory patient care*, San Diego: Western Schools, 1994.

- Get the patient to a place of safety and protect her privacy and confidentiality. Do not leave her alone; persons who have been sexually assaulted are frequently emotionally distraught, and their behavior may be unpredictable. The patient also may be afraid that the attacker will return.

- Do not examine the patient at the trauma scene unless a condition such as obvious excessive vaginal bleeding or complaints of pain lead you to believe she has a serious injury. Examination at the scene is emotionally distressing to the patient, is unnecessary in most cases, and may spoil valuable forensic evidence needed for prosecution of the attacker.

- Do not catheterize the patient unless absolutely necessary; catheterization may destroy evidence and aggravate injuries.

- Know beforehand your facility's policy on the care and treatment of persons who have been sexually assaulted. This helps avoid delays in the patient's care and ensures that protocols are followed in the collection of forensic evidence.

- Discourage the patient from brushing her teeth, urinating or defecating, bathing, washing her hands, changing her clothes, or eating or drinking. Her body cavities will be examined and swabbed for possible collection of evidence, and her clothing will be needed by the police for examination. Eating or drinking could destroy evidence and, if surgery is necessary, increase the patient's chances of serious complications under anesthesia. You cannot, however, force the patient to comply with your instructions.

- Provide support and empathy. Do not, simply out of curiosity, quiz the patient about the exact events surrounding the assault. This may deepen her emotional distress and make her feel as if she is being judged by the circumstances of the attack.

# SUMMARY

Trauma for two is the challenge in caring for a patient with obstetric trauma. The goal is to reduce mortality and morbidity for both the mother and the fetus by maintaining the mother's oxygenation and perfusion. Gynecologic trauma often occurs during sexual assault, and other injuries may be present also. The sensitivity displayed by those involved in caring for a patient who has been sexually assaulted will have a dramatic effect on the patient's psychologic and emotional recovery from the trauma.

# CRITICAL CONCEPTS

- A patient who is pregnant is at an increased risk of aspiration pneumonia because of delayed gastric emptying and other changes that occur during pregnancy. Apply cricoid pressure during manual ventilation until a tracheal tube with an inflated cuff is in place.

- With pregnant trauma patients, assess and stabilize the airway, breathing, and circulation first, because the patient will not survive without oxygenation and perfusion.

- Displace the gravid uterus with manual pressure or by tilting the spine board to the left to prevent aortocaval compression, which could impair blood circulation in both mother and fetus.

- Continue CPR of a pregnant patient even if she appears to be mortally wounded. It is slightly possible that the fetus might survive after an emergency cesarean delivery.

- Be aware that your actions and comments will have a dramatic effect on any patient's psychologic and emotional recovery from sexual assault.

# GLOSSARY

**Aortocaval syndrome:** Compression of the aorta and vena cava by the gravid uterus. Compression impedes circulation, which can cause supine hypotension syndrome.

**Abruptio placentae:** Partial or complete premature separation of the placenta from the uterine wall; may be the result of trauma.

**Cricoid pressure:** Pressure applied over the cricoid cartilage in the neck for the purpose of reducing the prevalence of aspiration of stomach contents during artificial ventilation or intubation.

**Rape-trauma syndrome:** The physical and emotional trauma that occurs as a result of sexual assault. Emotional reactions such as anger, embarrassment, fear, humiliation, and self-blame are common. Multiple physical signs and symptoms are also often noted, such as genitourinary discomfort, gastrointestinal upset, and sleep disturbances (Sparks & Taylor, 1991).

**Uterine rupture:** Bursting of the uterus. In obstetric trauma, uterine rupture most often occurs in response to severe blunt abdominal trauma in the last trimester of pregnancy and is a grave event, with significant morbidity and mortality.

# EXAM QUESTIONS

## Chapter 15

### Questions 72 - 76

72. A common nursing diagnosis for a patient with obstetric trauma might be:

    a. Cardiac output, decreased
    b. Mobility impairment
    c. Role performance alteration
    d. Sexuality pattern alteration

73. Cricoid pressure is applied in pregnant trauma patients in hopes of preventing:

    a. Hypovolemia
    b. Aspiration
    c. Cervical spine injury
    d. Hemorrhage

74. You are at a stop light when a car swerves through the intersection, striking another car head on. You get out and find an unrestrained near-term pregnant female behind the steering wheel, clutching her abdomen. Blood is rapidly staining her slacks and dripping down the seat, and she is moaning about severe abdominal pain. Which of the following injuries is most likely?

    a. Placenta previa
    b. Rupture of the amniotic sac
    c. Bladder perforation
    d. Uterine rupture

75. A common nursing diagnosis for a patient who has been sexually assaulted might be:

    a. Powerlessness
    b. Self-esteem, chronic low
    c. Health maintenance alteration
    d. Noncompliance

76. Which of the following are common physiologic changes during pregnancy?

    a. Decreased plasma volume and higher hematocrit
    b. Increased cardiac output and decreased blood pressure
    c. Decreased heart rate and delayed blood clotting
    d. Decreased renal blood flow

# CHAPTER 16

# PEDIATRIC TRAUMA

## CHAPTER OBJECTIVE

After completing this chapter, the reader should be able to specify the normal anatomy and physiology of infants and children, recognize common causes of trauma in this age group, and select nursing diagnoses and plan interventions for infants and children with trauma.

## LEARNING OBJECTIVES

After studying this chapter, the reader should be able to

1. Recognize the yearly incidence of reported child abuse in the United States.

2. Recognize normal physiologic parameters in infants and children.

3. Select the most common cause of trauma in children.

## INTRODUCTION

Knowledge of the basics of trauma care for infants and children is essential to nurses because injury is the leading cause of death in this age group. Between 800,000 and 1 million admissions for major trauma each year are infants and children (Sheehy & Jimmerson, 1994). According to the Justice Department, the most common victims of violent crime in the United States are young people 12-17 years old (Thomas, 1994). These children are raped, robbed, and assaulted five times as often as adults 35 years and over.

Basic trauma nursing skills are complicated even more by the fact that the injured person is an infant or a child; many nurses find themselves flooded with emotions ranging from sorrow and pity to anger when they are confronted with a traumatized infant or child. Yet, most nurses will be asked to intervene with an injured infant or child at some point in their careers. This chapter is designed to help develop the knowledge and skills necessary to meet the challenge of caring for such patients. The primary goals in caring for infants and children with trauma are to preserve the patient's life and transfer the infant or child to a pediatric trauma facility in order to reduce mortality and morbidity. A secondary goal is to provide emotional support for the parents.

This chapter reviews the normal anatomy and physiology of infants and children and describes common types of trauma in this age group. It also describes nursing strategies for the care of infants and children with trauma and discusses issues of child abuse.

# NORMAL ANATOMY AND PHYSIOLOGY IN INFANTS AND CHILDREN

Children and infants are not miniature adults. Anatomic and physiologic differences exist between the bodies of infants and children and adults. For example, the nares (nostrils) of a child are narrow; thus, use of a nasal airway is inappropriate in most cases. Some of the common differences between adults and infants and children are described here. Terms used include *neonate,* a newborn infant in the first 30 days of life, and *infant,* a child in the first year of life.

## Cardiovascular Differences

Unless he or she was born with a congenital heart defect, a child's heart is generally healthy and strong, so cardiogenic sources of shock are seldom seen as they are in adults.

**Blood volume.** Because of their smaller size, children can afford to lose less blood before shock and death result. Thus, an injury that might not cause shock in an adult, such as a scalp laceration, can cause shock and hypotension in a child. With a blood volume of about 80 ml/kg, a 10-month-old infant weighing 8 kg (17.6 lb) would have a total blood volume of 640 ml. Injuries causing a hemorrhage of 40% and symptoms of shock would mean a blood loss of only 256 ml. This lower blood volume and smaller size of a child also reduce the margin of error when fluids and medications are administered.

**Blood pressure.** Blood pressure generally increases as a child grows older. Systolic pressures of 50-60 mm Hg are normal in a neonate but indicate hypotension in a school-age child. Table 16-1 gives the normal ranges for vital signs in children.

**Heart rate.** Normal heart rate in a neonate is 120-160 beats per minute, but the heart rate decreases as the child grows older. In general, the younger a child is, the higher the heart rate is.

## Respiratory Differences

**Airway.** A jaw thrust or chin lift will often open the airway in an infant or child. Because the nostrils are narrower than in an adult, nasal airways are not usually appropriate or effective for a child. An infant's neck is short, and the tongue is large. The cricoid ring

### Table 16-1
### Normal Ranges of Vital Signs in Children

| Age | Pulse (beats per minute) | Respiration (breaths/min) | Systolic Blood Pressure (mm Hg) |
|---|---|---|---|
| 0–2 months | 120–140 | 30–50 | 50–60 |
| 2 months–1 year | 110–130 | 25–40 | 70–80 |
| 1–3 years | 100–110 | 20–30 | 80 |
| 3–5 years | 90–100 | 20–30 | 80–90 |
| More than 5 years | 80–100 | 15–30 | 90–100 |

Reprinted by permission from Kitt, S., & Kaiser, J. *Emergency nursing: A physiologic and clinical perspective.* Philadelphia: Saunders, 1990.

is the narrowest part of the airway in an infant; the glottis is narrow.

**Respiratory rate.** Generally, the younger the child is, the higher the respiratory rate is.

**Thorax.** The chest wall of infants and children is compliant and quite flexible. Rib and sternal fractures are less common than in adults, but the organs and structures usually protected by the rib cage are more vulnerable to blunt trauma because of this elasticity of the chest wall.

## Metabolic Differences

Children have an elevated basal metabolic rate, making their oxygen requirements higher than those of the typical adult.

## Renal Differences

The kidneys in a neonate are often immature and unable to handle large shifts in volume.

## Thermoregulatory Differences

The thermoregulatory mechanisms in infants and children are not as well developed as those in adults, and infants and children are prone to hypothermia. With their large surface-to-mass ratio, children are less able to maintain their body temperature.

# MECHANISM OF INJURY

Children are most frequently injured in the summer months during the daylight hours. Almost half of all trauma in infants and children involves motor vehicle accidents in which the child is a pedestrian, bicyclist, or passenger. Head injury is the most common type of trauma. Seventy-five percent of infants and chil-

dren who have multiple trauma have head injuries (Kitt & Kaiser, 1990). Falls, especially from urban high-rise buildings, are the second most common cause of injury in infants and children.

According to Sheehy & Jimmerson (1994), penetrating trauma (12%) in infants and children is not nearly as common as blunt trauma (84%). Of children who die of trauma, 75% die at the scene. Most of these deaths are due to an obstructed airway; the remainder, to blood loss. The other 25% die at a hospital after central nervous system injury.

Penetrating trauma in infants and children is usually due to assault (gunshot wounds) or accidents (impalement). As mentioned in the introduction, juveniles are frequent victims of violent crime; 1.5 million violent crimes against juveniles were recorded in 1992 ("Violent Crime Hits Young," 1994). Campbell (1988) lists the following as mechanisms of severe injury in infants and children:

- Falls from 20 ft (6 m) or higher.
- Motor vehicle accidents with associated fatalities.
- Ejection from an automobile in a motor vehicle accident.
- Being hit by a car while bicycling or on foot.
- Fractures in more than one extremity.
- Significant injury to more than one system.

# ASSESSMENT OF TRAUMA IN INFANTS AND CHILDREN

Assessment of an infant or a child who has a traumatic injury should follow the standard ABC plan given in chapter 2. Evaluate the airway, breathing and circulation. Assessment may be hampered because the patient may be unable to cooperate or communicate with you, and parents or caretakers may lose control because of their own stress at seeing the infant or child injured.

Observe the scene of the accident and elicit a history of the injury while assessing the patient. Try to obtain information from the parent or bystanders. Information from those at the trauma scene can provide clues about the nature of the injury and help guide assessment. Knowledge of the patient's age and of any preexisting medical conditions is obviously helpful.

Signs of trauma to look for include the following:

- **Hypovolemic shock:** Blood pressure is generally lower in infants and children than in adults, and the pulse rate is usually faster. Although head injuries in adults seldom cause enough blood loss to result in hypovolemic shock, head injuries in an infant can result in blood loss severe enough to cause shock.

- **Loss of consciousness:** Any loss of consciousness should be viewed as serious, and the patient should be transported to a hospital immediately.

- **Obvious injuries with deformities:** Any obvious injuries such as abrasions, contusions, avulsions, lacerations, and fractures should be evaluated by a pediatrician.

- **Respiratory distress:** Newborns may make grunting sounds on expiration; the ribs may seem to be drawn deeply in on inspiration in a phenomenon called retractions. Flaring of the nostrils may be another sign of respiratory distress.

# COMMON TRAUMA IN INFANTS AND CHILDREN

The summer months bring an increase in trauma in infants and children because children are out of school, riding bikes, and playing. Motor vehicle accidents remain the most common cause of injury, whether the child is a passenger, a pedestrian, or a bicyclist.

## Head Trauma

Because the head is disproportionately large in a child, it tends to contact surfaces first after impact; children who fall from high-rise buildings often land on their heads. Head injuries are also common in unrestrained children involved in motor vehicle accidents.

## Abdominal Trauma

Blunt trauma from a motor vehicle accident or a blow or kick to the abdomen can cause compression and subsequent rupture of the internal organs; the liver is most vulnerable. Campbell (1988) lists rupture of the liver as the second leading cause of death in traumatized children. Children restrained only by a seat belt without a shoulder harness may sustain abdominal trauma from the compression force of the belt in a motor vehicle accident.

## Chest Trauma

Because the chest is so compliant in infants and children, rib and sternal fractures are not common in young children. Blunt chest trauma in a child may cause a pneumothorax, but other thoracic injuries such as flail chest or rupture of great vessels are not as common as in adults because the ribs and chest wall are more flexible.

## Fractures

Participation in sports and routine play can result in fractures, as can child abuse. Any child with a fracture or suspected fracture should be transported to the hospital for examination by a pediatric orthopedic surgeon. Disability and deformity can result from improper care and treatment of fractures.

## Burns

Burns in a child can be serious and should be evaluated by a physician. Unless the source is obvious, such as a house fire, suspect possible child abuse. Children are commonly abused by being held in scalding water or being burned by cigarettes.

## Multiple Trauma

One of the most common causes of multiple trauma in children is a motor vehicle accident in which a child is struck by a car. Campbell (1988) reports that most children are hit on their left side by the right side of a car, causing a set of injuries known as Waddell's triad: fracture of the left femur from contact with the bumper; splenic injury from contact with the fender; and trauma to the right side of the head, which strikes the pavement when the child lands after impact. In this situation, assess the child for injuries to the femur, spleen, and head.

# NURSING STRATEGIES FOR INFANTS AND CHILDREN WITH TRAUMA

The primary goals in caring for infants and children with trauma are to preserve the patient's life and transfer the infant or child to a pediatric trauma facility in order to reduce mortality and morbidity. A secondary goal is to provide emotional support for the parents. In general, time is not spent at the trauma scene securing intravenous access or intubating unless it is deemed essential. These procedures are performed at the hospital or en route to the hospital.

Table 16-2 gives potential nursing diagnoses and interventions for the care of infants and children with trauma. The following strategies may also be useful. It is presumed with each that the airway, breathing, and circulation are already established. Your interventions should be within the scope of your professional license; commensurate with your skill and training; consistent with your state's nurse practice act; and when performed in a health care institution, adherent to that facility's standards of practice.

- Administer oxygen. Some children will not allow a mask on their face when they are conscious. In this case, have another rescuer direct the high flows of oxygen over the child's face when possible.

- Use the car seat of a child involved in a motor vehicle accident to transport the child to the hospital unless other injuries necessitate removing the child from the car seat. The child's head can be immobilized by taping it to the seat.

- Immobilize the head of a child or an infant in case the cervical spine is injured. This should be done even though injuries to the cervical spine

**Table 16-2**

**Potential Nursing Diagnoses and Interventions for Infants and Children with Trauma**

| Diagnosis | Interventions |
| --- | --- |
| Fear r/t unfamiliarity | Acknowledge the child's fear. Do not offer false reassurances that everything will be okay or that nothing will hurt. Get down on the child's eye level when possible so you will be perceived as less threatening. Allow and encourage parents or caretakers to be with the child as much as possible. Orient the child to sights and sounds; offer explanations appropriate to the patient's age and development. Allow the child to take a favorite toy or blanket to the hospital. |
| Aspiration, potential | Check the patient's mouth and sweep out and save any loose teeth; otherwise these teeth may be inhaled into the lungs. Monitor the status of loose teeth, and report their presence to the next caregiver. Have suction available. Do not offer the patient anything by mouth until cleared by a physician. |
| Fluid volume deficit r/t active loss from trauma | Infants and children have a smaller blood volume than adults, and shock and hypovolemia may develop quickly. This also reduces the margin of error for fluid administration. Stop active bleeding with pressure. Anticipate the intravenous or intraosseous administration of crystalloids or volume expanders in any patient who is hypovolemic. Determine the patient's weight as accurately as possible, because resuscitation medications and fluids are based on this. Monitor intake and output meticulously; use an intravenous fluid pump or a volume chamber to prevent inadvertent fluid overload. |
| Verbal communication impairment r/t age | Have parents or caretaker present when possible to help explain procedures to any child who is conscious. Allow the child an opportunity to ask questions, and respond with simple answers. |
| Parenting alteration r/t child abuse | Report suspected child abuse to the authorities, as is required by law. Establish an open and accepting relationship with parents so they may express feelings. Help parents identify deficits in their parenting skills and what is expected of them. Refer the family to appropriate social, counseling, and support resources. |
| Parental role conflict r/t child's hospitalization | Orient parents and family to the hospital. Allow open expression of feelings in a nonjudgmental atmosphere. Facilitate open communication to express feelings of guilt, blame, helplessness, anger, or fear. Explore coping techniques that have been helpful in the past. Refer the family to social agencies, counselors, ministers, or support groups as indicated. |

Note.—This is a sample of potential nursing diagnoses. It is not presented as or intended to be a complete care plan for the trauma patient. More complete information can be found in a medical-surgical nursing course and textbook. r/t = related to.
Adapted from Sparks, S. and Taylor, C. M. *Nursing diagnosis reference manual,* Springhouse, PA: Springhouse Corp., 1991, and Chitwood, L. *Ambulatory patient care,* San Diego: Western Schools, 1994.

are less common in infants and children than in adults.

- Be aware that improper management of fractures in a growing child can lead to permanent disability and deformity.

- Do not overlook the needs of the parent at the time of trauma; children often reflect their parents' emotions.

- Remember that bradycardia is a warning of serious hypoxia. Although a pulse rate of 80 beats per minute is normal in an adult, the same rate in a newborn is an ominous sign, and immediate intervention is required to prevent imminent brain damage and death.

- Guard against hypothermia by covering the child and protecting against heat loss when possible. Hypothermia depresses cardiac function; prolongs acidosis; diminishes the effectiveness of CPR; increases oxygen consumption while decreasing oxygen delivery to the tissues; and impairs platelet functions, which leads to increased bleeding times (Badgwell, 1993).

- Identify yourself to the child and the child's parent or guardian, and explain that you are there to help.

- Do not ask the child questions that can be answered with a no, because you will then have to force your plans on the child. Simply tell the child what you are going to do and then do it.

- Restrain your frustration with an uncooperative child by remembering that pain, fright, and hypoxia can prevent a child from cooperating with you.

- Do not chastise a child for crying; children cry when they are hurt and frightened. Chastising or ridiculing the child will not halt the tears. It may raise the child's stress level, and it usually will result in a child who is less cooperative.

- Offer children the chance to make minor inconsequential decisions whenever possible so they will at least perceive that they have retained some degree of control.

- Be professional and calm at the trauma scene (even if you feel neither) to help gain the confidence of the patient and the parent or caretaker.

- Accept the parent's or your ability to distract or comfort an injured child as evidence that cerebral perfusion is adequate (Campbell, 1988). A child cannot respond if circulation and perfusion of the brain are inadequate.

- Send another rescuer to search for the patient's parent or guardian if that person is not already present. Although an emergency in general implies consent to treatment, make every effort to locate the parent or guardian in order to obtain consent before treating or transporting a child.

- Note that intraosseous infusion (Figure 16-1) performed by those skilled and trained in the technique is gaining acceptance in the treatment of critically injured infants and children, especially when securing intravenous access is difficult or impossible. This technique involves boring a sturdy needle through the skin and into the bone marrow, connecting intravenous tubing, and giving fluid through the tubing. Most fluids, medications, and blood can be administered in this fashion. The tibia is the most frequently chosen site.

- Transport the patient to a pediatric facility whenever possible. Facilities designed and prepared for adult patients are less likely to have the complete services, supplies, and staff necessary to meet the needs of an injured infant or child.

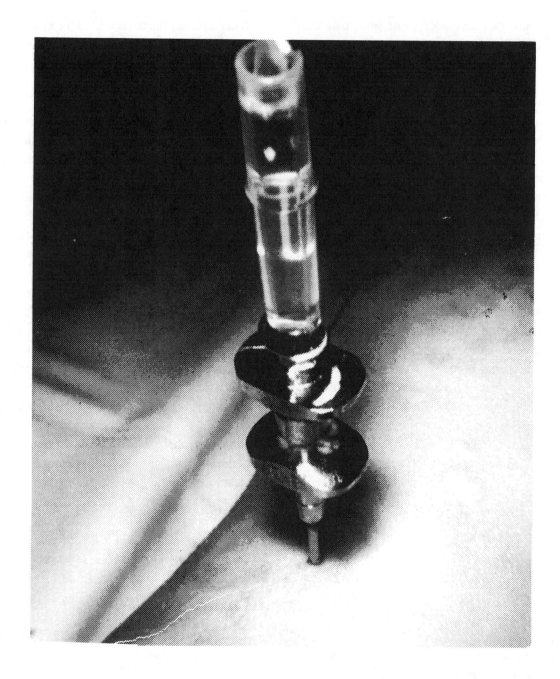

**Figure 16-1. Intraosseous infusion.** Reprinted by permission from Campbell, J. *Basic trauma life support: Advanced prehospital care* (2nd ed.). Englewood Cliffs, NJ: Prentice-Hall, 1988.

- Do not allow the patient to eat or drink until he or she is seen by a pediatrician. Immediate surgical intervention may be indicated, and oral intake increases the risk of a fatal aspiration during the perioperative period.

- Reassure the patient and the parents or guardian that everything possible is being done for the patient, as injuries distress both patients and parents.

- Be aware that the infants and children with trauma may become restless and agitated and pull out intravenous lines, endotracheal tubes, or monitors. Secure tubes and lines adequately.

- Keep pediatric emergency equipment available if you work in an emergency clinic, because airways and catheters suitable for adults will not work on a child.

- Do not move a child who has fallen from a structure unless it is necessary to establish breathing and circulation or to escape imminent danger. Stay with the child and call for assistance. Apply pressure to sites of bleeding as indicated; administer oxygen at the earliest opportunity.

- Uncuffed endotracheal tubes are generally used in infants and children less than 6-8 years old, and these tubes are even more easily dislodged than cuffed tubes. Always auscultate for breath sounds after intubation to determine equality. Listen in the midaxillary line; listening in the midclavicular line can result in your hearing sounds referred from the other side. Endotracheal tubes inserted too far may be pushed into the right bronchus so only the right lung is ventilated. This can significantly increase mortality and morbidity.

- Do not use an esophageal obturator airway on children, especially those less than 12 years old.

- When possible, keep an infant or child who has trauma from seeing other trauma patients or frightening circumstances to prevent compounding the infant's or child's psychic trauma.

- Transport any child with blunt abdominal trauma to the hospital immediately, as shock may ensue. Fluid resuscitation may be necessary en route; pediatric pneumatic antishock trousers may be used.

# CHILD ABUSE

In the United States, about 3 million cases of child abuse are reported each year, but it is suspected that many more cases go unreported. Approximately 14 children die each day at the hands of their caretakers. The National Committee to Prevent Child Abuse (NCPCA) defines child abuse as a nonaccidental injury or pattern of injuries to a child (*Think You Know*, 1993). Child abuse includes nonaccidental physical injury, neglect, sexual molestation, and emotional abuse (Table 16-3). Recent legal actions have also expanded child abuse to include drug-addicted pregnant women who deliver drugs to their fetuses.

The family is becoming a nucleus of violent activity; most women and children are attacked not by strangers but by persons they know. The perpetrator of child sexual abuse is most likely the father or father-figure to the child; abuse by strangers is rare (Smith & Goretsky, 1992). Prosecutors are also reporting more cases involving younger children.

Child abuse crosses all social, ethnic, and racial borders. Risk factors for child abuse include unemployment and related financial difficulties; alcohol or other drug abuse; legal problems; overcrowding, extreme poverty, and inadequate housing; social isolation and lack of social supports or social networks that set good examples of proper parenting; and a

---

**Table 16-3**
**Definitions of Child Abuse**

| Type of Abuse | Definition |
|---|---|
| Nonaccidental physical injury | An injury to a child for which there is no "reasonable" explanation. May include severe beatings, burns, strangulation, or human bites. |
| Neglect | Failure to provide a child with the basic necessities of life, including refusal or delay in providing food, clothing, shelter, medical care, and education as well as abandonment and inadequate supervision. |
| Sexual molestation | The exploitation of a child for the sexual gratification of an adult, as in rape, incest, fondling of the genitals, or exhibitionism. (Author's note: Authorities also consider many nontouching offenses to be sexual molestation. Examples include forcing a child to watch sexual activity, making obscene telephone calls to a child, and forcing a child to undress for an adult voyeur.) |
| Emotional abuse | A pattern of behavior that attacks a child's self-worth. Examples include constant criticizing; belittling; insulting; rejecting; and providing no love, support, or guidance. |

From *Think you know something about child abuse?* [Booklet]. Chicago: National Committee to Prevent Child Abuse, 1993.

---

history of child abuse in the family (*Think You Know,* 1993).

Triggering factors for child abuse include major or minor crises such as social or economic problems, illness, noise, breakdown in family structure or relations, and everyday mishaps such as spilling food or soiling clothes. Infants are most often assaulted for inconsolable crying; preschoolers and young children, for inappropriate elimination.

Types of trauma closely linked with child abuse include the following:

- Head injuries in the absence of an obvious accident such as a motor vehicle accident. These injuries may result from the child being beaten by fists or blunt objects or being violently shaken by an adult.

- Burns from scalding or cigarettes.

- Fractures.

- Internal injuries caused by blows to the abdomen.

- Genital injuries, including lacerations.

- Cuts, bruises, and swollen eyes.

In general, almost any injury can be caused intentionally, so you must learn to look for certain clues (Table 16-4) that the child's injury was not caused by an accident.

If you suspect child abuse, Grant et al. (1990) advise that you do the following:

## Table 16-4
## Indications of Possible Abuse

- Repeated responses to provide care for the same child or children in a family.

- Indications of past injuries. This is why you must do a physical examination and why you must remove articles of clothing. Pay special attention to the back and buttocks of the child.

- Poorly healing wounds or improperly healed fractures. It is extremely rare for a child to receive a fracture, be given proper orthopedic care, and then show angulations and large "bumps" and "knots" of bone at the "healed" injury site.

- Indications of past burns or fresh bilateral burns. Children seldom put both hands on a hot object or touch the same hot object again (true, some do, . . . this is only an indication, not proof). Some types of burns are almost always linked to child abuse, such as cigarette burns to the body and burns to the buttocks and lower extremities that result from the child being dipped in hot water.

- Many different types of injuries to both sides or the front and back of the body. This gains even more importance if the adults on the scene keep insisting that the child "falls a lot."

- Fear on the part of the child to tell you how he was injured. Combine this with the adults on the scene indicating they do not wish to leave you alone with the child, parents who tell conflicting or changing stories, or parents who overwhelm you with their explanations of the cause of the injury.

From Grant, H. D., Murray, R. H., Jr., & Bergeron, J. D. (Eds.). *Brady emergency care* (5th ed.). Englewood Cliffs, NJ: Prentice-Hall, 1990

- Treat the child but do not confront or accuse the parents at the scene or try to extract information from the child.

- Notify the authorities of your suspicions as soon as possible. Most metropolitan areas have teams with special training and skills to manage this situation. All states require certain persons to report suspected child abuse. Failure to report can result in penalties.

- Transport the child to the hospital for further evaluation of the injuries, even if the injuries under other circumstances would not seem to warrant it.

- Do not divulge your suspicions to anyone other than the appropriate authorities. This is privileged medical information.

- Keep accurate records, and document your findings and actions.

# SUMMARY

An infant or child with trauma presents the challenge of caring not only for the patient but also for grieving, shocked, or angry parents. The primary goals are to preserve the patient's life and transport the infant or child to an appropriate facility in order to reduce mortality and morbidity. A secondary goal is to aid the parents in instituting coping skills to deal with stress and anxiety caused by the accident. More than size distinguishes an infant or child from an adult. Knowledge of the basics of trauma nursing for infants and children is essential, because injury is the leading cause of death in children. Because children are quite resilient, outcome is often good with appropriate intervention.

# CRITICAL CONCEPTS

- Guard against hypothermia in any infant or child with trauma.

- Injury is the leading cause of death in children.

- Almost one-half of all trauma in children involves motor vehicle accidents in which the child is a passenger, pedestrian, or bicyclist.

- Intraosseous infusion is gaining rapid acceptance for volume replacement and administration of medications in infants and children with trauma.

- Report any suspected child abuse to the proper authorities. If in doubt, err in favor of the child.

# GLOSSARY

**Child abuse:** A nonaccidental injury or pattern of injuries to a child. Child abuse includes not only non-accidental physical injury but also neglect, sexual molestation, and emotional abuse.

**Intraosseous infusion:** Placement of a needle into the bone marrow, usually of the tibia in the lower leg, for infusion of fluids, medications, and blood products.

**Waddell's triad:** Fracture of the femur coupled with blunt trauma to the spleen and head; seen as a classic set of injuries in children hit by a car.

# EXAM QUESTIONS

## Chapter 16

## Questions 77 - 80

77. About how many cases of child abuse are reported each year in the United States?

    a.  3 million
    b.  1 million
    c.  250,000
    d.  100,000

78. What is a normal range of heart rate for a newborn?

    a.  120–140 beats per minute
    b.  90–120 beats per minute
    c.  80–100 beats per minute
    d.  80–100 beats per minute

79. What is the likely blood volume of a child who weighs 15 kg (34 lb)?

    a.  2000 ml
    b.  1200 ml
    c.  900 ml
    d.  450 ml

80. The most common cause of trauma in infants and children is:

    a.  Burns
    b.  Falls
    c.  Motor vehicle accidents
    d.  Sports accidents

# CHAPTER 17

# MULTIPLE PATIENTS AND TRIAGE

## CHAPTER OBJECTIVE

After completing this chapter, the reader should be able to plan care when several patients are present at a trauma scene.

## LEARNING OBJECTIVES

After studying this chapter, the reader should be able to

1. List two classifications of disaster.

2. Differentiate between three classifications of a patient's condition: immediate, urgent, and nonurgent.

3. Select potential nursing diagnoses for a disaster victim.

4. Recognize concerns in securing a disaster scene.

## INTRODUCTION

Generally, only one or two trauma patients require attention at the same time. However, when more than one patient has been injured in the same accident or assault, the challenge of multiple trauma pa-

tients exists. There may be two patients, or there may be hundreds. Weather-related disasters, earthquakes, transportation accidents, industrial accidents, occupational accidents, and environmental disasters may result in multiple patients with injuries ranging from minor to life threatening. The nurse's goals are to evaluate the scene, set priorities, organize resources, classify victims according to severity of injury, intervene as indicated, stabilize the patients, and plan transport to the most appropriate facility. With an understanding of basic trauma nursing skills and proper planning, the nurse generally can expect to improve the patients' outcome.

This chapter discusses evaluation of the trauma scene, including access and personal safety, and describes the two classifications of disasters: localized and compartmentalized. It also reviews triage, assessment of patients and management of the trauma scene, and hospital and community disaster planning.

## DISASTERS

Disasters are sudden events that substantially damage property and harm people. Sheehy and Jimmerson (1994) also define disasters as events "in which the capacity of the daily operating system of care is exceeded." Disasters tax or overwhelm the capabilities of the local health care delivery system, so planning and rehearsing for such events are essential functions of health care professionals, hospitals, and community agencies. Personnel reinforcements may be necessary to meet the needs of the injured. Coordination of care is essential at this time even though communications may be limited and resources few. Confusion can reign; the patients ultimately suffer. Even while facing their own concerns about the status of their families and friends, nurses frequently find themselves called on to intervene and provide basic trauma nursing care to the victims. An understanding of the types and phases of disasters will help you prepare for one of the greatest challenges a nurse can face: multiple patients.

## Phases of Disasters

Grant et al. (1990) describe seven phases of a disaster. Knowledge of these phases can provide tips to patients' potential behavior.

1.  **Warning period:** Not all disasters give warning. Tornadoes and floods, however, are precipitated by certain weather conditions, and likely victims may have an opportunity to seek safety. Unfortunately, persons often ignore or do not receive the warning. Other disasters, such as a train wreck or an airplane crash, are sudden and unpredictable.

2.  **Threat period:** When a warning of potential disaster has been issued or a threat is perceived, those affected must take action to avoid harm. This period is a critical, decision-making time that some may not be able to face effectively, especially those whose coping mechanisms are not well developed.

3.  **Impact period:** The impact period includes the period when the disaster actually strikes, battering people and property. Both the injured and uninjured may be immobilized by the reality of impact.

4.  **Inventory period:** After the impact of the disaster, most survivors take stock of the damage, activate coping skills, and begin purposeful activity designed to assess their

situation and restore order. Others will continue to be immobilized by injury and fear; psychologic decompensation may manifest itself as hysteria, anger, or other emotional outbursts.

5.  **Rescue period:** During the rescue period, intervention begins as the survivors set priorities, begin to help the injured, and meet immediate concerns.

6.  **Remedy period:** The remedy period is often the longest phase after a disaster. Teamwork among the survivors fuels the drive to reconstruct the disaster area and help the victims.

7.  **Restoration period:** In the restoration period, the disaster area is rebuilt and returned to its predisaster level of functioning. The type of disaster and the resources available influence the level of restoration.

## Classification of Disasters

The Society of Orange County Emergency Physicians and the Orange County Emergency Medical Services Agency developed two classifications of disasters (Bade, 1990):

1.  **Localized disaster:** When the event is localized to a specific geographic area and involves large numbers of casualties, a localized disaster exists. An airliner crash into a housing development or a terrorist bombing of a restaurant is an example. Because the localized disaster occurs in a well-defined area, access to the victims is generally not restricted, and community resources can be tapped for assistance. Local disaster plans are implemented, and most health care professionals can be mobilized for service within the plan.

2. **Compartmentalized disaster:** When the event is widespread, and the victims are isolated from one another, a compartmentalized disaster exists. A serious earthquake is an example of a compartmentalized disaster. Compartmentalized disasters can fragment care because the persons who were integral to the disaster plan may also be victims of the disaster. For example, a hospital may be destroyed, or nurses and other rescuers may be trapped in their own homes. Both transportation routes and communication may be impaired.

# TRIAGE

As health care professionals, nurses are trained to care for the sick and injured. When presented with more than one patient requiring attention at a chaotic trauma scene, a nurse must be able to assess the situation, set priorities, and begin rapid interventions if any of the victims are to survive. The challenge is to sort through a barrage of information, extract critical data, and react. An essential skill for the management of more than one patient is triage, from the French word "to sort."

Triage is a system for assigning priority of care to the injured. The goal is to maximize use of available resources and promote optimal outcome for all the trauma victims. Figure 17-1 shows a typical triage tag that is affixed to trauma patients. Triage is not a one-time task. Patients must be reassessed as often as possible, because their condition may deteriorate quickly.

Although a uniform system of triage is not in place, with most disaster triage systems, patients are classified, labeled, and transported according to the patients' status. Two systems are described here. In the first, patients are classified as immediate, delayed, and nonurgent. The second, the simple triage and rapid treatment (START) system, is based on these classifications.

## The Immediate, Delayed, Nonurgent System

When a patient is classified as having an immediate need for intervention by a health care professional, that patient is expected to receive treatment and transport to a health care facility before other classifications of patients. Patients in this category include those who have the following:

- Complete or partial obstruction of the airway.
- Respiratory arrest.
- Severe bleeding or shock.
- Fractured femur or femurs.
- Major burns.
- Cervical spine injury.
- Tension pneumothorax.
- Severe head injuries.
- Serious long-bone or open fractures.
- Witnessed cardiac arrest.

Patients classified as urgent require intervention as soon as possible but are thought to be stable for the moment. Patients who might be classified as urgent include those who have the following:

- Major but stable injuries (some types of abdominal trauma, open fractures, burns, moderate degree of blood loss).
- Eye injuries.
- Spinal cord injuries.

Patients classified as nonurgent will receive attention and transport after patients in the other two classifications are treated and transported. Nonurgent patients may have the following:

- Simple cuts, lacerations, or bruises.
- Sprains and strains.

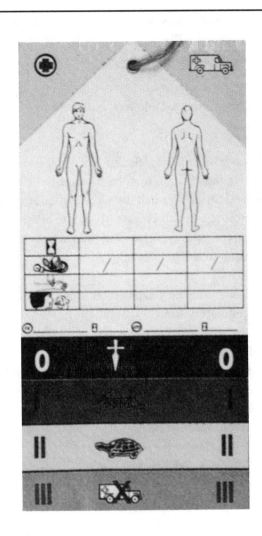

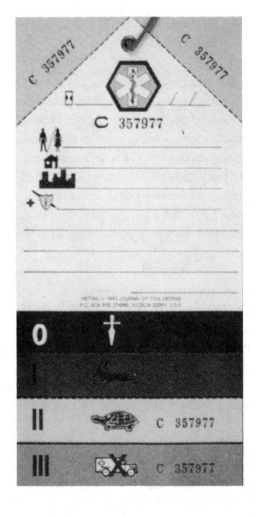

**Figure 17-1. The Mettag system.** Typical triage tags used to identify highest priority, second-priority, and lowest-priority patients. Reprinted by permission from Grant, H. D., Murray, R. H., Jr., & Bergeron, J. D. (Eds.). *Brady emergency care* (5th ed.). Englewood Cliffs, NJ: Prentice-Hall, 1990.

• Injuries that are not generally compatible with life, including extensive burns and multiple severe trauma in cases in which the hope of survival is remote. These patients are considered nonurgent so that other patients who do have hope of survival can receive the limited resources available at the time.

## The START System

The START system is a triage system for rapid review of multiple patients at a trauma scene (Grant et al., 1990). It is based on having the first rescuers on the scene quickly assess and sort patients. This system gets assistance flowing to the injured and facilitates their treatment as more professionals arrive on the scene. In the START system, patients are tagged and classified as delayed (lowest priority for care), immediate (highest priority for care), and dead (nonsalvageable); see Table 17-1. The following is a brief overview of the four steps of the START system:

1. **Determination of delayed patients:** Direct all patients who can walk to one area and categorize them as delayed. Then move on to those patients who cannot walk.

2. **Respiration check:** Check the respirations of each patient who cannot walk. Open the airway as necessary; enlist the aid of conscious ambulatory patients when possible to keep the airway open. Quickly *estimate* respiratory rate and tag those with respirations greater than 30 breaths/min as immediate. Consider those with respirations less than 30 breaths/min as delayed, and continue to the next step. Note those patients who are nonsalvageable or dead.

3. **Perfusion assessment:** Now check both the immediate and delayed patients for adequate perfusion. Palpate the radial pulse. If it is palpable, assume that perfusion is adequate and consider the patient as delayed. If the radial pulse is not palpable, tag the patient as immediate, and raise the patient's legs to increase venous return to the heart. Apply pressure to major bleeding sites, or ask a walking patient to do this for you.

4. **Brain injury assessment:** If the patient has adequate respirations and perfusion and can follow simple commands such as opening the eyes, assume the patient has adequate mental function and tag him or her as de-

---

## Table 17-1
## The START Plan for Triage

| Immediate | Delayed | Dead |
|---|---|---|
| Respirations more than 30/min | Walking wounded | No respirations |
| Respirations less than 30/min, no radial pulse | Respirations less than 30/min, radial pulse | |
| Adequate respirations and perfusion, unable to follow directions | Adequate respirations and perfusion, able to follow directions | |

Note.—START = **Simple triage and rapid treatment.** From Grant, H. D., Murray, R. H., Jr., & Bergeron, J. D. (Eds.). *Brady emergency care* (5th ed.). Englewood Cliffs, NJ: Prentice-Hall, 1990.

layed. Tag as immediate patients who cannot respond.

# NURSING STRATEGIES FOR MULTIPLE TRAUMA PATIENTS AND TRIAGE

The needs and conditions of multiple trauma patients vary; the resources available at disaster scenes are unpredictable. The ability to adapt and improvise is essential under these circumstances. Table 17-2 gives potential nursing diagnoses and interventions for disaster victims. The following strategies may also be useful. Your intervention in any disaster or trauma situation involving multiple patients should be within the scope of your professional license; commensurate with your skills and training; consistent with your state's nurse practice act; and when performed in a health care setting, adherent to that facility's standards of practice.

- While approaching the trauma scene, assess it to detect any threats to your own safety; do not enter a trauma scene only to become another victim. Note hazards such as downed power lines, fires or potential explosive situations, inadequate building supports or foundations, and gases in the air.

- Approach the first victim and begin triage if the area is safe to enter. If you are alone, do the best you can until help arrives; recognize that you will probably not be able to help every patient. If you are not alone, work with other professionals to secure the scene and triage the patients.

- Do not leave a trauma scene with multiple patients to transport any patient until the scene is stabilized. Stay to assist those who need your care and wait for the arrival of emergency teams who can transport patients. Whoever arrives first should begin triage until additional qualified rescuers are on the scene.

- Enlist responsible bystanders or walking patients to apply pressure to bleeding sites, comfort hysterical patients, control traffic, call for assistance, and perform other simple tasks.

- Reassess patients as frequently as possible, because conditions may deteriorate quickly.

- Be aware of the psychological impact of disaster. Counselors are frequently called to a disaster scene or the receiving facility to help both victims and rescuers cope with emotional reactions. Posttraumatic stress disorder may develop in those involved in the disaster; this condition often requires professional intervention.

- Help ensure the security of the disaster scene and the delivery of care by cooperating with security personnel and by reporting intruders. Those who are not actively involved in the rescue should not be at the site, because their presence can delay rescues.

- Protect patients' confidentiality and privacy by shielding them from reporters, photographers, and curious bystanders. Check identification of those inquiring about or wanting to visit disaster victims in the hospital; refer the press and legal representatives to the proper public relations department in the facility.

# DISASTER PLANNING

Preparation and planning are the keys to meeting the needs of disaster victims. Most communities have dis-

**Table 17-2**
**Potential Nursing Diagnoses and Interventions for Disaster Victims**

| Diagnosis | Interventions |
|---|---|
| Posttrauma response r/t disaster | Provide emotional support. Allow victims to express emotions and feelings without fear of judgment. Refer patients to mental health professionals and support groups. Explain the posttrauma response to patients' family members Listen and help patients (if possible) in the way they think will be most helpful. |
| Powerlessness | Orient the patient to surroundings frequently. Explain who you are, what has happened, what you are doing, and what to expect. Allow the patient to make decisions when possible to give some feeling of control. |
| Fear | Reassure the patient that the trauma event is over and that you are there to help; explain to the patient that he or she is safe now. Answer the patient's questions about family and loved ones as honestly as you can. Offer support and empathy Call clergy or counselors to be present to assist the patient and the patient's family as needed. |
| Spiritual distress r/t disaster | Talk to the patient about the grief process and encourage him or her to discuss concerns with clergy or spiritual advisors. Provide privacy if the patient wishes to see a minister; allow expression of spiritual concerns in an atmosphere of acceptance. |
| Injury, potential | Assess victims frequently and be prepared to change their triage status and intervene if their condition has deteriorated. |

Note.—This is a sample of potential nursing diagnoses. It is not presented as or intended to be a complete care plan for the trauma patient. More complete information can be found in a medical-surgical nursing course and textbook. r/t = related to.

Adapted from Sparks, S. and Taylor, C. M. *Nursing diagnosis reference manual*, Springhouse, PA: Springhouse Corp., 1991, and Chitwood, L., *Ambulatory patient care*, San Diego: Western Schools, 1994.

aster planning committees; most hospitals have plans for meeting the needs of disaster victims. Nurses can act as leaders in disaster planning by serving on committees, lending professional expertise to public disaster planning, and participating in disaster drills. An awareness of a facility's disaster plans is essential for nurses employed there. Nurses should also maintain certification in basic life support skills, heed warnings of impending disasters (such as weather reports or bulletins), and take advantage of opportunities to educate patients and the public about disaster planning.

# SUMMARY

Trauma involving multiple patients means that care must be provided for more than one patient who has been injured in an accident or assault. Whenever multiple patients are present at a trauma scene, the rescuers must set priorities, organize resources, and begin interventions. Nurses must be able to assess and classify patients quickly. With an understanding of basic trauma nursing skills and proper planning, nurses can affect the outcome of any disaster or trauma event involving multiple patients. Because of their background and training, nurses are often called on to meet the needs of disaster victims. Staying current on basic life support and trauma skills, participating in disaster planning, teaching patients and the public about disaster preparedness, and heeding warnings of disaster are methods of meeting the challenges posed by disasters.

# CRITICAL CONCEPTS

- Do not enter a trauma scene when your own safety is threatened. You may become another victim and thus delay rescue of the original victims.

- Recognize that when several patients are injured in the same event, some critically injured patients will be deemed nonsalvageable under the circumstances and will have to be passed by in order to care for those whose chances of survival are greater.

- Reassess patients as frequently as possible, because their conditions can deteriorate quickly.

- Be aware of the impact that your own emotions and distress may have at the time of a disaster.

- Stay current on basic life and trauma support skills and participate in disaster training drills to help prepare for potential disasters.

# GLOSSARY

**Compartmentalized disaster:** A widespread catastrophic event in which victims are isolated from one another and communication and transportation are disrupted. An example is an earthquake.

**Disasters:** Sudden catastrophic events that substantially damage property and harm persons or overwhelm the ability of the health care delivery system to provide care.

**Localized disaster:** A catastrophic event that is localized to a specific geographic area and involves large numbers of casualties. An example is an airplane crash.

**Triage:** A system for classifying patients for priority of care according to the nature of their injuries. The goal is to maximize use of available resources and promote optimal outcome for all the patients.

# EXAM QUESTIONS

## Chapter 17

## Questions 81 - 86

81. Which of the following would be described as a compartmentalized disaster?

    a. Small aircraft crash
    b. House fire
    c. Statewide flood
    d. Chemical plant explosion

82. Which of the following is an example of a localized disaster?

    a. Earthquake in five counties
    b. Ice storm covering half a state
    c. Fire covering six square city blocks
    d. Blizzard covering four states

83. You are at a wreck between a bus and a tanker truck. You quickly assess the first victim and note an open fracture of a femur. The patient is unconscious and has no palpable radial pulse. Respirations are 40 breaths/min. The triage classification for this patient is:

    a. Immediate
    b. Urgent
    c. Nonurgent
    d. Delayed

84. Common potential nursing diagnoses for victims and rescuers involved in disaster situations might include emotional turmoil and:

    a. Neglect, unilateral
    b. Self-esteem, chronic low
    c. Posttrauma response
    d. Personal identity disturbance

85. You are helping triage victims at the scene of a train and truck collision. A man who is neither a victim nor a rescuer puts his card into your pocket and tells you he will pay you to refer victims to his law office. Which of the following actions should you take?

    a. Ask him how much money he can get for the victims.
    b. Gather patients' names and fax the names to his office that afternoon.
    c. Continue working while calling for police to remove him.
    d. Determine his sincerity in wanting to help the victims with recompense.

86. A 15-car collision has occurred on the interstate. At the scene, you have a patient who can respond to simple commands, has a palpable radial pulse and a respiratory rate of 20 breaths/min. The patient has a facial laceration and cannot walk because of a possible ankle fracture. The triage classification for this patient is:

    a. Nonurgent
    b. Immediate
    c. Urgent
    d Delayed

# CHAPTER 18

# ORGAN DONATION

## CHAPTER OBJECTIVE

After completing this chapter, the reader should be able to recognize the nationwide need for donated organs and formulate an intervention plan for trauma patients who are potential donors.

## LEARNING OBJECTIVES

After studying this chapter, the reader should be able to

1. Recognize the criteria for donation of organs or tissues.

2. List the steps involved in organ donation.

3. Specify the purposes of the Uniform Anatomical Gift Act, the Required Request Act, and the United Network for Organ Sharing.

4. Select potential nursing diagnoses for the family of a potential organ and tissue donor.

## INTRODUCTION

When a trauma patient sustains a fatal injury, it is sometimes possible to turn this tragedy into a gift of life for another patient. Nursing interventions include recognizing trauma patients who may be potential donors, beginning the steps for the donation of organs and tissues, and preserving the organs for transplantation. This chapter provides guidelines for preparing the donor and the family for transplantation. It also discusses the need for the donation of organs and tissues, reviews the laws regulating donations, describes determination of potential donors, and presents nursing diagnoses and interventions for families of organ donors.

## THE NEED FOR DONATED ORGANS

Since the first reported kidney transplant occurred in 1954 in Boston, and the first reported heart transplant took place in South Africa in 1967, transplantation has evolved into a sophisticated and life-saving procedure. Patients whose illnesses are life threatening or debilitating are assessed as potential transplant recipients and then registered on waiting lists for donated organs.

Although the number of organs suitable for transplantation is more than adequate, the number of these actually offered for donation falls far short of need. Nurses can form a critical link in transplantation by determining if a trauma patient meets criteria for donation and by starting the process that leads to successful transplantation. It is estimated that 20,000 patients become potential donors each year, but only 4,000 organs were offered for transplantation in 1988

(*A Guide to the Recognition*, 1988). Transplant teams think that more organs would be donated if professionals knew how to recognize donors and understood the transplantation process better. A 1987 Gallup poll indicated that 74% of Americans say they would consent to donate organs from a family member when asked.

It appears that greater awareness among health care professionals is the key to procuring donor organs. Also, in many cases, talking with the patient's family about donation is not just a humanitarian gesture anymore; it is the law. Congress passed the Required Request law in 1986; this directs all hospitals receiving Medicare funds to ask surviving family members for organ donation.

Basic components of the Required Request law include the following:

- The attending physician can secure consent for organ donation.

- Next of kin must be asked to consent to organ donation.

- Discretion and sensitivity to the family's emotional state are expected, and deference is given to the donor's religious beliefs.

- Notification must be made to the Organ Procurement Organization.

Organs that may be transplanted include the heart and heart valves, lungs, liver, kidney, pancreas, and eyes. Tissues that may be donated include skin, bone, blood vessels, corneas, cartilage, and fascia. The U.S. Department of Health and Human Services (*Statistical Abstract*, 1990) reports the following:

- More than 13,000 persons are waiting for kidney transplants, a procedure with a greater than 90% success rate.

- More than 1,200 persons need heart transplants.

- More than 1,000 persons need a liver transplant.

- About 250 persons need a heart-lung transplant.

- About 200 persons need a pancreas transplant.

- More than 4,000 persons need corneas.

The process of matching donors and recipients and evaluating patient need for organs has been assigned to the United Network for Organ Sharing (UNOS), a nationwide, nonprofit organization for the procurement of organs. Table 18-1 presents more statistics on organ transplantation.

# REGULATION OF ORGAN TRANSPLANTATION

To better coordinate the nationwide harvest and transplantation of organs, the federal government in 1986 awarded a contract to UNOS to promote, facilitate, and scientifically advance procurement and transplantation of organs. The Uniform Anatomical Gift Act (UAGA) was enacted into law in 1969 in all 50 states. The basic components of this act include the following:

- Anyone more than 18 years old has the right to donate any part or all of his or her body for transplantation or research. Intention to donate should be indicated on a Uniform Organ Donor card.

- Even when a person has signed a donor card, the person's family still is asked for consent to remove organs for donation. The order for giving consent is spouse, adult son or daughter, parent,

## Table 18-1
### Organ and Tissue Transplantation in the United States

| Organ or Tissue | No. of Transplants in 1987 | No. Waiting (March 1991) |
|---|---|---|
| Kidney | 8,940 | 18.163 |
| Heart | 1,688 | 1,884 |
| Liver | 2,190 | 1.344 |
| Pancreas | 418 | 516 |
| Heart-lung | 67 | 182 |
| Lung | 91 | 394 |

From United Network for Organ Sharing, Richmond, VA.

adult sibling, legal guardian, anyone else obligated to dispose of the body.

• Preferably, consent is obtained in person, but it may be granted by telephone.

• The physician who pronounces death should not be a member of the team that removes organs from the patient.

• Health care professionals who act in good faith in accordance with the UAGA are protected from civil and criminal liability for their role in the transplantation.

Despite the UAGA, some aspects of the laws involving transplantation vary from state to state, as do the regulations of individual institutions. You should familiarize yourself with your own institutional policies and state laws. You can telephone UNOS at 1-800-24-DONOR if you need more information.

The federal government in 1990 passed a law requiring that Medicare and Medicaid patients be informed of their right to make choices about their treatment. This is known as advance directive notification. This gives persons the opportunity to decide in advance what kind of treatment they want or would refuse in the event of illness. This law requires all health care providers who accept Medicare and Medicaid patients to tell patients about the patients' rights regarding treatment. State laws vary on these rights. Many states allow two types of advance directives: the living will and the durable power of attorney for health care. Patients who have executed these documents generally have already indicated their preferences on organ donation; this facilitates the process. Nurses should be familiar with their state's laws and institution's policy on advance directives.

# RECOGNITION AND REFERRAL OF POTENTIAL ORGAN AND TISSUE DONORS

Early recognition of a potential organ or tissue donor frequently begins with a nurse. The best organ and tissue donor is a person who was in good health when a serious injury resulted in brain death. Many donors are victims of severe head trauma. Other donors have had cerebral hemorrhage, smoke inhalation, or brain hypoxia from drowning. When determining if a patient is a potential donor, do not forget that body tissues such as skin, heart valves, and veins can be donated as well as organs such as the pancreas or heart.

In some states, victims of fatal trauma must be evaluated by the medical examiner or the coroner's office; check your state and institutional guidelines. Also, restrictions on the age of the donor vary widely among transplant teams, and donors often are assessed on a case-by-case basis, with the planned recipient in mind. The physiologic condition of the donor, rather than the chronologic age, is often of greater concern to the transplant team.

## Criteria for Donors

At a minimum, the potential organ donor should have cessation of brain function, have a beating heart, and be dependent on a respirator. Thus, the three criteria are brain death, intact circulation, and cessation of respirations. Whenever a patient meets these criteria, explore the potential for organ donation. Tissue donors are not required to have a heartbeat; certain tissues remain viable for several hours after circulation stops.

**Brain death.** Because brain death is an elusive and somewhat esoteric concept that is often misunderstood by the lay public, nurses should have an understanding of this fundamental requirement for organ donors. The cause of the cessation of brain function, such as head trauma, must be known before the patient can become a donor. In general, the diagnosis of brain death is based on these signs:

- Deep coma.

- No spontaneous movements.

- No response to stimuli.

- Apnea.

- No reflexes other than spinal reflexes.

- No indication of reversible causes (such as drug overdose or hypothermia) of a nonfunctioning brain.

When brain death is confirmed, the patient is considered to be dead. Many families perceive that the patient is being "kept alive" by machines, but this is incorrect: The patient is dead. The ventilator and fluids or drugs are merely maintaining the circulation.

Neurologists and other specialists typically are consulted to diagnose or confirm brain death. Remember, the UAGA advises that the physician who diagnoses brain death should not participate in the removal or transplantation of organs from the patient.

Some tests used to determine brain death include the following:

- Electroencephalogram to evaluate electrical activity in the brain.

- Studies of blood flow in the brain, including cerebral radionuclide scans and arteriograms.

- Computed tomography to evaluate the brain tissue.

Intact circulation. An organ donor must have a beating heart; oxygenation of the organs is not possible otherwise. A tissue donor may not be required to have an intact circulation because certain tissues remain viable for a period without circulation. Even if cardiac arrest occurs, a patient still can be an organ donor if the circulation is restored soon enough.

**Cessation of respirations.** An organ donor must not breathe spontaneously; doing so would imply that the brainstem is still functioning, and the patient would, of course, not be considered brain dead. A potential donor must be dependent on a mechanical respirator for oxygenation and removal of carbon dioxide from the bloodstream. Transplant teams often assess the patient by turning off the ventilator for a brief period while measuring the carbon dioxide tension (pCO2) in the blood and looking for any spontaneous effort at inspiration by the patient.

If these three criteria are met, the patient may be a suitable organ donor. However, it is essential to check facility guidelines and the potential transplant team's requirements for donors. As technology advances, transplant teams are accepting organs and tissues from donors of wider age ranges; research continually changes the requirements for donor organs and tissues.

## Contraindications to Organ Donation

In general, to be considered as an organ or tissue donor, the patient must not have any of the following:

- Any transmittable disease, such as bacterial, fungal, or viral infections; this includes patients in a high-risk category for acquired immune deficiency syndrome.

- Malignant tumors (except certain brain tumors).

- Diabetes mellitus.

- History of chronic or intravenous drug abuse.

- Severe preexisting hypertension.

- A period of prolonged hypotension.

Once it is determined that a patient is a potential donor, the nurse can mention the possibility of organ and tissue donation to the attending physician, who may ask someone to contact UNOS or the local or regional transplant team. Most professionals are relieved to know that the transplant team usually will take over from there, offering guidance, support, and advice throughout the transplantation process.

Sheehy and Jimmerson (1994) list four steps that must be followed for donation to take place:

1. Determination of death based on an accepted protocol.

2. Pronouncement of death.

3. Consent from next of kin for donation.

4. Approval by the state medical examiner in accordance with state law.

# THE PROCESS FOR TRANSPLANTATION

## Approaching the Family

Once it is determined that a patient is an acceptable donor, the patient's family is asked to consider donating organs or tissues. This frequently is handled by the transplant team or the physician in charge. In general, it is best to allow the family a chance to grieve, express anger, and confront the tragedy of their loss before proposing organ donation. The request for donation may be made by a nurse, physician, social worker, or clergyperson.

Nurses can provide support by answering the family's questions. Facts to know include the following:

- The donor's condition and care are always the first priority. Transplantation is never started until the donor has been pronounced legally dead.

- All the major religions in the United States support organ and tissue donation.

- The donor will not be obligated to pay any charges related to transplantation. These fees are paid by the recipient.

- Recovery of the organs is done in a dignified manner under sterile conditions in the operating room. Once the organs and/or tissues are harvested, the ventilator is shut off, the wounds are closed, and the donor's body is released to the morgue.

- The donor will not be disfigured by organ donation and still can have an open-casket funeral service.

- The identities of the donor and recipient are not revealed. The donor's family will be told only general information, such as age, sex, and general geographic location of the recipient.

### Caring for the Donor

Care of the donor usually proceeds from an intensive care unit. The transplant team will direct management of the patient once death has been pronounced. Common actions for the donor include the following:

- Maintaining adequate oxygenation and perfusion of the organs. Inotropic agents may be necessary to maintain a normotensive state. Dopamine or dobutamine are the drugs of choice; metaraminol, norepinephrine, and epinephrine are contraindicated (Strange, 1987).

- Regulating body temperature with warming or cooling measures as necessary.

- Maintaining fluid and electrolyte balance and adequate urinary output.

- Protecting the organs or tissues to be donated by using routine nursing care measures such as taping the eyes shut to protect the corneas.

- Ensuring that the donor continues to be treated with respect even in death.

# NURSING STRATEGIES FOR ORGAN DONATION

Caring for an organ donor and the donor's family is both a challenge and a privilege. It requires both technical expertise and deep compassion. One must be sensitive to both the family's and the donor's needs. Table 18-2 presents potential nursing diagnoses and interventions for families of organ donors. The following nursing strategies may also be useful. However, each case is unique and should be approached as such. The important thing to remember is that transplant teams are skilled in these matters and are generally excellent resources; indeed, most teams will shoulder much of the burden and provide astute guidance.

Your nursing interventions in organ and tissue donation should be within the scope of your professional license, commensurate with your skills and training, consistent with your state's nurse practice act, and adherent to your facility's standards of practice.

- Contact UNOS at 1-800-24-DONOR or your local transplant center for more information on organ and tissue donation. These groups provide literature and guidelines for both professionals and the public on organ donation. Ask a member of a local transplant team to come and speak at your facility about the issues involved in organ and tissue donation.

- Familiarize yourself with your institution's policies and procedures on organ donation in advance of need so you will be able to respond accurately and promptly. Wasted time can mean the loss of an organ donation.

## Table 18-2
## Potential Nursing Diagnoses and Interventions for Families of Organ Donors

| Diagnosis | Interventions |
|---|---|
| Knowledge deficit r/t lack of exposure | Explain organ and tissue donation in simple terms. Allow the donor's family members and/or significant others to ask questions and have those questions answered to their satisfaction. Many persons have been exposed to myths and fallacies about organ donation; debunk those myths and provide written information when possible to reinforce your teaching. Common misconceptions include the belief that the donor's family must pay part of the costs of the transplantation and the belief that the donor's body is disfigured by the procedure. |
| Spiritual distress r/t situational crisis | Facilitate visits from clergy or spiritual leaders to aid the donor's family in making decisions about organ or tissue donation. Provide a private place for this meeting, and encourage family members to be candid with their minister or advisor. When possible, provide for religious rituals or practices the family desires before transplantation and removal of equipment and agents sustaining circulation and ventilation. |
| Fear r/t unfamiliarity | Orient the donor's family to anticipated events associated with the transplantation. Answer questions in simple language, and be prepared to repeat the answers as needed. When possible, assign the same nurse to be with the family members as they make the decision for transplantation or wait for the organs or tissues to be removed. Provide privacy for the family. Accept without judgment the family's decision to refuse to allow donation. |
| Grieving, anticipatory, r/t loss of loved one (donor) | Allow family members and designated significant others adequate private time with the donor before the donor is transferred to the operating suite for removal of organs or tissues. Recognize that families may have difficulty accepting the patient as dead when they can see electrocardiographic evidence of a heartbeat. Explain that the patient is dead; the equipment and drugs are only maintaining the circulation. Explain the grieving process, and encourage the family to use other family members, friends, and support systems to enhance their coping. Help them formulate a plan for functioning through the next few days; provide for follow-up and referral to mental health professionals or support groups as necessary. |

Note.—This is a sample of potential nursing diagnoses. It is not presented as or intended to be a complete care plan for the trauma patient. More complete information can be found in a medical-surgical nursing course and textbook. r/t = related to.

Adapted from Sparks, S. and Taylor, C. M. *Nursing diagnosis reference manual*, Springhouse, PA: Springhouse Corp., 1991, and Chitwood, L., *Ambulatory patient care*, San Diego: Western Schools, 1994

- Encourage your family members and friends to discuss organ donation with loved ones and spiritual leaders to make sure wishes about donation are known before the need arises.

- Familiarize yourself with the general steps to organ donation (Figure 18-1). Appendix C contains sample forms.

- Accept the family's decision to refuse tissue and organ donation. This is an intensely personal decision based on the family's beliefs and value system and is also affected at times by religious beliefs.

- Provide for follow-up with the donor's family if the transplant team does not. This will allow the family to ask questions that may be unanswered and to express concerns that may have developed since the patient's death. Refer them to support groups as necessary.

- Be aware that organ transplantation is expensive and therefore is falling under scrutiny by insurers and the government. This is a difficult ethical issue, and patients may wish to have this concern addressed.

# SUMMARY

Organ and tissue donation enables health care professionals to transform the tragedy of death into a gift of life for another, but this process requires sensitivity as well as technical expertise. Nurses often are the professionals who begin the transplantation cycle. However, nurses should familiarize themselves with their own institutional policies and state laws before acting. UNOS and local transplant teams are excellent resources for information about organ and tissue donation.

# CRITICAL CONCEPTS

- Consider as a potential organ donor any trauma patient who has cessation of brain function, has a beating heart, and is dependent on a ventilator.

- The death of a potential donor should not be pronounced by a member of the team that will remove organs from the donor.

- Acting in good faith in accordance with the UAGA generally affords you protection from civil and criminal liability for your role in transplantation.

- Consider a trauma patient as a potential organ donor even if cardiac arrest has occurred if oxygenation and circulation were restored promptly.

# GLOSSARY

**Brain death:** Cessation of brain function. Signs include apnea, coma, and unresponsiveness. Diagnosis is based on the results of objective testing and subjective assessment of the patient.

**Required Request Act:** A 1986 law that requires hospitals receiving Medicare funds to ask surviving family members for organ donation from any trauma patient who has died.

**UAGA:** Acronym for Uniform Anatomical Gift Act, a federal law enacted in 1969 to promote standards for the donation of body parts.

**UNOS:** Acronym for United Network for Organ Sharing, a nonprofit organization for the procurement of organs for transplantation.

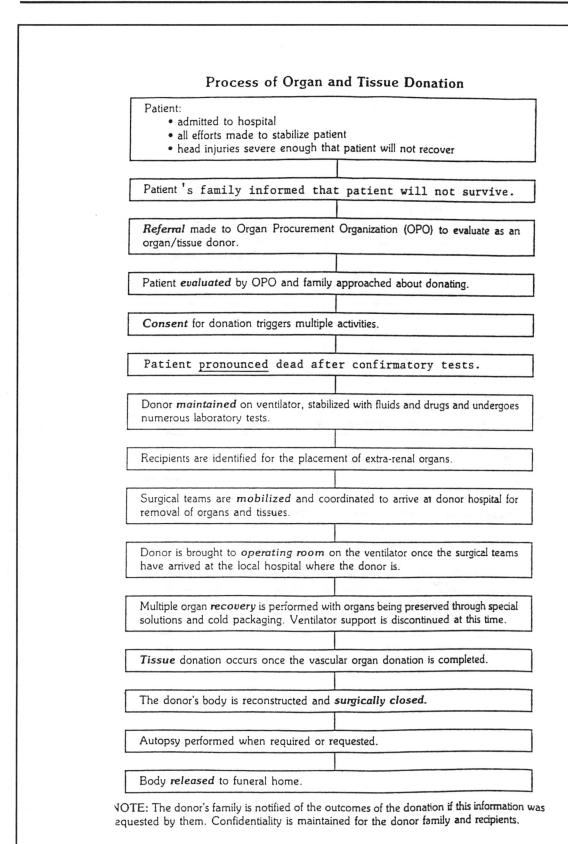

Figure 18-1. Flow chart of key activities that take place during organ and tissue donations.

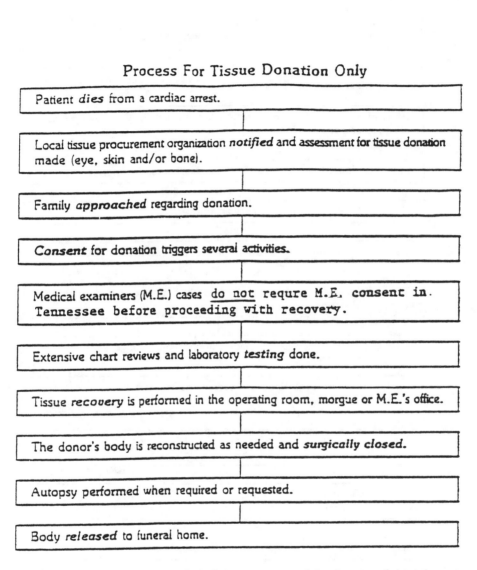

## Process For Tissue Donation Only

Patient *dies* from a cardiac arrest.

Local tissue procurement organization *notified* and assessment for tissue donation made (eye, skin and/or bone).

Family *approached* regarding donation.

*Consent* for donation triggers several activities.

Medical examiners (M.E.) cases do not requre M.E. consent in Tennessee before proceeding with recovery.

Extensive chart reviews and laboratory *testing* done.

Tissue *recovery* is performed in the operating room, morgue or M.E.'s office.

The donor's body is reconstructed as needed and *surgically closed*.

Autopsy performed when required or requested.

Body *released* to funeral home.

NOTE: The donor's family is notified of the outcomes of the donation if this information vas requested by them. Confidentiality is maintained for the donor family and recipients.

**Figure 18-1, continued**. Reprinted by permission from Pierce, J. M. *Regional Medical Center at Memphis acute ambulatory care survival guide.* Memphis: University of Tennessee, Department of Medicine, Division of Emergency Medicine, 1990.

# EXAM QUESTIONS

## Chapter 18

## Questions 87 - 91

87. The 1986 law that requires hospitals receiving Medicare funds to ask surviving family members for organ donation from trauma patients is the:

   a. Medicare Procurement Act
   b. Uniform Anatomical Gift Act
   c. Required Request Act
   d. Medicare Organ Sharing Act

88. The three minimum criteria for organ donation are brain death, cessation of respiration, and:

   a. Intact circulation
   b. Normothermia
   c. Completed organ donor card
   d. Flat line on an electroencephalogram

89. A common potential nursing diagnosis for an organ or tissue donor's family would be:

   a. Airway clearance, ineffective
   b. Knowledge deficit
   c. Adjustment impairment
   d. Body image disturbance

90. Your 30-year-old divorced patient has signed a donor card, but your institution's policy still requires consent or the family. Which of the following persons will be asked to give consent?

   a. Former spouse
   b. Oldest child
   c. Parent
   d. Sibling

91. Which of the following would in general be considered a contraindication to organ donation?

   a. Malignant brain tumor
   b. Viral infection
   c. Brief witnessed cardiac arrest
   d. Cessation of brain function

# CHAPTER 19

# PSYCHOSOCIAL ASPECTS OF TRAUMA

## CHAPTER OBJECTIVE

After completing this chapter, the reader should understand basic psychosocial responses to the crisis created by trauma and know how to plan interventions and referrals for trauma patients and their families.

## LEARNING OBJECTIVES

After studying this chapter, the reader should be able to

1. List the five stages, as outlined by Kubler-Ross, that most persons go through when confronted with a loss or a potential loss.

2. Characterize posttraumatic stress disorder.

3. Specify a type of psychologic disturbance that may be seen in a trauma survivor.

4. Recognize concerns and needs of the rescuers of trauma patients.

5. Suggest potential nursing diagnoses related to the psychosocial needs of a trauma patient.

## INTRODUCTION

This chapter provides guides for understanding the psychosocial responses of patients and their families when trauma turns their lives into turmoil. It reviews crisis intervention theory, presents specific strategies for supporting trauma patients' families, and discusses the special needs of some patients. Appendix A lists referral resources and support groups that help patients and their families achieve maximum recovery.

## TRAUMA AND STRESS

What if, one day, instead of arriving safely at work, you suddenly find yourself lying on the freeway while rescuers splint your fractures and cool your burns. Behind you, firemen douse the blazing wreckage of your car. You get a glimpse of your son as he's loaded into the helicopter, but the only thing your rescuers will say is, "They're doing everything they can for him." Imagine hearing the fading roar of the helicopter as your child is rushed ahead of you to the hospital. Feel the pain that strikes with each breath you take. Sense the dizziness, nausea, and visual changes that accompany the drop in your blood pressure. You will yourself to remain conscious, but you cannot. When you open your eyes again, you have lost 2 days of your life. Your son has lost his life. You will not walk again for 6 months. Your face is scarred and disfigured. How will your family respond when the police call to tell them you've been critically injured and are under treatment in a shock trauma unit?

If this seems a bit melodramatic, remember that trauma happens everyday. Trauma disrupts lives, and nurses are some of the first care providers. Trauma disrupts the order we cherish in our lives and throws us into turmoil. Most of us have routines and rituals that are part of our daily lives: Dress the kids for school, feed the dog, drive to work, run to the bank, buy the groceries, meet with colleagues, socialize with friends, visit family. When this daily routine is disrupted even by something as minor as a flat tire, many of us tend to act and feel a little unnerved. We call this stress.

Stress results from events that challenge the host's steady state. Stress requires adaptation and the implementation of coping mechanisms to return the host to a steady state, or a state of equilibrium. Trauma causes stress not only to the persons who are injured but also to their families and friends. Trauma may disrupt a family's structure, function, routines, and income. Some patients and families are not able to adapt to the stress of trauma, and they may react with anger and violence, or even physical signs such as tachycardia, syncope, hypertension, and physical violence. Imagine your response to the stress of a disruption of your life that is due to trauma as opposed to a flat tire.

# CRISIS INTERVENTION THEORY

A crisis is a situation resulting in turmoil and distress that disrupts the equilibrium of a person's life. Trauma is a situation that results in crisis because it is a sudden, unanticipated event that affects both the person who experiences it and those concerned for

that person. Crisis intervention is often necessary to help all concerned cope.

Persons in crisis may lack sufficient coping skills to master this turmoil and restore stability and order to their lives. Even the nurse caring for a trauma patient can be thrown into a state of crisis when facing horrible injuries and hysterical families. Yet, the nurse often must fill a gap in the foundation of support of the patient and the patient's family. The goal is to avoid collapse and breakdown while helping the patient and his or her family rally their own resources. Although a study of crisis intervention is beyond the scope of this book, the following is an overview of crisis intervention theory and techniques for trauma patients and their families. No one crisis intervention theory is best, and each patient's crisis situation should be considered unique.

A crisis generally consists of three phases: a precrisis phase, impact of the crisis, and the postcrisis phase. Nurses intervene in all three phases by teaching patients, families, friends, and colleagues to avoid injury; helping at the trauma scene; and counseling or referring for recovery. When you encounter someone in crisis, Sheehy and Jimmerson (1994) recommend that you assess the person, help the person define the crisis, allow the person to express feelings about the incident, explain hospital procedures, and provide support.

# RESPONSES OF THE PATIENT AND THE PATIENT'S FAMILY TO TRAUMA

Because accidents and assaults disrupt life-styles and cause crisis situations, trauma patients and their families appear distressed. Trauma nurses also find that the typical trauma patient comes complete with family and friends who, in fact, become the nurses' patients also. Trauma nurses not only must care for the patient but also must deal with acute stress reactions on the part of the patient's family and friends and sometimes even bystanders. Acute stress reactions that may occur in family and friends include syncope, hypertensive crisis, and myocardial infarction.

Elisabeth Kubler-Ross (1974) identified the five stages that most persons go through when confronted with a loss or potential loss:

1. **Denial:** The patient and/or the patient's family may deny the extent of the injuries or even pretend that nothing has happened.

2. **Anger:** Most nurses have at some point felt the wrath of a patient or a patient's family. Anger may be expressed for the accident or assault that caused the injury, it may be directed at the patient, or it may be directed at hospital personnel. Anger is often a manifestation of some type of hurt, frustration, or emotional wound.

3. **Bargaining:** In desperation, the distressed person offers an exchange in a final attempt to recoup the loss. Bargaining is often carried out with a perceived higher being. For example, someone in the patient's family may say, "God, if you let him live, I'll give my life savings to charity."

4. **Depression and guilt:** In this difficult stage, patients and their families feel remorse for the trauma and speculate with "if onlys" about how they could have prevented the accident.

5. **Acceptance:** In the final phase, acceptance, patients and their families come to grips

with the tragedy, repair their lives, and begin to move forward again.

Table 19-1, which is from the American Heart Association's text on advanced cardiac life support (Cummins, 1994), offers guidelines that are useful when a patient's family is to be informed of the patient's death. It can be modified for use when a patient has a critical injury.

The body's response to physical trauma is not limited to physical signs and symptoms. The mind and spirit also react to the event. According to Herman (1992), the "ordinary human response to danger is a complex, integrated system of reactions, encompassing both body and mind. Threat initially arouses the sympathetic nervous system, causing the person in danger to feel an adrenalin rush and go into a state of alert. Threat also concentrates a person's attention on the immediate situation. In addition, threat may alter ordinary perceptions: people in danger are often able to disregard hunger, fatigue, or pain." Trauma may also leave a person crippled by posttraumatic stress disorder, a reaction seen in veterans of the war in Vietnam and in survivors of disasters, assaults, or traumatic events.

A woman whose last glimpse of her son was as he was airlifted from an accident will most likely experience intrusive thoughts based on "the indelible imprint of the traumatic moment" and constriction, an altered state of consciousness manifested by psychic numbing and surrender. In this state, a person may feel as though the event is not happening to him or her. It is as if it is happening to someone else; it's like watching a movie (Herman, 1992). Trauma survivors may also feel that the traumatic event is recurring; this is called a flashback. A flashback is terrifying to the patient and calls for calm reassurance from the nurse (Cumbie, 1994). It is clear that the trauma team must not neglect the care of the mind and spirit after life-threatening or terrifying events. Specialists in posttraumatic stress disorder, such as mental health professionals or the clergy, may be called to help

## Table 19-1
## Conveying News of Sudden Death to Family Members

- Remember: the moment you stop resuscitative efforts on a person, you acquire a new set of patients—the family and loved ones.

- Call the family if they have not been notified. Explain that their loved one has been admitted to the emergency department and that the situation is serious. In general, survivors should be told of a death face-to-face, not over the telephone.

- Obtain as much information as possible about the patient and the circumstances surrounding the death. Carefully go over the events as they happened in the emergency department.

- Ask someone to take family members to a private area. Walk in, introduce yourself, and sit down. Address the closest relative.

- Briefly describe the circumstances leading to the death. Go over the sequence of events in the emergency department. Avoid euphemisms such as "he's passed on," "she is no longer with us," or "he's left us." Instead use the words "death," "dying," or "dead."

- Allow time for the shock to be absorbed. Make eye contact. Consider touching the family member and sharing your feelings. Convey your feelings with a phrase such as "You have my (our) sincere sympathy" rather than "I am (we are) sorry."

- Allow as much time as necessary for questions and discussion. Go over the events several times to make sure everything is understood and to facilitate further questions.

- Allow the family the opportunity to see their relative. If equipment is still connected, let the family know in advance.

- Know in advance what happens next and who will sign the death certificate. Physicians may impose burdens on staff and family if they fail to understand policies about death certification and disposition of the body. Know the answers to these questions before meeting the family. One of the survivors will surely ask, "What do we do next?" Be prepared with a proper answer.

- Enlist the aid of a social worker or the clergy if not already present.

- Offer to contact the patient's attending or family physician and be available if there are further questions. Arrange for follow-up and continued support during the grieving period.

- 

Reproduced with permission. *Textbook of advanced cardiac life support*, 1994. Copyright American Heart Association.

trauma patients heal spiritually during recovery from the physical injuries.

Appendix A provides a list of referral and resource groups for trauma patients. Social workers and local or hospital libraries offer valuable assistance in locating peer support groups and resources.

To review, the basics of crisis intervention are as follows:

- Allow the patient and the patient's family to express their feelings.

- Provide information in simple, honest, and direct terms.

- Do not overwhelm the patient and the patient's family with details.

- Repeat explanations often.

- React as a professional to the concerns of the patient and the patient's family.

Patients may experience lingering or long-term effects from a traumatic event, and referral to specialists can be helpful in recovery.

# FOR THE HEALER

The needs of the rescue team members are not to be overlooked after the trauma patient is stabilized and the emergency phase has ended. This is a period when the adrenaline rush diminishes and the team members take stock of their role in the rescue. Team members should have an opportunity to look back at their actions, consider whether to modify their interventions in the future, and reflect on their emotions after the rescue. Burnout can develop rapidly in trauma care; aftercare for the healers or rescuers may help deflect their descent into cynicism, anger, depression, or other painful emotional states. The AHA (Cummins, 1994) recommends a "critical incident debriefing" for those involved in emergency therapeutic interventions (Table 19-2). This debriefing also allows the team to consider the ethical issues involved in the rescue.

---

## Table 19-2
## Critical Incident Debriefing

- The debriefing should occur as soon as possible after the event, with all team members present.

- Call the group together, preferably in the resuscitation room. State that you want to have a "code debriefing."

- Review the events and conduct of the code. Include the contributory pathophysiology leading to the code, the decision tree followed, and any variations.

- Analyze the things that were done wrong and especially the things that were done right. Allow free discussion.

- Ask for recommendations/suggestions for future resuscitative attempts. All team members should share their feelings, anxieties, anger and possible guilt.

- Team members unable to attend the debriefing should be informed of the process followed, the discussion generated, and the recommendations made.

- The team leader should encourage team members to contact him or her if questions arise later.

Reproduced with permission. *Textbook of advanced cardiac life support*, 1994. Copyright American Heart Association.

---

# SUICIDE AND SUICIDE ATTEMPTS

Suicide is the second leading cause of death in persons 15-24 years old. In addition, suicide is on the rise in older persons; elderly suicides are most often white men who were recently widowed. Each year, 25,000-30,000 Americans die of self-inflicted injuries. A firm tally of suicides is impossible, because not all suicides are reported as such. For example, single-car crashes and drug overdoses—are they accidents or suicides? As in accidental injuries, use of alcohol and firearms is prevalent in suicide.

The suicide survivor and the families of both suicide survivors and suicide victims warrant special attention. After all, some persons have trouble expressing sympathy for self-inflicted injuries, and the patient may not thank you for your rescue. Be nonjudgmental and accept the patient's feelings as real for that patient. Fortunately, counseling is usually offered to suicidal patients, and you can help see that follow-up care is provided.

# SPECIAL PATIENTS

Sometimes you will encounter patients with special circumstances: those who are blind, deaf, or disabled or those who do not speak English. Grant et al. (1990) suggest some actions that can be used to facilitate communication under these circumstances:

- **For a patient who is deaf:** Find out if the patient reads lips. If he or she does not, communicate in writing whenever possible. If he or she uses sign language, seek a person who also knows sign language to interpret. Remain face to face with the patient when possible, and use touch to communicate when feasible. Shouting at a deaf patient is ineffective and inappropriate.

- **For a patient who is blind:** Inasmuch as this patient can hear, communication should not be impaired. Shouting is inappropriate. Offer frequent explanations and descriptions.

- **For a patient who does not speak English:** Locate an interpreter when possible; see Appendix D for when an interpreter is not available. If you live or work in an area with large numbers of persons who do not speak English, learn some of the key phrases in the language or languages

usually spoken. Note that the most rapidly growing population group in the United States speaks Spanish.

- **For a patient who is disabled:** The physically disabled trauma patient presents a challenge, as you may not know what limitations existed before the trauma. In general, assume that an injury exists until it is proved otherwise. Do not use terms such as crippled or lame; let disabled patients do for themselves what they can and want to do.

# NURSING STRATEGIES FOR MEETING THE PSYCHOSOCIAL NEEDS OF TRAUMA PATIENTS

The nursing care of the mind and spirit of the trauma patient focuses on identifying the stressors, assessing the patient's psychosocial response to the traumatic event, supporting the patient, and guiding the patient to resources that can support his or her efforts at recovery. Do this within the limits of your skills and training. Table 19-3 outlines some common nursing diagnoses and nursing interventions for meeting the psychosocial needs of trauma patients. The following strategies may also be relevant:

- Remain calm and professional when caring for a trauma patient so the patient and the patient's family will perceive you as a knowledgeable and skilled provider.

- Be brief, honest, and to the point in your initial contact with the patient's family. Their capacity for comprehension will be initially limited.

**Table 19-3**

**Potential Nursing Diagnoses and Interventions**

**for Meeting the Psychosocial Needs of Trauma Patients**

| Diagnosis | Interventions |
|---|---|
| Posttraumatic response r/t accidental injury or assault | Provide emotional support and simply listen as the patient expresses feelings about the traumatic event. Respond empathetically. Do not insist that the patient talk about the event. Do not quiz for details about an assault. Reduce environmental stimuli, as these may trigger flashbacks to the traumatic event. Monitor mental status. As needed, consult with a physician about the need for specialists. |
| Anxiety r/t situational crisis | Listen to the patient and allow verbalization of concerns. Offer verbal reassurance and gentle touch as indicated. Alter the environment when possible to reduce stress: Reduce noise, provide privacy, and minimize traffic through the area used to care for patients. |
| Body image disturbance r/t injuries | Accept the patient's perception of himself or herself and offer an opportunity to express feelings. Refer the patient to a counselor or community resource such as a support group of persons with similar concerns (e.g., burns). Offer positive reinforcement of efforts at adaptation made by the patient and the patient's family. |
| Spiritual distress r/t situational crisis | Acknowledge the patient's concerns, and allow him or her to vent feelings. Consult clergy and provide privacy if the patient wishes to see a clergy member. Provide for continuation of patient's religious practices. |
| Knowledge deficit r/t lack of exposure | Give clear concise explanations and repeat them often. Use terms appropriate to the level of understanding of the patient and the patient's family. Provide written information as appropriate. Orient the patient to surroundings. Encourage the patient and the patient's family to ask questions. |

Note.—This is a sample of potential nursing diagnoses. It is not presented as or intended to be a complete care plan for the trauma patient. More complete information can be found in a medical-surgical nursing course and textbook. r/t = related to.

Adapted from Sparks, S. and Taylor, C. M. *Nursing diagnosis reference manual*, Springhouse, PA: Springhouse Corp., 1991, and Chitwood, L. *Ambulatory patient care*, San Diego: Western Schools, 1994

- Reassure the patient and the patient's family frequently and address their concerns. Offer simple, honest explanations and repeat them often.

- Accept that many of the patient's emotions and feelings result from stress and pain. Keep in mind that restlessness may be a sign of hypoxia.

- Understand that pain and stress often limit the ability of the patient and the patient's family to comprehend information; repeated explanations are usually necessary. Be patient and honest; use simple terms.

- Accept that patients and families under stress sometimes direct their frustrations and anxiety at the nearest available person; this is often the nurse. Allow them to vent their feelings, and then restate the facts in simple language. Avoid escalating their anxiety by responding with hostility.

- Reflect for a few moments on the situation of the patient and the patient's family: What would you do if the patient were your child? How would you react if it happened to your spouse? Reflecting may give you insight into the perspective of the patient and the patient's family. Do not forget that although you may go to the hospital (as a nurse) everyday, your patients do not; it is all new to them.

- Offer simple explanations in language the patient and the patient's family can understand. Do not say, "He's hypovolemic with bilateral femur fractures, and he has a fractured sternum with probable myocardial contusion. We're transferring him to a level 1 center." Instead, say, "Both of his thigh bones and his breastbone are broken, so he's lost a lot of blood, and his heart is probably bruised. These injuries are serious, so we need to get him to a special trauma hospital where they can offer him the best possible chance of survival."

- Be honest, sensitive, and prompt (Cummins, 1994) in dealing with the family and friends of a trauma patient. They are entitled to regular updates and to a private place to receive that information.

- Do not become so caught up in technology that you become oblivious to the fact that the patient and the patient's family are humans who have needs.

- Expedite the reunion between the trauma patient and his or her family or significant others (Strange, 1987). This gives them more accurate knowledge and helps dispel images that the fam-

ily may be harboring. It also facilitates the sorting out of their needs.

- Refer the patient and the patient's family to community resources and support groups as indicated.

Your interventions should be within the scope of your professional license; commensurate with your skills and training; consistent with your state's nurse practice act; and when performed in a health care institution, adherent to that facility's standards of practice

# CRITICAL CONCEPTS

- Trauma causes turmoil and subsequent stress in the lives of trauma patients and their families, and they may react with hostility and anger.

- Crisis develops in three stages: the precrisis phase, impact, and the postcrisis phase.

- Pain and stress often limit the ability of trauma patients and their families to comprehend information; repeated simple explanations are usually necessary.

- Patients and families under stress often direct their frustrations and anxiety at the nearest available person, often the nurse.

- Traumatic events can cause posttraumatic stress disorder; this often requires intervention by a mental health professional.

- The nurse's role is to help trauma patients and their families identify resources and implement coping strategies.

# GLOSSARY

**Crisis:** A situation resulting in turmoil and distress that disrupts homeostasis.

**Critical incident debriefing:** An opportunity for rescuers to look back at their actions, consider whether to modify their interventions in the future, and reflect on their emotions after the rescue.

**Posttraumatic stress disorder:** A psychologic response to trauma characterized by symptoms such as hyperarousal, intrusion, and constriction. The disorder may cause flashbacks, in which the person feels as if the traumatic event is recurring.

**Support group:** A gathering of persons with a common interest whose goal is to offer guidance and assistance to members of the group.

# EXAM QUESTIONS

## Chapter 19

## Questions 92 - 96

92. Persons with posttraumatic stress disorder may experience intrusion, constriction, and:

    a. Hyperarousal
    b. Flashbacks
    c. Psychosis
    d. Melancholia

93. Which of the following might be a nursing diagnosis related to the psychosocial needs of a trauma patient?

    a. Injury, potential
    b. Self-esteem, chronic low
    c. Posttraumatic response
    d. Hypothermia

94. A psychologic disorder that may develop as a result of trauma is:

    a. Endogenous depression
    b. Posttraumatic stress disorder
    c. Borderline personality disorder
    d. Agoraphobia

95. As outline by Elisabeth Kubler-Ross, what is the third of the five stages that persons go through when confronted with a loss or a potential loss?

    a. Acceptance
    b. Bargaining
    c. Denial
    d. Depression

96. What is the term used for a meeting held after a rescue when the members of the rescue team discuss the event, their responses, and their feelings?

    a. Critical incident debriefing
    b. Psychologic seminar
    c. Ethical debate
    d. Support group

# CHAPTER 20

# PREVENTION AND REHABILITATION

## CHAPTER OBJECTIVE

After completing this chapter, the reader should be able to educate patients in methods of minimizing the chance of trauma and begin planning for rehabilitation when trauma does occur.

## LEARNING OBJECTIVES

After studying this chapter, the reader should be able to

1. List strategies to prevent and reduce the occurrence of trauma.

2. Describe the factors that influence violent behavior.

3. Describe rehabilitation of trauma patients.

## INTRODUCTION

No study of trauma would be complete without a discussion of how to prevent trauma from happening in the first place. Injuries are not random, unpredictable accidents; like disease, they occur in predictable patterns and are often preventable (*Introductions Injury Prevention*, 1990).

The purpose of this chapter is to help you meet the challenge of preventing trauma by educating patients, their families, and the public. When trauma does occur, the goal is to return the patient to his or her maximum level of functioning. This chapter reviews common sources of trauma and describes methods to enhance safety and reduce the occurrence of trauma. After trauma occurs, the potential for rehabilitation must be explored, so the final section describes rehabilitation and directs you to the appropriate resources for times when more information is needed.

## PREVENTION OF TRAUMA

The ACS ("Resources for Optimal Care," 1990) has described three general strategies to prevent injuries:

1. Persuade those at risk of injury to alter their habits.

Example: In Memphis, Tennessee, nurses and others at the level 1 trauma center teamed up to bring a series of trauma prevention messages to the public. They focused specifically on drunk driving and use of safety restraints in vehicles.

2. Require changes in individual behavior by law or administrative rules such as restraint laws.

Example: Many states now have laws requiring the use of seat belts and child safety restraints in motor vehicles, but these laws often have a minimal fine and may not even be enforced unless an injury occurs. Laws against drunk driving, assault, homicide, and child or spouse abuse have been in place for years; some have minimal effect. Unfortunately, behavior is influenced by many factors. Those most likely to respond to rules or laws are often those who are already concerned and are already following current guidelines.

3.  Provide automatic protection by product and environment design.

Example: Manufacturers have built cars with automatic shoulder harnesses, air bags, and antilock brakes; motorized equipment is manufactured with increasingly sophisticated designs to provide protection against injury.

The Johns Hopkins Injury Prevention Center (*Introduction: Injury Prevention*, 1990) recommends that health professionals become aggressively involved in prevention efforts. Some of the center's suggestions for professionals include the following:

- **Define the problem:** Interview patients about their injuries and identify families or groups at risk.

- **Collect and analyze data:** Improve data collection. Record comprehensive data from patients' charts when noting injuries, and then combine this with research and reporting.

- **Design interventions:** Approaches are generally educational, legal, or technologic. They include writing to legislators, working with engineers to create safer products, and educating the public on how to prevent injuries.

In the final analysis, injury prevention will be probably be influenced most by personal decisions and personal responsibility for actions and behaviors. As indicated throughout this book, alcohol and drugs are significant factors in trauma. Alcohol is involved in about one half of all accidental deaths. The following is a review of some of the methods for reducing the occurrence of trauma.

## Motorized Vehicles

The safety of occupants of motorized vehicles is increasingly a concern of legislators, insurers, and the general public. Proposed changes include stricter laws against drunk driving, mandatory restraint laws for occupants, and restrictions on licenses for both teenagers and the elderly.

**Passenger vehicles.** More cars are being built with proved safety features such as air bags and antilock brakes. Nevertheless, simple use of seat belts and air bags together will reduce mortality and morbidity from automobile accidents by 40%. Advise patients that all occupants, including children, should be restrained anytime the engine in a passenger vehicle is running. Many states now have mandatory child restraint laws; advise patients to buy approved child safety seats for the car and to use them. A child held on an adult's lap is not adequately restrained. Remind patients to drive within the speed limit and observe the rules of the road.

**All-terrain vehicles.** Notoriously unstable, three-wheeled recreational vehicles are not appropriate for children. These vehicles account for substantial numbers of injuries and fatalities every year. Most injuries occur when the vehicle tips over on the occupants. If your patients insist on using these vehicles, recommend that adults supervise children closely and that all occupants wear helmets.

**Motorcycles.** Because motorcycles are less visible than the vehicles around them, they are involved in more accidents. Without the protection that the shell of a car affords, motorcycles can be deadly. Mandatory helmet laws, once uniform across the United

States, have been weakened by some states, despite evidence that helmets reduce head trauma. In 1988, Rivara et al. reported that public funds covered the average $26,276 charge for caring for injured motor-cyclists at one medical center, so the public has an interest in motorcycle safety. Advise patients to wear helmets and clothing that covers the extremities when they are motorcycling. Some states have laws requiring that motorcycles have the headlight turned on at all times to increase the vehicles' visibility to others.

## Air Travel

Air travel remains relatively safe, despite such safety concerns as overcrowded skies and overworked air traffic controllers. Advise patients to do the following:

- Listen carefully to the flight attendant's instructions before takeoff.

- Keep the seat belt fastened at all times.

- Wear natural, not synthetic, fibers when traveling by air. Natural fibers like cotton do not melt and stick to the skin the way synthetic fibers do in a fire.

- Count the number of rows of seats between their seat and the nearest exit in the event that the lights go out and the exit cannot be seen in an emergency situation.

- Avoid ingestion of alcohol or sedatives that could dull reaction time in an emergency situation.

## Pedestrian Safety

Teaching children about pedestrian safety should begin early. Show children how they should stop, look, and listen before they cross the street. You can also advise patients to do the following:

- Wear reflective clothing when walking.

- Stick to well-lighted streets.

- Avoid the use of headphones that block out warning signals from traffic.

- Walk facing oncoming traffic.

## Household Accidents

Safety in the home is an essential component of trauma prevention.

**Fire safety.** Smoke detectors can cut the risk of dying in a fire by 50%. Advise patients to establish and practice a fire emergency plan at their homes that includes planned escape routes and a predetermined gathering place. Remind them to check smoke detectors monthly and to keep a fire extinguisher in the house. Advise adults who continue to smoke tobacco that they must not smoke in bed and that smoking materials must be kept out of the reach of children.

**Falls.** Because the elderly are especially prone to falls, remind patients to secure all carpeting or use nonskid mats, install handrails on stairs, and add lighting as needed. Rails should be up on the beds of patients who are prone to falls; bed monitors may be needed. Baby-guard gates should be at the top of flights of stairs, and window guards should be in place whenever children live in high-rise buildings.

## Environmental Safety

Teach patients to heed weather warnings and take shelter as advised. Earthquakes, although rare, can cause widespread devastation. Advise patients to do the following to prepare for an earthquake:

- Stock bottled water and canned goods in their houses.

- Secure bookcases and pictures to the walls.

- Avoid placing heavy objects on upper shelves where the objects can fall on persons.

- Know how to turn off the gas and water supply to their homes.

Most fatalities during earthquakes occur as persons rush to get out of buildings. Teach patients to avoid that crush. In an earthquake, they should get under a sturdy object such as a desk and stay away from windows and glass. In tornadoes, it is best to seek shelter in a basement or in a windowless inner room on the ground floor of the house.

## Industrial Safety

Because on-the-job injuries are both tragic and costly, help patients identify hazards in the workplace, and encourage them to become involved in industrial safety by joining safety committees and by planning safer work areas.

## Child Safety

Accidents are the leading cause of death in children, so safety should be a top priority. A discussion of child safety is beyond the scope of this book, but the following are some common safety measures:

- Have children use the right equipment when they are playing sports. Do not allow a child to engage in a sport with equipment that has been altered.

- Be sure children always wear a helmet when they are bicycling.

- Restrain children in approved child safety seats in the car.

- Use plastic electrical outlet blockers to keep children from putting hairpins or metal into electrical sockets. Use child-proof locks to secure cabinet doors and drawers, and stove and oven knobs. Store unused refrigerators with the doors removed or facing the wall.

- Advise children to avoid abandoned buildings.

- Teach children that they should not approach or attempt to pet strange or stray animals.

- Teach children that they should not talk to or accept rides from strangers. Teach children to report any offers or unusual conduct by an adult to a parent, guardian, or teacher.

- Teach children to approach someone in uniform or a mother with children when they do need help.

- Tell children about "good touch" and "bad touch" (molestation), and tell them to inform a trusted adult if they experience bad touching. The child should continue to tell until an adult intervenes in the harmful situation.

- Teach children to stay away from water when they are alone.

- Do not let children play near or with lawn mowers.

- Teach children that they should not play with matches.

- Store poisons out of the reach of children. Use child-proof containers in the home if poisons cannot be eliminated

- Do not give balloons to unattended small children and infants.

- Do not keep firearms in the home if small or unsupervised children are present. If patients insist on having weapons in the house, advise them to investigate methods of locking up and securing the weapons so children will not be hurt.

## Violence

Violence in the United States is reaching epidemic proportions. Because most victims and assailants know each other, efforts at prevention may center on early intervention, conflict-resolution programs, and environmental changes. According to the Johns Hopkins Injury Prevention Center (*Introduction: Injury Prention*, 1990), "Violent behavior is influenced by the wider context in which it occurs: culture and attitudes, socioeconomic status, firearm availability, and drug and alcohol use." The following suggestions are adapted in part from that report:

- Dispel the image of violence as an acceptable and effective tool for solving problems.

- Identify victims of interpersonal violence, such as women and children who are repeatedly injured by the same person. Refer these victims to appropriate social and judicial systems for assistance in stopping the cycle of violence.

- Confront and alter attitudes about the way handguns and other firearms are used in the United States.

# REHABILITATION

Rehabilitation actually begins with the first contact with the patient, as the trauma patient's rescuers intervene to limit the injuries and promote a return to the best possible state of wellness. Rehabilitation is an integral aspect of trauma care that involves nurses, physicians, physical and occupational therapists, social workers, and other professionals. Restoring the patient's previous level of health may not be possible, but the team's efforts are directed at maximizing the patient's potential and assisting him or her to adapt to changes as necessary.

Numerous support groups have been formed for patients and families injured by specific types of trauma. If a social worker is unable or unavailable to guide a patient and the patient's family through the maze of paperwork and resources, check with some of the organizations listed in Appendix A. Many newspapers carry listings of free and low-cost services and groups; check your public or hospital library.

In the United States, only 1 in 10 severely injured patients has access to rehabilitation services after initial treatment, according to the ACS ("Resources for Optimal Care," 1990). Because rehabilitation is crucial in the battle against permanent disability or death, rehabilitation services must be made more available to trauma patients. That is why the nurse must explore the patient's and family's feelings and goals and then intervene as indicated. As so often happens when it comes to making a difference for a patient, it is up to the nurse.

# NURSING STRATEGIES FOR PREVENTION OF INJURY AND FOR REHABILITATION OF TRAUMA PATIENTS

Table 20-1 gives common nursing diagnoses for counseling patients about injury prevention and about rehabilitation.

# CRITICAL CONCEPTS

- Rehabilitation begins as the rescuers reach the patient and attempt to limit injury and establish conditions conducive to full recovery.

**Table 20-1**

**Potential Nursing Diagnoses and Interventions for Prevention of Injury and for Rehabilitation of Trauma Patients**

| Diagnosis | Interventions |
|---|---|
| Violence, potential, other directed, r/t excitement or antisocial behavior | Refer patients to appropriate and specialized long-term treatment programs, such as for drug or alcohol abuse. Follow hospital policy to prevent violent patients or family members from injuring themselves or others. Teach the public via community meetings and seminars about the causes of violence. Help victims of violence (most know their attacker) get out of the relationship with the abusive person by referral to appropriate social and legal agencies. |
| Violence, potential, self-directed, r/t suicide attempt | Ask the patient directly, "Have you thought about killing yourself?" Make appropriate referrals to mental health professionals and social service agencies. Use a warm, compassionate, and nonjudgmental attitude to show your concern. Advise patient's family members or partner how to secure the environment to reduce suicide attempts (e.g., removing firearms from the home). |
| Injury, potential, r/t lack of awareness of environmental hazards | Help patients detect home hazards that could cause accidents. Encourage patients to make repairs and remove safety hazards. Tell parents to teach children safety principles and safe behavior. Talk to parents about child abuse, and make referrals when appropriate. Report suspected spouse and child abuse. Make referrals to community resources. |
| Knowledge deficit r/t lack of exposure (to safe living practices) | Counsel patients about potential hazards in their homes. Develop protocols to detect, counsel, and refer at-risk patients such as battered women and children. Teach CPR; train paramedics; educate other professionals in injury prevention. Educate the public about the needs for specific laws; appear on radio and talk shows; write letters to the editor of your local newspaper; write your legislator. Counsel patients and families about what to expect during rehabilitation; act as an advocate during transition to a rehabilitation facility; communicate information as necessary. |
| Trauma, potential, r/t external factors | Teach patients, patients' families, and the public about health hazards; instruct them in safety practices. Counsel industry about safe employee practices. Remind patients to use seat belts; restrain children in cars at all times; obey traffic laws; reduce or eliminate alcohol or drug ingestion; and eliminate operation of motorized vehicles, boats, or machinery when drinking or using drugs. Teach families about preventing falls. |
| Home maintenance management impairment r/t support system and functioning | Help patients and their families explore strengths, options, and available resources. Detect discharge needs, and facilitate transition from hospital to home or rehabilitation institute. Refer patients to appropriate social service agencies. Discuss obstacles to rehabilitation. Counsel families and guide them to appropriate expectations; encourage regular meetings to discuss concerns. |
| Poisoning, potential, r/t external factors | Teach about child safety and safe home practices. Counsel parents and families to remove dangerous products from their homes. Provide families with information about home safety. |

Note.—This is a sample of potential nursing diagnoses. It is not presented as or intended to be a complete care plan. More complete information can be found in a medical-surgical nursing course and textbook. r/t = related to.

Adapted from Sparks, S. and Taylor, C. M. *Nursing diagnosis reference manual*, Springhouse, PA: Springhouse Corp., 1991, and Chitwood, L., *Ambulatory patient care*, San Diego: Western Schools, 1994.

- Injuries are not random, unpredictable accidents; like disease, they occur in predictable patterns and are often preventable.

- Alcohol is involved in about half of all deaths from injury.

- Children should never be left unattended.

- Smoke detectors cut the risk of dying in a fire in half.

- Use of seat belts and air bags reduces mortality and serious injuries from car crashes by about 40%.

# GLOSSARY

Rehabilitation: A process of returning a patient after an injury to his or her previous or highest possible level of wellness.

Safety: Prevention of accidents and injury; best accomplished through education.

Support group: A gathering of persons with a common interest whose goal is to offer guidance and assistance to members of the group.

# EXAM QUESTIONS

## Chapter 20

## Questions 97 - 100

97. The American College of Surgeons recommends three strategies to prevent injuries: persuading those at risk to alter their habits, requiring changes in individual behavior by laws, and:

    a. Establishing a national registry of accidental injuries
    b. Sponsoring legislation requiring stricter compliance with safety requirements
    c. Providing automatic protection by product design
    d. Offering insurance discounts to those who live safely

98. The Johns Hopkins Injury Prevention Center recommends three actions to prevent injury: define the problem, collect and analyze data, and:

    a. Write to legislators.
    b. Seek out funding.
    c. Design interventions.
    d. Perform research.

99. Violence is influenced by cultures and attitudes, availability of firearms, use of drugs and alcohol, and:

    a. Epidemiologic status
    b. Technologic advances
    c. Socioeconomic status
    d. Community organization

100. When does rehabilitation of the trauma patient begin?

    a. As rescuers reach the patient at the trauma scene
    b. When the social worker evaluates the patient at the hospital
    c. At the first interdisciplinary care planning conference
    d. When the patient enters a rehabilitation institute

# APPENDIX A

# Professional Resources

## Injury Control & Emergency Health Services

American Public Health Association Membership Office
1015 15th St. N.W.
Washington, DC 20005
(202) 789-5600

## Emergency Nurses Cancel Alcohol Related Emergencies, Inc. (C.A.R.E.)

18 Lyman St.
Westborough, MA 01581
(508) 753-7222

## The American Trauma Society

8903 Presidential Parkway, Ste. 512
Upper Marlboro, MD 20772
(800) 556-7890

## American Association of Critical-Care Nurses

101 Columbia
Aliso Viejo, CA 92656
(800) 899-AACN

## American Nurses' Association

600 Maryland Ave. S.W., # 100 West
Washington, DC 20024-2571
(202) 554-4444

## American Association of Nurse Anesthetists

222 S. Prospect Ave.
Park Ridge, IL 60068-4001
(708) 692-7050

## American Association of Occupational Health Nurses, Inc.

50 Lenox Pointe
Atlanta, GA 30324
(404) 262-1162

## American Society of Ophthalmic Registered Nurses, Inc.

P. O. Box 193030
San Francisco, CA 94119
(415) 561-8513

## American Society of Plastic & Reconstructive Surgical Nurses, Inc.

N. Woodbury Rd.
Box 56
Pitman, NJ 08071
(609) 256-2340

## American Thoracic Society, Section on Nursing

1740 Broadway
New York, NY 10019-4374
(212) 315-8700

**Association of Operating Room Nurses**

21770 S. Parker, Ste. 300
Denver, CO 80231-5711
(303) 755-6300

**Association of Rehabilitation Nurses**

5700 Old Orchard Rd.
Skokie, IL 60077
(708) 966-3433

**Emergency Nurses Association**

216 Higgins Rd.
Park Ridge, IL 60068
(708) 698-9400

**National Association of Orthopaedic Nurses, Inc.**

N. Woodbury Rd.
Box 56
Pitman, NJ 08071
(609) 256-2310

**National Association of Pediatric Nurse Associates and Practitioners**

1101 Kings Hwy. N., Ste. 206
Cherry Hill, NJ 08034
(609) 667-1773

**National Association of School Nurses**

P. O. Box 1300
Lamplighter Lane
Scarborough, ME 04074
(207) 883-2117

**National Flight Nurses Association**

6900 Grove Rd.
Thorofare, NJ 08086
(609) 848-1000

**North American Nursing Diagnosis Association**

3525 Caroline St.
St. Louis, MO 63104

**Society of Gastroenterology Nurses and Associates, Inc.**

1070 Sibley Tower
Rochester, NY 14604
(716) 546-7241

**Society of Otorhinolaryngology and Head/Neck Nurses**

116 Canal St., Ste. A
New Smyrna Beach, FL 32168
(904) 428-1695

# APPENDIX B

**REGIONAL MEDICAL CENTER AT MEMPHIS**

### TRAUMA ASSESSMENT
### NURSES' NOTES

| DATE: | CLOTHING DISPOSITION: | IV FLUIDS |||||
|---|---|---|---|---|---|---|
| | ☐ Family ☐ Patient ☐ Storage ☐ Disposal | TIME | SIZE | SITE | SOLUTION | AMT |
| ALLERGIES: | ☐ Police ☐ None | | | | | |
| PAST MEDICAL HISTORY: | VALUABLES DISPOSITION: | | | | | |
| | ☐ Family ☐ Patient ☐ Police ☐ None | | | | | |
| PATIENT MEDICATIONS: | ☐ Security Envelope # | | | | | |
| LAST TETANUS: | PROCEDURES ||| | | | |

| | PROCEDURES | | | | |
|---|---|---|---|---|---|
| | TIME | | SIZE | INT | |
| WRIST BAND NUMBER: | 12 Lead EKG | | | | |
| | Backboard | | | | |
| POLICE NOTIFICATION: ☐ Yes ☐ No | C-Collar | | | | |
| Time: Officer: | Cardiac Monitoring | | | | |
| | Cast Application | | | | |
| DISCHARGE INSTRUCTIONS: | Catheter - Foley | | | | |
| ☐ Discharge instructions given | Catheter - In & Out | | | | |
| ☐ Time: | Chest Tube ☐ R ☐ L | | | | |
| ☐ Discharge Vital Signs: | CVP Line | | | | |
| P: R: B/P: | Lab drawn | | | | |
| ☐ Patient verbalized understanding | N/G Tube | | | | |
| ☐ Unable to comprehend | O₂ BNC @ | | | | |
| ☐ Instructions given to: | O₂ NRB Mask @ | | | | |
| ☐ Ambulatory ☐ W/C ☐ Stretcher | Peritoneal Lavage | | | | |
| ☐ Instructions given by: | Sorenson ☐ R ☐ L | | | | |
| | Suturing | | | | |

**IV FLUIDS** — TOTAL

**OUTPUT**

| TIME | TYPE | AMT |
|---|---|---|
| | | |
| | | |
| | | |

TOTAL

**RADIOLOGY**

☐ Ambulatory ☐ W/C ☐ Stretcher

| X-RAY: | To: | From: |
|---|---|---|
| ☐ Returned: | To: | From: |
| ☐ Returned: | To: | From: |
| CT SCAN: | To: | From: |
| ☐ Returned: | To: | From: |
| ☐ Returned: | To: | From: |
| ARTERIOGRAM: | To: | From: |

| VITAL SIGNS ||||||| TIME | NURSING OBSERVATIONS |
|---|---|---|---|---|---|---|---|
| TIME | T | P | R | B/P | O₂ SAT | | |
| | | | | | | | |
| | | | | | | | |
| | | | | | | | |
| | | | | | | | |
| | | | | | | | |
| | | | | | | | |
| | | | | | | | |
| | | | | | | | |

| MEDICATIONS |||| | |
|---|---|---|---|---|---|
| TIME | INT | DRUG/DOSAGE | ROUTE | | |
| | | 0.5cc Tetanus Toxoid | IM | | |
| | | Lot # | | | |
| | | Exp: | | | |
| | | | | | |
| | | | | | |
| | | | | | |
| | | | | | |
| | | | | | |
| | | | | | |

| RN SIGNATURE | INITIALS | RN SIGNATURE | INITIALS | RN SIGNATURE | INITIALS | RN SIGNATURE | INITIALS |
|---|---|---|---|---|---|---|---|
| | | | | | | | |

WHITE-Chart Copy      YELLOW-Dept. Copy                      FORM 6233.001

**Trauma Assessment Nurses' Notes.**

Reprinted with permission. The Elvis Presley Memorial Trauma Center. A division of The Regional Medical Center at Memphis (THE MED).

REGIONAL MEDICAL CENTER AT MEMPHIS

## ELVIS PRESLEY MEMORIAL TRAUMA CENTER
### SHOCK TRAUMA FLOWSHEET

**PATIENT INFORMATION:**

Age _____ Sex _____

Last Tetanus _____

Allergies _____

_____

Medications _____

_____

Past Medical History _____

_____

_____

Last Meal _____

Wrist Band # _____

**EVENTS:**

Mechanism of Injury _____

Time of Injury (est.) _____

Mode of Arrival _____

Time of Arrival _____

**PREHOSPITAL CARE:**

VS            B/P _____ P _____ R _____

Cervical Collar            ☐ Yes    ☐ No

Spineboard            ☐ Yes    ☐ No

Mast Trousers            ☐ Yes - Time _____ ☐ No

Splints            ☐ Yes   Type _____

☐ No   Location _____

IVF's _____

**MEDICATIONS PTA:**

Chest Tube  ☐ PTA

**INJURIES:**

**FAMILY NOTIFICATION:**

Here        ☐        Time _____

Called      ☐        Time _____

Phone ( ____ ) _____
          A.C.

Person Contacted _____

**VALUABLES:**

Family  ☐            Security  ☐

Police  ☐            Envelope # _____

Other  ☐            None  ☐

**CLOTHING:**

Family  ☐            Storage  ☐            None  ☐

Police  ☐            Other  ☐            Disposal  ☐

**POLICE NOTIFICATION:**        ☐ Yes      ☐ No        528-2222
                                                           or
                                                           Ext. 7947

Time _____ Officer _____

**SHOCK TRAUMA DEATH OR IMPENDING DEATH:**

Shock Trauma Death        ☐ Yes      ☐ No
Impending Death        ☐ Yes      ☐ No
Notification of Mid-South Transplant Foundation        ☐ Yes      ☐ No
(901) 528-5923 or (901) 577-1727

Nurse Responsible For Contact _____

**Shock Trauma Flowsheet.**

## VITAL SIGNS

| Time | | | | | | | | | | | |
|---|---|---|---|---|---|---|---|---|---|---|---|
| BP (ART. LINE) | | | | | | | | | | | |
| BP (CUFF) | | | | | | | | | | | |
| HEART RATE | | | | | | | | | | | |
| RESPIRATIONS | | | | | | | | | | | |
| TEMPERATURE | | | | | | | | | | | |
| CVP 3-15 CM | | | | | | | | | | | |
| $O_2$ SAT | | | | | | | | | | | |
| ETCO$_2$ | | | | | | | | | | | |
| CPR | | | | | | | | | | | |
| MAST | | | | | | | | | | | |
| | | | | | | | | | | | |

**① Pupil Reaction/Size**

S-Sluggish      B-Brisk      N-Nonreactive

Pupil sizes: 2 3 4 5 6 7 8

| | ① R | ① L | ② | ③ | ④ | Glascow | ⑤ | ⑥ | Trauma Score |
|---|---|---|---|---|---|---|---|---|---|
| Admission | | | | | | | | | |
| Discharge | | | | | | | | | |

| Skin Color | | Skin Temperature | | Skin Moisture | | Pulses | Absent R | Absent L | Present R | Present L |
|---|---|---|---|---|---|---|---|---|---|---|
| Normal | ☐ | Normal | ☐ | Normal | ☐ | Cartoid | ☐ | ☐ | ☐ | ☐ |
| Cyanotic | ☐ | Hot | ☐ | Dry | ☐ | Radial | ☐ | ☐ | ☐ | ☐ |
| Pale | ☐ | Cool | ☐ | Diaphoretic | ☐ | Femoral | ☐ | ☐ | ☐ | ☐ |
| Ashen | ☐ | Cold | ☐ | | | Post. Tibial | ☐ | ☐ | ☐ | ☐ |
| Flushed | ☐ | | | | | Pedal | ☐ | ☐ | ☐ | ☐ |

**Glascow**

| | | |
|---|---|---|
| Eye Opening ② | Spontaneous | 4 |
| | Verbal | 3 |
| | To Pain | 2 |
| | None | 1 |
| Verbal Response ③ | Oriented | 5 |
| | Disoriented | 4 |
| | Inappropriate | 3 |
| | Incomprehensible | 2 |
| | None | 1 |
| Motor Response ④ | Obeys Command | 6 |
| | Localize Pain | 5 |
| | Flexion-Withdrawal | 4 |
| | Flexion-Abnormal | 3 |
| | Extension (pain) | 2 |
| | None | 1 |

**Trauma**

| | | |
|---|---|---|
| Respiratory Rate ⑤ | 10-29 | 4 |
| | 29 | 3 |
| | 6-9 | 2 |
| | 1-5 | 1 |
| | 0 | 0 |
| Systolic Blood Pressure ⑥ | 89 | 4 |
| | 76-89 | 3 |
| | 50-75 | 2 |
| | 1-49 | 1 |
| | 0 | 0 |
| | 13-15 | 4 |
| | 9-12 | 3 |
| | 6-8 | 2 |
| | 4-5 | 1 |
| | 0-3 | 0 |

## PROCEDURES

| | | Size | Time | | | Time |
|---|---|---|---|---|---|---|
| ETT | | | | Cardiac Monitoring | | |
| Chest Tube: | R / L | | | Pericardiocentesis | | |
| Foley | | | | ABD Tap: IN OUT | | |
| CVP | | | | ☐ Bloody ☐ Pink ☐ Clear | | |
| N/G Tube | | | | Crico | | |
| Arterial Line | | | | Thoracotomy R / L | | |
| 12-Lead EKG | | | | Autotransfusion | | |

## OXYGEN/VENTILATOR SETTINGS

| | Setting/Time | Setting/Time | Setting/Time |
|---|---|---|---|
| FiO$_2$ | | | |
| T.V. | | | |
| Rate | | | |
| PEEP | | | |
| Mode | | | |
| BNC | | | |
| NRB Mask | | | |

**Shock Trauma Flowsheet. (Cont.)**

**MEDICATIONS**

| Time | Drug/Dose/Route | Site | Given By |
|------|-----------------|------|----------|
|  |  |  |  |
|  |  |  |  |
|  |  |  |  |
|  |  |  |  |
|  |  |  |  |
|  |  |  |  |
|  |  |  |  |
|  |  |  |  |
|  |  |  |  |
|  |  |  |  |
|  |  |  |  |
|  |  |  |  |
|  |  |  |  |
|  |  |  |  |
|  |  |  |  |
|  |  |  |  |
|  |  |  |  |
|  |  |  |  |
|  |  |  |  |
|  |  |  |  |
|  |  |  |  |

**INTRAVENOUS FLUIDS - CRYSTALLOIDS**

| Time | Type & Amount | Site | Amount Infused |
|------|---------------|------|----------------|
|  |  |  |  |
|  |  |  |  |
|  |  |  |  |
|  |  |  |  |
|  |  |  |  |
|  |  |  |  |
|  |  |  |  |
|  |  |  |  |
|  |  |  |  |
|  |  |  |  |
|  |  |  |  |
|  |  |  |  |
|  |  |  |  |
|  |  |  |  |
|  |  |  |  |
|  |  |  |  |
|  |  |  |  |
|  |  |  |  |
| **TOTAL** |  |  |  |

| INTAKE TOTALS | | OUTPUT TOTALS | |
|---------------|--|---------------|--|
| Field |  | Urine |  |
| IV |  | N/G |  |
| Blood |  | Chest Tube R |  |
| Lavage |  | Chest Tube L |  |
| Other |  | Lavage |  |
| TOTAL |  | TOTAL |  |

| RADIOLOGY | ORDERED | RADIOLOGY | ORDERED |
|-----------|---------|-----------|---------|
| Laterial C-spine |  | Leg • R • L |  |
| Swimmers |  | CT of Head |  |
| T-spine |  | CT of Abdomen |  |
| LS-spine |  | CT of Pelvis |  |
| Chest |  | CT of |  |
| KUB |  | IVP/Cysto |  |
| Pelvis |  | Arteriogram |  |
| Arm • R • L |  | Other: |  |

**INTRAVENOUS FLUIDS - COLLOIDS/BLOOD**

| Time | Type & Amount | Donor # | Amount Infused |
|------|---------------|---------|----------------|
|  |  |  |  |
|  |  |  |  |
|  |  |  |  |
|  |  |  |  |
|  |  |  |  |
|  |  |  |  |
|  |  |  |  |
|  |  |  |  |
|  |  |  |  |
|  |  |  |  |
|  |  |  |  |
|  |  |  |  |
|  |  |  |  |
|  | **TOTAL** |  |  |

| | | |
|--|--|--|
| R ANTE - Right Antecubital | L ANTE - Left Antecubital | RW - Right Wrist |
| LW - Left Wrist | RF - Right Forearm | LF - Left Forearm |
| EJ - External Jugular | FL - Femoral Line | CD - Cut Down |
| SL - Subclavian | | |

**Shock Trauma Flowsheet. (Cont.)**

| DATE | TIME | NURSING OBSERVATIONS |
|------|------|----------------------|
|      |      |                      |
|      |      |                      |
|      |      |                      |
|      |      |                      |
|      |      |                      |
|      |      |                      |
|      |      |                      |
|      |      |                      |
|      |      |                      |
|      |      |                      |
|      |      |                      |
|      |      |                      |
|      |      |                      |
|      |      |                      |
|      |      |                      |
|      |      |                      |
|      |      |                      |
|      |      |                      |
|      |      |                      |
|      |      |                      |
|      |      |                      |
|      |      |                      |
|      |      |                      |
|      |      |                      |
|      |      |                      |
|      |      |                      |
|      |      |                      |
|      |      |                      |
|      |      |                      |
|      |      |                      |
|      |      |                      |
|      |      |                      |
|      |      |                      |
|      |      |                      |
|      |      |                      |
|      |      |                      |
|      |      |                      |
|      |      |                      |
|      |      |                      |

Patient Disposition _____          Team Leader _____

Time of Discharge _____          Primary Nurse _____

Condition _____          Recorder _____

Total Time in Shock Trauma _____

Nurse Signatures

_____          _____

_____          _____

**Shock Trauma Flowsheet. (Cont.)**
Reprinted with permission. The Elvis Presley Memorial Trauma Center. A division of The Regional Medical Center at Memphis (THE MED).

# APPENDIX C

**MASSACHUSETTS GENERAL HOSPITAL**

## REPORT OF DEATH

(Fill in immediately and completely and deliver to Admitting Office
with Patient's Medical Record.)

DATE

| 1. PATIENT LOCATION | BLDG. | ROOM NO. | PRIVATE PATIENT OF DR. |
|---|---|---|---|

| DATE OF ADMISSION | DATE OF DEATH | HOUR | AM PM |
|---|---|---|---|

**2. IS THIS A MEDICO-LEGAL CASE REPORTABLE TO MEDICAL EXAMINER?**
This includes all deaths due to/or influenced by other than natural causes — includes death resulting from trauma, accidents, suicide, or environmental exposure; within 24 hours of admission, of persons suffering from chronic substance abuse or acute intoxications, following accidents in the hospital, during surgery or procedures of any sort, of children less than 2 years of age unless that patient is in the terminal phase of a well-documented natural disease and death is expected, of persons with no known serious medical conditions (i.e. upon arrival), or of a person admitted to the hospital in a coma who never regained consciousness, outside the hospital or in an institution, public place, or correctional facility, within 90 days following delivery or abortion. IF UNSURE, CALL MEDICAL EXAMINER 267-6767.

No ☐   Yes ☐   (specify) _____

Reported to Medical Examiner _____ by _____ Title _____ Date _____
(M.E. NAME)

Jurisdiction ☐ Accepted ☐ Declined by_____ Time _____ Date _____
(M.E. NAME)

**3. REQUEST TO CONSIDER ORGAN AND TISSUE DONATION FOR TRANSPLANTATION — NOTE: THIS IS NOT OFFICIAL CONSENT**
By law, a request for organ and tissue donation must be made to next of kin of deceased. The New England Organ Bank should be contacted to come in and talk with the next of kin of deceased to obtain official consent.

Was consent granted to contact     To
New England Organ Bank           Discuss ►

**TISSUE DONATION REQUEST**
(includes eyes, skin, bone, heart valves) Yes ☐ No ☐
**ORGAN DONATION REQUEST**
(heart, liver, pancreas, lungs, kidney) Yes ☐ No ☐

Yes ☐  No ☐

Relationship to
the deceased _____

By whom (name) _____
New England Organ Bank (617 277-8500) to be contacted if consent granted — was this done? Yes ☐ No ☐

If no family request made, why?   Medical unsuitability of deceased ☐   (Check one or both)
                                 Undue emotional stress to family ☐

**4. REQUEST FOR POST-MORTEM EXAMINATION** (Do not request if this is a Medical Examiner case.).

Permission for autopsy   Received ☐   Refused ☐

Name of deceased_____
I, (an adult) hereby authorize physicians of the Massachusetts General Hospital to conduct a post-mortem examination of the above-named deceased with generally accepted methods and customary extent of dissection to determine the cause of death, extent of disease, presence of any associated conditions, or the answers to other uncertainties concerning the deceased's physical condition. Tissues exposed in the course of such an examination may be retained for scientific investigation after the examination is completed.

Restrictions   None ☐   Yes ☐   (please specify) _____

_____

Signed: _____ Relationship to deceased: _____

Address: _____

Permission received by: _____
                       Doctor's Signature
**Telephone Consent:**
If permission is obtained by telephone, the entire conversation must be witnessed by a third party listening in.

NAME OF WITNESS: _____ SIGNATURE OF WITNESS _____

If permission received from other than nearest relative, state reason: _____

If NO next of kin: Autopsy authorization granted by J. Robert Buchanan, M.D., General Director per_____
                                                                        (Assistant Director or his designee)

**5. READ CAREFULLY BEFORE COMPLETING**

**A.** This section is similar to standard Medical Certificate of Death used in practice outside of the hospital. Before completing, see ''Death Certificates'' section of the House Officers' Manual. Use terminology of International List of Causes of Death.

Do not enter more than one cause for each of (a), (b) and (c)

*This does not mean the mode of dying, such as heart failure, asthenia, etc. It means the disease, or complications which caused death.*

*Morbid conditions, if any, giving rise to the above cause (a) stating the underlying cause last.*

*Conditions contributing to the death but not related to the disease or condition causing death.*

|  |  | Interval between Onset and Death (estimate days, months, years or unknown) |
|---|---|---|
| DISEASE OR CONDITION DIRECTLY LEADING TO DEATH (a) _____ |  |  |
| ANTE CEDENT CAUSES | (The above was) Due to: (b) _____ |  |
|  | (The above was) Due to: (c) _____ |  |
| OTHER SIGNIFICANT CONDITIONS _____ |  |  |

_____

_____

OPERATIONS (This WITH DATES admission) _____

COMPLETED BY _____ M.D. TIME: _____ DATE: _____
(Attending Physician, Resident, Asst. Resident)

**B. * THIS SECTION TO BE COMPLETED BY PATHOLOGY SERVICE.**

**CAUSES STATED BELOW ARE TO DUPLICATE THOSE ON THE OFFICIAL DEATH CERTIFICATE AS ISSUED TO THE FUNERAL DIRECTOR.**

Do not enter more than one cause for each of (a), (b) and (c)

*This does not mean the mode of dying, such as heart failure, asthenia, etc. It means the disease, or complications which caused death.*

*Morbid conditions, if any, giving rise to the above cause (a) stating the underlying cause last.*

*Conditions contributing to the death but not related to the disease or condition causing death.*

This part is similar to standard Medical Certificate of Death used in practice outside the Hospital. Before completing it, see ''Death Certificates'' section of House Officers' Manual, unless you are familar with it. Use terminology of International List of Causes of Death.

|  |  | Interval between Onset and Death (estimate days, months, years or unknown) |
|---|---|---|
| DISEASE OR CONDITION DIRECTLY LEADING TO DEATH (a) _____ |  |  |
| ANTE CEDENT CAUSES | (The above was) Due to: (b) _____ |  |
|  | (The above was) Due to: (c) _____ |  |
| OTHER SIGNIFICANT CONDITIONS _____ |  |  |

_____

_____

**Maryland Anatomical Gift Act**
**Uniform Disposition Form**

**Decedent Information**

Name _____

History No. _____

NAME OF HOSPITAL

Sex _____ Age _____ Date of Request _____ Time of Request _____

CITY

In order that humanity may benefit, I _____ being the:

☐ spouse, ☐ adult son or daughter, ☐ parent, ☐ adult brother or sister, ☐ person authorized or responsible for

the disposition of _____

give to the herein named hospital and/or the appropriate organ or tissue procurement agency/s
for: ☐ any purpose allowed by law, ☐ transplantation, ☐ medical research and education — the following:

**ORGANS**     (heart, lung, liver, kidneys, pancreas) subject to the following restriction:

_____     ☐ Declined     ☐ Not Suitable
(IF NO RESTRICTIONS WRITE NONE)

**TISSUES**     (eyes, skin, bone, inner ear, heart valves, connective) subject to the following restrictions:

_____     ☐ Declined     ☐ Not Suitable
(IF NO RESTRICTIONS WRITE NONE)

**Post Mortem**     I authorize the representatives of this hospital to perform a complete autopsy on the deceased,
**Examination**     including examination of the central nervous system, and to remove and retain such organs and tissues
as required for proper diagnosis.

_____     ☐ Declined     ☐ Not Suitable
(IF NO RESTRICTIONS WRITE NONE)

I certify that I bear the above noted relationship to the decedent, that I am unaware of any objection by the decedent regarding
the making of this anatomical gift and that I fully understand this form.

_____     _____     _____
WITNESS     DATE     SIGNATURE

_____     _____     _____
WITNESS     DATE     ADDRESS

_____
CITY     STATE     ZIP

**For Hospital Use Only**

**Medical**     Does this patient's death fall within the jurisdiction of the Medical Examiner? ☐ No  ☐ Yes
**Examiner**
**Information**     If yes has the Medical Examiner been informed? ☐ No ☐ Yes by _____

Have the above procedures been authorized? ☐ Yes Authorized by: _____

**Anatomical**
**Gift Information:** ☐ Donor ☐ Non-donor ☐ Medically unsuitable: _____
(SEE ABOVE)                                                             COMMENTS

☐ Family Unavailable ☐ Family Declined: _____
COMMENTS

Request Made by: _____     Position: _____

# APPENDIX D

| English | French | German | Spanish | Italian |
|---------|--------|--------|---------|---------|
| Hello | Bonjour | Guten Tag | ¡Hola! | Pronto |
| My name is | Je m'appelle | Ich heisse | Mi nombre es (Me llamo) | Mi chiamo |
| I am an emergency technician | Je suis infirmier de salle d'urgence | Ich bin Medizin-Techniker für Notfälle | Yo soy un enfermero (una enfermera) | Sono un tecnico del pronto soccorso |
| I am here to help you | Je suis ici pour vous aider | Ich bin hier um Ihnen zu helfen | Estoy aquí para ayudarle | Sono qui per aiutarLa |
| Do you understand? | Comprenez-vous? | Verstehen Sie? | ¿Me comprende? | Comprende? |
| I do not understand | Je ne comprends pas | Nein, ich verstehe Sie nicht | ¡No comprendo! | No, non capisco |
| What is your name? | Comment vous appelez-vous? | Wie heissen Sie? | ¿Cuál es su nombre? (¿Cómo se llama usted?) | Come si chiama (Lei)? |
| Mr. | Monsieur | Herr | Señor | Signore |
| Mrs. | Madame | Frau | Señora | Signora |
| Miss | Mademoiselle | Fräulein | Señorita | Signorina |
| Are you sick? | Etes-vous malade? | Sind Sie krank? | ¿Está usted enfermo? (enferma) | È malato(a)? |
| Are you injured? | Etes-vous blessé? | Sind Sie verletzt? | ¿Está usted herido? (herida) | È ferito(a)? |
| Are you a diabetic? | Etes-vous diabétique? | Sind Sie zuckerkrank? | ¿Es usted diabético? (diabética) | È diabetico(a)? |
| Yes/No | Oui/Non | Ja/Nein | Si/No | Si/No |
| Do you have a doctor? | Avez-vous un docteur? | Haben Sie einen Hausarzt? | ¿Tiene usted un doctor? | Ha un medico di famiglia? |
| Who is your doctor? | Qui est votre docteur? | Wer ist Ihr Arzt? | ¿Quién es su doctor? | Chi è il Suo dottore? |
| Where do you live? | Où habitez-vous? | Wo wohnen Sie? | ¿Dónde vive usted? | Dove abita (Lei)? |

Translation by Denise Guback, Translator, University of Illinois-Champaign.

| English | French | German | Spanish | Italian |
|---|---|---|---|---|
| What is your telephone number? | Quel est votre numéro de téléphone? | Was ist Ihre Telefonnummer? | ¿Cuál es el número de su teléfono? | Qual 'è il Suo numero di telefono? |
| Do you have a priest? (Rabbi? Minister?) | Avez-vous un prêtre? (un rabbin, un pasteur?) | Haben Sie einen Priester? (Rabiner, Pastor) | ¿Conoce usted un sacerdote? (Rabbi, pastor) | Conosce un sacerdote? (rabbino, ministro?) |
| I need to examine you for injuries | J'ai besoin de voir vos blessures | Ich muss Ihre Verletzungen untersuchen | Tengo que examinarle para ver si tiene heridas | Devo esaminarLa per eventuali ferite. |
| Is that all right? | D'accord? | Sind Sie damit einverstanden? | ¿Está de acuerdo? | Va bene? |
| I am going to measure your blood pressure | Je vais prendre votre tension artérielle | Ich nehme Ihren Blutdruck | Le voy a tomar la presión arterial | Devo misurarLe la pressione del sangue |
| I need to adjust your clothing | J'ai besoin d'ajuster vos vêtements | Ich muss Ihre Kleider lockern | Necesito quitarle (sacarle) parte de la ropa | Devo sbottonarLe il vestito |
| I am going to touch the injury site. It may cause pain. Do you understand? | Je vais toucher l'endroit de vos blessures. Cela peut faire mal. Comprenez vous? | Ich werde Ihre Wunde anfassen. Es wird Ihnen vielleicht weh tun. Verstehen Sie? | Le voy a tocar la parte herida y tal vez le cause dolor. ¿Me comprende? | Ora devo toccare la ferita. Potrebbe sentire dolore. Comprende? |
| Does this hurt? | Cela fait mal? | Tut es weh? | ¿Le duele ésto? | Fa male? |
| Can you move your foot? (leg, hand) | Pouvez-vous remuer le pied? (la jambe, la main?) | Können Sie Ihren Fuss bewegen? (Ihr Bein, Ihre Hand) | ¿Puede usted mover el pie? (la mano) | Può muovere il piede? (la gamba, la mano?) |
| Can you feel that? | Pouvez-vous sentir cela? | Fühlen Sie das? | ¿Siente usted cuando le toco? | Sente dove La tocco? |
| I have finished the examination. Can I go ahead with emergency care procedures? | J'ai terminé mon examen. Puis-je continuer avec les premiers soins d'urgence? | Ich habe die Untersuchung durchgeführt. Kann ich jetzt mit der Erstversorgung beginnen? | He terminado de examinarle. ¿Puedo comenzar con los tratamientos de emergencia? | Ho finito la visita. Posso cominciare con le procedure d'emergenza? |
| Don't move! | Ne bougez pas! | Bleiben Sie still! | ¡No se mueva! | Non ti muovere! |

# BIBLIOGRAPHY

Aehlert, B. (1992). *ACLS quick review study guide*. St. Louis: Mosby–Year Book.

Anthony, C. P., & Kolthoff, N. J. (1975). *Textbook of anatomy and physiology*. St. Louis: Mosby.

Bade, R. (1990, May). Mass casualty: Are you ready? Paper presented at a meeting in Santa Ana, CA.

Badgwell, J. M. (1993). *Anesthetic considerations for major pediatric trauma*, (Vol. 21, Chapter 17) [Audiotape]. In P. Barash (Ed.). Refresher courses in anesthesiology. Park Ridge, IL: American Society of Anesthesiologists.

Barker-Stotts, K. (1988). Hyphema: Prepare yourself now for a serious injury. *Nursing 88, 18*(12), 33.

Bartkiw, T. P., & Pynn, B. R. (1993). Close-up on mandible fracture. *Nursing 93, 23*(12), 42.

Berg, E. (1983). Emergency treatment of open and closed fractures. *Current Concepts in Trauma Care, 6*(4), 9–11.

Bobo, L., Burlew, B., Hackman, B., et al. (1990). *Regional Medical Center at Memphis medicine observation survival guide*. Memphis: University of Tennessee, Department of Medicine, Division of Emergency Medicine.

Bonica, J. J. (Ed.). (1980). *Obstetric analgesia and anesthesia* (2nd ed. rev.). Amsterdam: World Federation of Societies of Anesthesiologists.

Cales, R. H., & Heilig, R. W. (1986). *Trauma care systems: A guide to planning, implementation, operation and evaluation*. Rockville, MD: Aspen.

Campbell, J. (1988). *Basic trauma life support: Advanced prehospital care* (2nd ed.). Englewood Cliffs, NJ: Prentice-Hall.

Cardona, V. D. (1985). *Trauma nursing*. Oradell, NJ: Medical Economics.

Centers for Disease Control and Prevention. (1994). *Violence and injury*. Paper presented at a meeting in Washington, DC.

Chadwick, A. T., & Oesting, H. H. (1989). Not for specialists only: Caring for patients with spinal cord injuries. *Nursing 89, 19*(9), 53–56.

Christensen, J. B., & Telford, I. R. (1982). *Synopsis of gross anatomy*. New York: Harper & Row.

Coursin, D. B. (1993). *Perioperative care of the trauma patient* (Vol. 35, No. 15) [Audiotape]. Glendale, CA: Audio-Digest Foundation.

Cumbie, B. (1994). Treating a PTSD flashback. *Nursing 94, 24*(2), 33.

Cummins, R. O. (Ed.). (1994). *Textbook of advanced cardiac life support*. Dallas: American Heart Association.

Cushing, M. (1989). Finding fault when patients fall. *American Journal of Nursing, 89*(6), 808–809.

Dallaire, L. B., & Burke, E. V. (1989). A new program for reducing patient falls. *Nursing 89, 19*(1), 65.

*The donor family: Obtaining consent for post-mortem donation* [Pamphlet]. (1988). Memphis: Mid-South Transplant Foundation.

Dripps, R. D., Eckenhoff, J. E., & Vandam, L. D. (1982). *Introduction to anesthesia: The principles of safe practice.* Philadelphia: Saunders.

Edlich, R. F., Glassberg, H. H., & Tobiasen, J. A. (1994). Abbreviated burn severity index. *Current Concepts in Trauma Care, 7*(1), 20.

*Emergency burn care for first responders.* (1987). Oklahoma City: Baptist Medical Burn Center.

Fabian, T. C., Mangiante, E. C., Patterson, C. R., Payne, L. W., & Isaacson, M. L. (1988). Myocardial contusion in blunt trauma: Clinical characteristics, means of diagnosis, and implications for patient management. *Journal of Trauma, 28*(1), 50–57.

Fabian, T. C., & Patterson, R. (1985). Staving off serious injury during pregnancy. *Contemporary OB/GYN, 17,* 159.

Fleming, A. (Ed.). (1993). *Facts, 1993.* Arlington, VA: Insurance Institute for Highway Safety.

Grant, H. D., Murray, R. H., Jr., Bergeron, J. D. (Eds.). (1990). *Brady emergency care* (5th ed.). Englewood Cliffs, NJ: Prentice-Hall.

Guerriero, W. G. (1984). Management of urologic injuries. *Trauma Quarterly, 1*(1), 52–65.

Guerriero, W. G., & Devine, C. J., Jr. (1984). *Urologic injuries.* East Norwalk, CT: Appleton-Century-Crofts.

*A guide to the recognition and referral of post-mortem organ donors* [Pamphlet]. (1988). Memphis: Mid-South Transplant Foundation.

Guss, D. A. (1985). The head-injured patient: Pre-hospital care. *Trauma Quarterly, 2*(1), 1–7.

Hamelberg, W., & Bosomworth, P. B. (1968). *Aspiration pneumonitis.* Springfield, IL: Charles C Thomas.

Harris, B. H. (1984). Pediatric multisystem trauma management. *Trauma Quarterly, 1*(1), 79–85.

Henderson, V. J., Smith, R. S., Fry, W. R., Morabito, D., Peskin, G. W., Barkan, H., & Organ, C. H. (1994). Cardiac injuries: Analysis of an unselected series of 251 cases. *Journal of Trauma, 36*(3), 341–348.

Herman, J. L. (1992). *Trauma and recovery.* New York: Basic Books.

Hoyt, D. B., Shackford, S. R., & Marshall, L. F. (1985). Initial resuscitation: The trauma surgeon and neurosurgeon—a combined perspective. *Trauma Quarterly, 2*(1), 8–19.

Injury prevention: Meeting the challenge [Supplement]. (1989). *American Journal of Preventive Medicine, 5*(3).

*Introduction: Injury prevention for health professionals.* (1990). Newton, MA: Education Development Center, Inc., & The Johns Hopkins Injury Prevention Center.

Jacobs, L. M. (1984). Initial management of severe trauma. *Trauma Quarterly, 1*(1), 1–15.

Jubeck, M. E. (1994). Teaching the elderly: A commonsense approach. *Nursing 94, 24,* 70–71.

Jurkovich, G. J., & Moore, E. E. (1984). Thoracic trauma. *Trauma Quarterly, 1*(1), 37–51.

Kitt, S., & Kaiser, J. (1990). *Emergency nursing: A physiologic and clinical perspective.* Philadelphia: Saunders.

Kubler-Ross, E. (1974). *On death and dying.* New York: Collier.

Lerer, L. B., & Knottenbelt, J. D. (1994). Preventable mortality following sharp penetrating chest trauma. *Journal of Trauma, 37*(1), 9–12.

*The lifeline to organ donation* [Pamphlet]. (1990). Wilmington, DE: Du Pont Pharmaceuticals.

McAlary, B. G. (1994). *Anesthesiology and trauma care* (Vol. 36, No. 14) [Audiotape]. Glendale, CA: Audio-Digest Foundation.

Miller, B. F., & Keane, C. B. (1972). *Encyclopedia and dictionary of medicine and nursing.* Philadelphia: Saunders.

Miller, R. (Ed.). (1981). *Anesthesia* (2nd ed., Vol. 2). New York: Churchill Livingstone.

Miller, R. (Ed.). (1990). *Anesthesia* (3rd ed.). New York: Churchill Livingstone.

Morton, D. (1989). Five years of fewer falls. *American Journal of Nursing, 89*(2), 204–205.

National Spinal Cord Injury Association. (1988). *Fact sheet No. 2: Spinal cord injury statistical information.* Woburn, MA: Author.

Norton, D. J. (1990). Helping patients give the gift of life. *RN, 53*(12), 30–33.

Oakes, A. R. (1981). *Critical care nursing of children and adolescents.* Philadelphia: Saunders.

Ordog, G. J., Balasubramanium, S., Wasserberger, J., Kram, H., Bishop, M., & Shoemaker, W. (1994). Extremity gunshot wounds: Part 1. Identification and treatment of patients at high risk of vascular injury. *Journal of Trauma, 36*(3), 358–368.

Ordog, G. J., Wasserberger, J., Balasubramanium, S., & Shoemaker, W. (1994). Asymptomatic stab wounds of the chest. *Journal of Trauma, 36*(5), 680–684.

Peters, T. G. (1990). Organ donation and emergency medicine: The golden hour. *Topics in Emergency Medicine, 12*(4), 63–70.

Pierce, J. M. (1990). *Regional Medical Center at Memphis acute ambulatory care survival guide.* Memphis: University of Tennessee, Department of Medicine, Division of Emergency Medicine.

Reeder, S., Mastroianni, L., Jr., Martin, L. L., & Fitzpatrick, E. (1976). *Maternity nursing* (13th ed.). Philadelphia: Lippincott.

Resources for optimal care of the injured patient: An update. (1990). *American College of Surgeons Bulletin, 75*(9).

Rivara, F. P., Dicker, B. G., Bergman, A. B., Dacey, R., & Herman, C. (1988). The public cost of motorcycle trauma. *Journal of the American Medical Association, 258,* 221–223.

Roy-Shapira, A., Levi, I., Khoda, J. (1994). Sternal fractures: A red flag or a red herring? *Journal of Trauma, 37*(1), 59–62.

Russell, C. A. (1989, October 17). Accidents happen—or do they? *Washington Post Health,* pp. 14–17.

Russell, S. (1994). Hypovolemic shock. *Nursing 94, 24*(4), 34–39.

Shea, J. F. (1985). *Assessment of the spinal cord injured patient.* Lecture presented at Loyola University, Maywood, IL.

Sheehy, S. B., & Jimmerson, C. L. (1994). *Manual of clinical trauma care: The first hour.* St. Louis: Mosby–Year Book.

Sherman, D. W. (1990). Managing an acute head injury. *Nursing 90, 20*(4), 47–51.

Shnider, S. M., & Levinson, G. (1979). *Anesthesia for obstetrics.* Baltimore: Williams & Wilkins.

Smith, B. E., & Goretsky, S. R. (1992). Prosecutors surveyed on sex abuse cases. *Tennessee Networker, 3*(4), 9–10.

Sommers, M. (1990). Rapid fluid resuscitation: How to correct dangerous deficits. *Nursing 90, 20*(1), 52–59.

Sophie, L. R., Salloway, J. C., Sorock, G., Volek, P., & Merkel, F. K. (1983). Intensive care nurses' perceptions of cadaver organ procurement. *Heart and Lung, 12*(3), 261–266.

Sparks, S. M., & Taylor, C. M. (1991). *Nursing diagnosis reference manual.* Springhouse, PA: Springhouse Corp.

*Statistical abstract of the United States (110th ed.).* (1990). U. S. Department of Commerce, U.S. Bureau of the Census.

Strange, J. M. (1987). *Shock trauma care plans.* Springhouse, PA: Springhouse Corp.

Synder, L. A., & Peter, N. K. (1989). How to manage organ donation. *American Journal of Nursing, 89,* 1294–1299.

*Think you know something about child abuse?* [Pamphlet]. (1993). Chicago: National Committee to Prevent Child Abuse.

Thomas, P. (1994, June 23). Study finds rape of young girls is common. *Washington Post,* reprinted in *The Commercial Appeal,* pp. A1–A5.

Trunkey, D. D. (1985). *Advanced trauma life support course for physicians.* Chicago: American College of Surgeons, Committee on Trauma.

Vachss, A. (1993). Rapists are single-minded. *Parade,* pp. 4–6.

Violent crime hits young most often. (1994, July 18). *The Commercial Appeal,* p. 2.

Walz, J. A. (1989). A simulated disaster drill. *American Journal of Nursing, 89*(3), 301–303.

West, R. J., Mangiante, E. C., & Fabian, T. C. (1986). Penetrating cardiac wounds. *Journal of the Tennessee Medical Association, 68,*32–33.

Williams D. A., & Powers, I. (1994). Preventing violent outbreaks. *Nursing 94, 24*(5), 32O–32P.

Wilson, H. S., & Kneisl, C. R. (1979). *Psychiatric nursing.* Menlo Park, CA: Addison-Wesley.

Wilson, M. T. (1988). Setting up an effective E.D. triage system. *Nursing 88, 88*(12), 55–56.

Wreckreation. (1994, June 20). *Newsweek,* p. 6.

# SUGGESTED READING

Barker, E., & Higgins, R. (1989). Rescuing an SCI victim from a pool. *Nursing 89, 19*(5), 58–64.

Barker-Stotts, K. (1989). Strangulation: Prepare yourself now for a life-or-death crisis. *Nursing 89, 19*(3), 33.

Coolican, M. B. (1987). Katie's legacy. *American Journal of Nursing, 87*(4), 483–485.

Deaton, H. L., & Hensley, J. (1990). Taking the terror out of transport. *American Journal of Nursing, 90,* 58–60.

Emergency Nurses Association. (1991). *Standards of Emergency Nursing Practice* (2nd ed.). St. Louis: Mosby–Year Book.

Goldsmith, J., & Montefusco, C. M. (1988). Nursing care of the potential organ donor. *Critical Care Nurse, 5*(6), 22–29.

Hopkins, T. K. (1990). A different kind of recovery. *RN, 53*(12), 35–36.

Jarlsberg, C. R. (1990). Neck and chest burns: How to maintain a patient airway and prevent shock when a patient is severely burned. *Nursing 90, 20*(1), 33.

Jordan, K. (1990). Chest trauma: How to detect and react to serious trouble. *Nursing 90, 20*(9), 34–41.

Layendecker, M., Turcke, S., Will, J., & Barker, E. (1989). Rescuing a multiple trauma victim. *Nursing 89, 19*(10), 54–61.

Miracle, V. A., & Allnutt, D. R. (1990). How to perform basic airway management. *Nursing 90, 20*(4), 55–60.

Norris, R. M. (1989). Common sense tips for working with blind patients. *American Journal of Nursing, 89,* 360–361.

Northrop, C. E. (1990). How good samaritan laws do and don't protect you. *Nursing 90, 20*(2), 50–51.

Perkins, S. B., & Kennally, K. M. (1989). The hidden danger of internal hemorrhage. *Nursing 89, 19*(7), 34–41.

Redheffer, G. (1989). Treating wounds on the scene: Part 1. *Nursing 89, 19*(7), 51–57.

Redheffer, G. (1989). Treating wounds on the scene: Part 2. *Nursing 89, 19*(8), 47–51.

Redheffer, G., & Bailey, M. (1989). Assessing and splinting fractures. *Nursing 89, 19*(6), 51–59.

Reimer, M. (1989). Head-injured patients: How to detect early signs of trouble. *Nursing 89, 19*(3), 34–41.

Shubin, S. (1990). Offer families hope . . . or help them let go? The story of Anna, a brain-injured patient. *Nursing 90, 20*(3), 45–49.

Smith, G. A., & Savinski-Bozinko, G. (1989). Giving emergency care for burns. *Nursing 89, 19*(9), 55–62.

# GLOSSARY

**ABC:** Acronym for airway, breathing, and circulation; the first priority in attending a trauma patient.

**Amniotic sac:** The membrane that holds the fluid in which the fetus floats. The amniotic sac and fluid are commonly called the "bag of water."

**Bladder:** A muscular hollow sac that collects, stores, and expels urine.

**Brain:** A spongy mass that weighs about 3 lb (1.4 kg) and rests in the skull; it is a vital organ and the body's control center.

**Cerebrospinal fluid (CSF):** A clear, straw-colored fluid that bathes the brain and spinal cord, providing a cushion of support and offering protection against some harmful substances.

**CPR:** Acronym for cardiopulmonary resuscitation.

**Diaphragm:** The muscle separating the chest from the abdomen. Attached to the ribs, sternum, and spine, the diaphragm contracts to allow inspiration of air into the lungs.

**Dislocation:** Displacement from the normal position of the bone in the joint.

**Distributive shock:** Shock that results when the circulating volume is adequate but the distribution is impaired. Two types are neurogenic shock and septic shock.

**Dura:** The toughest and outermost of the meninges; it covers the brain.

**Epidermis:** The outer thin layer of skin that you can see and touch.

**Fetus:** The developing human offspring that evolves from an embryo into a fetus at about 6 weeks' gestation and is referred to as a fetus until birth.

**Flow obstruction shock:** Shock caused by impeded ejection of blood from the heart. An example is cardiac tamponade.

**Fracture:** Disruption in the continuity of a bone.

**Gestation:** Pregnancy; usually 40 weeks. Fetuses may survive when born as early as 24–26 weeks of gestation.

**Hemothorax:** A collection of blood in the pleural cavity.

**Homeostasis:** A trend to normalcy and stability by resistance to disruption and stress.

**Hyoid bone:** A U-shaped bone that is attached to the tongue; it may play a role in airway obstruction.

**Infant:** A child in the first year of life.

**Kidneys:** Bean-shaped vital organs that perform the life-saving functions of filtering wastes from the blood, maintaining acid-base balance, and regulating sodium and water balance in the body.

**Larynx:** A series of cartilages and muscles that assist in speech; its most critical function is as an air passage.

**Liver:** The largest of the abdominal organs; the liver is solid and highly vascular.

**Manual ventilating bag:** A pliable reservoir or bag-valve-mask device connected to a source of oxygen; squeezing it generates positive pressure and delivers a breath to the patient; often referred to as an "ambu bag."

**Meninges:** The three fibrous membranes that cover the brain and spinal cord.

**Neonate:** An infant from birth to 1 month of age.

**Osteoporosis:** Loss of bone mass and density that occurs with aging; most common in elderly white females but occurs to some degree in most elderly persons.

**Pancreas:** A solid organ located behind and beneath the stomach and the liver and commonly injured by blunt trauma; aids in digestion and carbohydrate metabolism.

**Paraplegia:** Loss of sensation and function from about the level of the waist down.

**Pharynx:** A muscular structure referred to as the throat; it performs double duty as a passage for air and food and is subject to obstruction from trauma.

**Philadelphia collar:** A firm collar that encircles the neck to enhance stability and reduce movement of the head and neck; also called a cervical immobilizer.

**Placenta:** A structure that embeds in the wall of the uterus and functions in metabolic exchange (e.g., oxygen, carbon dioxide, and nutrients) between the fetus and the mother; commonly referred to as the afterbirth.

**Pulse pressure:** The difference between the diastolic pressure (the lower number in a blood pressure reading) and systolic pressure (upper number). The pulse pressure narrows in hemorrhagic shock.

**Quadriplegia:** Loss of sensation and function from about the level of the shoulders down. Quadriplegics may require artificial respiration for the rest of their lives.

**Rigid cervical immobilizer:** A firm collar that encircles the neck to enhance stability and reduce movement of the head and neck; also called a Philadelphia collar.

**Skull:** The bony structure that forms the cranium and holds the brain.

**Spinal column:** A bony structure that protects the spinal cord and gives humans the ability to walk upright; formed from 33 individual bones called vertebrae. Each vertebra forms a protective ring through which the spinal cord runs. Commonly referred to as the spine.

**Spinal cord:** A soft tissue housed in the spinal column; a critical part of the body's neural network because it controls movement and sensation in many parts of the body.

**Spleen:** A solid, highly vascular organ located on the left side of the body; participates in blood production, blood destruction, and defense against disease.

**Stress:** Events that challenge the host's steady state and require adaptation and the implementation of coping mechanisms to return the host to steady state.

**Teeth:** Hard, bonelike structures emanating from the mandible and maxillae.

**Trachea:** The air passage from the throat to the left and right bronchus; composed of C-shaped rings of cartilage joined by tough membranes; commonly called the windpipe.

**Umbilical cord:** The collection of vessels that exchange blood between the fetus and the mother.

**Upper part of the airway:** The air passages that begin at the nose and lips and end at the epiglottis.

**Ureters:** Tubular, muscular structures that propel urine produced by each kidney down to the bladder.

**Urethra:** The passageway for urine from the bladder to the outside of the body and the final structure in the urinary system.

# INDEX

# PRETEST ANSWER KEY

| | | |
|---|---|---|
| 1. | B | Chapter 1 |
| 2. | A | Chapter 1 |
| 3. | B | Chapter 2 |
| 4. | A | Chapter 3 |
| 5. | A | Chapter 4 |
| 6. | A | Chapter 4 |
| 7. | B | Chapter 5 |
| 8. | B | Chapter 6 |
| 9. | B | Chapter 7 |
| 10. | B | Chapter 7 |
| 11. | B | Chapter 8 |
| 12. | A | Chapter 9 |
| 13. | A | Chapter 10 |
| 14. | A | Chapter 11 |
| 15. | B | Chapter 12 |
| 16. | B | Chapter 13 |
| 17. | A | Chapter 13 |
| 18. | B | Chapter 14 |
| 19. | A | Chapter 15 |
| 20. | A | Chapter 16 |
| 21. | B | Chapter 17 |
| 22. | B | Chapter 17 |
| 23. | A | Chapter 18 |
| 24. | A | Chapter 19 |
| 25. | A | Chapter 20 |